Power, Suffering, and
the Struggle for Dignity

PENNSYLVANIA STUDIES IN HUMAN RIGHTS

Bert B. Lockwood, Jr., Series Editor

A complete list of books in the series is available from the publisher.

Power, Suffering, and the Struggle for Dignity

Human Rights Frameworks for Health and Why They Matter

Alicia Ely Yamin

Foreword by Paul Farmer

PENN

UNIVERSITY OF PENNSYLVANIA PRESS

PHILADELPHIA

Published by
University of Pennsylvania Press
Philadelphia, Pennsylvania 19104-4112
www.upenn.edu/pennpress

Printed in the United States of America
on acid-free paper

10 9 8 7 6 5 4 3 2 1

Library of Congress Cataloging-in-Publication Data
Yamin, Alicia Ely, author.
    Power, suffering, and the struggle for dignity : human rights frameworks for health and why they matter / Alicia Ely Yamin.
        pages cm. — (Pennsylvania studies in human rights)
    Includes bibliographical references and index.
    ISBN 978-0-8122-4774-9 (alk. paper)
 1. Right to health. 2. Human rights—Health aspects. 3. Health services accessibility. 4. Medical policy—Moral and ethical aspects. 5. Public health—Moral and ethical aspects. 6. Women—Medical care. 7. Poor—Medical care.
I. Farmer, Paul, 1959– writer of preface. II. Title. III. Series: Pennsylvania studies in human rights.
    K3260.3.Y26 2016
    323—dc23
                                                                    2015017697

Contents

My profound admiration and respect for Alicia Ely Yamin and her work in health and human rights goes back many years, beginning well before our work together as editors of the journal *Health and Human Rights*. But when we each penned our first contributions as editors for the journal in 2007, our shared experiences, indignation, and understandings about the inequities in the world became even more evident.

Alicia is not just an extraordinary leader in the field but someone who has been in the trenches. She speaks authoritatively because she understands the ways in which cycles of poverty and disease become ingrained in poor communities across the globe, as the stories in this remarkable new book attest. Too often I have found that many human rights lawyers remain in the realm of the abstract, failing to address the realities of what health practitioners—and impoverished patients—face every day. In *Power, Suffering, and the Struggle for Dignity*, Alicia does exactly this, showing us what a human rights framework can and should mean.

Alicia and I, along with many of our colleagues, share the same sense of outrage at global inequities, and the need to enact transformative change. In our first issue of the journal, I wrote about having been "part of an effort to provide basic services—medical care, primary education, clean water, even exhumation and proper burial for the victims of mass violence—in Latin America, Siberia, and inner-city Boston. The people we served had neither a language nor a culture in common. What they had in common, by and large, was poverty." Alicia may not have provided direct services, but it is apparent from this text how much time she has spent with impoverished women in labor and delivery rooms throughout the world, as well as in their communities and homes.

Our shared perspective on national and global inequities, on the "pathologies of power" as I have called them and the suffering they produce reaches beyond outrage to the desire to forge solutions. Although working in different professions, we both remain committed to the conviction that the root causes of poverty and ill health are inextricably linked to questions of justice, including the right to health. We share deep frustration with those limited conceptions of justice which would restrict the domain of human rights to a slim portion of civil and political liberties. But importantly, Alicia's critiques of traditional human rights theory in *Power, Suffering, and the Struggle for Dignity*, emerge from within and propose alternative pathways for moving beyond frameworks that, in her words, "sit all too easily with neoliberalism."

This theme of the connection between the power relations between the so-called "North" and "South" runs throughout Alicia's profoundly moving book. Alicia describes this text as a call to remake our institutions and our social and legal arrangements at national and global levels. We owe as much to one another as human beings with equal dignity. This book deftly illustrates the core purpose of a human rights-based approach—eradicating the suffering arising from dramatic inequality within and between nations.

In *Power, Suffering, and the Struggle for Dignity*, Alicia makes the argument that the divide between theory and practice is deeply misleading; rather, she shows us repeatedly that the ways in which we think about global health problems shapes what we do about them—both in terms of substance and process. Alicia is quick to note that many human rights-based approaches have "only brought about incremental changes." But she explains that incremental changes need not be a sign of failure, because a small change in a relationship of power can "trigger a cascade of changes, which create meaningful improvements in the effective enjoyment of health and other rights by many other people."

Power, Suffering, and the Struggle for Dignity, achieves an accessibility rare in academic literature. Her writing transcends the academy and, true to human rights practice, reaches out to an audience that does not need to be privileged to be included. Her stories highlight the social construction of power; they illustrate how the unequal share of wealth, knowledge, and health care is socially and politically determined. They illustrate power relations in the government, in the home, and in relationships. Her text brings a frank reframing of the dynamics of *power* and of *suffering*.

Power, Suffering, and the Struggle for Dignity, is not, as Alicia notes, a manual on human rights-based approaches to health. Those of us working in medicine and public health know that manuals offering technocratic solutions to deeply entrenched inequitable systems do not work. Rather— ranging from Colombia to Uganda and Peru to South Africa—Alicia provides examples of how human rights-based approaches can be applied to "destabilize and disentrench" practices and systems that perpetuate inequality and injustice. She calls on readers to combat the apathy that so often engulfs us and to question the inevitability of institutional arrangements and approaches to health and development, as well as approaches to human rights. It is not a newly envisioned world that *Power, Suffering, and the Struggle for Dignity,* leads us toward; rather, it is the world imagined when the Universal Declaration of Human Rights was drafted nearly seventy years ago: a social and international order in which everyone can enjoy health and other essential rights.

Paul Farmer, M.D.

Growing up, I often thought about the day my mother was born. My mother was an extraordinarily beautiful woman and it was only when I would sit on the edge of the tub in her bathroom, watching her get ready to go out and as she brushed her hair, and the light shifted, that the telltale scars of the forceps on her forehead were visible, evoking thoughts of the struggle her mother must have had. She'd told me the story so many times that I knew it by heart. The pregnancy had been relatively easy and nothing portended how unimaginably awful the delivery was to be. My grandfather was a tall, sturdy man. But my grandmother was a petite woman and her pelvis simply couldn't open broadly enough for my mother to emerge well. She had what we would call now a protracted labor, which seems an unduly cold and clinical term for the agony she must have felt, pushing for hours, hours turning into days, feeling as though her body were breaking in two, the child inside her slowly being starved of oxygen, the odor of blood mixed with fear-drenched sweat and feces overcoming my grandmother who was, in every other respect, the daintiest and most proper of women. It was before the advent of cesarean sections or my mother would have been born that way, but finally the doctor must have been able to reach up far enough to grab her forehead with the long tongs of the forceps, pulling and guiding her into the world. My grandmother had lost a lot of blood; she'd come very close to dying. She was told she could never have another child. That was my mother's original sin—her size, her very birth—and of course the fact that she was a girl.

At the time, I had no idea so much of my life would be devoted to advancing women's sexual and reproductive health and rights, and maternal health in particular. But the toll of that near-miss and the context of both a family and a world that continue to value male children more than female children played a tremendous role in my grandmother's life, my mother's life, and my own.

This book is in many ways a narrative birthed in anger. It is a book saturated with indignation at the fact that so many girls across the global South continue to be robbed of basic life choices; that women everywhere continue to be defined not by their humanness but by their sexual otherness; and that, across the globe, so many girls' and women's voices still are not heard and their dignity not valued—simply because they were born female.

These pages are also filled with outrage at the scandalous disparities in health and other fundamental rights that plague the globe, as well as at the enormous suffering wrought by avoidable poverty-related conditions. No issue demonstrates this more than maternal mortality, which shows the greatest disparities between the global South and the economic North—much greater than HIV/AIDS or child mortality, for example. Poor women in poor, and lower middle-income countries are overwhelmingly the ones who die from maternal causes.

But this book is also filled with hope. I deeply believe that we can transform our world and, indeed, that combining the tools of human rights and public health can help us to do so. I have witnessed the impacts that applying human rights frameworks and strategies can have on people's health—and lives—and I share some of those insights in these pages. I have no doubt we can achieve far more social justice in this world if and when human rights are widely applied to health issues in bold and transformative ways.

The initial idea for this book grew out of a series of articles that I published as executive editor for the Critical Concepts section of *Health and Human Rights: An International Journal* (hereafter referred to as the *Health and Human Rights* journal) between 2008 and 2010. In 1994, Jonathan Mann, the founding director of the François-Xavier Bagnoud Center for Health and Human Rights at Harvard University, launched the *Health and Human Rights* journal to provide an inclusive forum for rigorous discussion and debate on the relationships between health and human rights. Over the following two decades, so-called human rights–based approaches (HRBAs) flourished in health and development organizations and the normative development of health rights advanced tremendously. In 2007, Paul Farmer had the bold vision of adopting a new format for the *Health and Human Rights* journal, converting it into an online forum for activists, scholars, and practitioners to continue the sort of dialogue that Mann had envisioned. I was privileged to be invited to be part of that undertaking.

With Farmer and the other editors, I proposed that we explore the elements of HRBAs to health systematically in the first set of issues under this new leadership, and examine more broadly what it could mean to apply a human rights framework to health. The impetus for reshaping the *Health and Human Rights* journal and adopting this approach was the paradox that the world faced, and continues to face. On the one hand, human rights is now the dominant language for claims of human emancipation around the world, and human rights theory and practice have permeated many domains beyond the law, including health. On the other hand, as already noted, the landscape of global health is marked by vast inequities and brutal deprivation, and it is not yet clear to policy makers and health practitioners, or to those affected, how applying human rights concepts and strategies will change the lives of the millions of people who are suffering.

I believed then, and I continue to believe, that human rights provides one—but certainly not the only—critical framework through which to advance social transformation, and social justice in health in particular. In those initial issues of the revamped *Health and Human Rights* journal we explored the implications of adopting human rights frameworks relating to health for policy makers and programmers, for activists and advocates, for researchers and service providers, and for the many different communities and people around the world whose lives are affected. In my Critical Concepts articles—which became the basis for this book—I sought to inspire critical thinking not just about the fields of medicine and public health but also about how to adapt and expand traditional human rights frameworks and tools to meaningfully advance people's health at national and global levels. Human rights means many things to many people and, as I reiterate throughout this book, we need to hold onto bold rights claims to transform the world and not allow HRBAs to become yet another formulaic approach to health programming.

Although this book is a continuation of the thinking that I began in those journal articles, it also draws heavily on other conceptual thinking and work that I have done in the field. Consequently, there is a much greater emphasis here on women's and children's health and rights, and on sexual and reproductive, and maternal health in particular, because during the more than twenty years that I have been in this field, I have worked overwhelmingly on these issues. I have added to the themes addressed in the journal articles by including five new chapters and by substantially revising the articles that were originally published in the journal.

This book speaks in a much more personal voice than did the Critical Concepts articles. Throughout these pages, I have included stories from my personal experience because I believe the universal elements of what it means to apply a rights framework to health—the multidimensional and embedded aspects of rights enjoyment, as well as deprivations—can frequently be better understood through the stories of particular individuals than through the staggering, and often numbing, statistics of global inequalities. And sometimes identifying with others' stories enables us to piece together our own stories and in turn to understand more clearly what applying human rights requires of each of us in terms of being ethical individuals in this interconnected world.

I have spent much of my professional life interviewing victims of human rights deprivations, among other things, in an effort to understand better what leads to women dying in pregnancy and childbirth and what happens to the families when they do die of maternal causes. My own grandmother easily could have died when she was giving birth to my mother, and I have often thought of that, of how different my own family's story could have been, when interviewing others.

I thought of this again when I met Rediet in Ethiopia, who, at the age of eleven, had lost her mother, Meron. In 2013, Rediet, now eighteen, was stunningly beautiful, with high cheekbones setting off her large, dark eyes and perfectly shaped lips. Over a couple of hours, she and her brother spoke disconsolately about everything they had lost when their mother died, including their sense of themselves and their dreams for their lives. They both had to drop out of school, Rediet's brother forsaking hopes of being a civil servant and Rediet marrying a man she had no fondness for and bearing his child to spare the family the expense of having to feed her. Rediet and her brother also went on at length about how beautiful Meron had been, and when I noted I was sure her mother would have told her how beautiful she too was, Rediet burst into tears I recognized well, tears of grief mixed with love, of hope she had buried long ago mixed with irredeemable loss. We talked for quite a while longer about being daughters, and mothers, and women who both wanted agency and dignity in our lives. The injustice in her life was unbearable to us both, and we cried together—so much so that the young Ethiopian data collectors I was training asked how I could do this kind of work for so long if it affected me so deeply. "It's when it stops affecting you, when you stop thinking of them as people, and only as research subjects, that you should stop doing this work," I replied.

It is indeed a peculiar kind of work though, to spend so much time listening to the stories of people's anguish and suffering and to have strangers from very different backgrounds share some of the most intimate and painful details of their lives. It is not a privilege or a responsibility that I take lightly. It is no exaggeration to say that these stories are from some of the women, men, and children who have taught me what the condition of being human means. And it is through the experiences they have shared with me that I have come to believe that in a real sense having and exercising *rights* makes us fully human. If only by telling some of their stories in these pages, I hope I can give these different individuals and their families some small recognition.

An asterisk beside an abbreviation indicates that the term also appears with a fuller explanation in the Glossary.

*AAAQ	availability, accessibility, acceptability, and quality (of health facilities, goods, and services)
ANC	African National Congress
ARV	antiretroviral
CCBRT	comprehensive community based rehabilitation
CBA	cost-benefit analysis
CCM	Chama Cha Mapinduzi
*CEA	cost-effectiveness analysis
*CEDAW	Convention on the Elimination of All Forms of Discrimination Against Women
*CEDAW Committee	UN Committee on the Elimination of Discrimination Against Women
*CESCR	UN Committee on Economic, Social and Cultural Rights
CESR	Center for Economic and Social Rights
CLAS	Committees for the Local Administration of Health Care
*CP	civil and political
*CRPD	Convention on the Rights of Persons with Disabilities
CRR	Center for Reproductive Rights
*DALYs	disability-adjusted life years
DFID	British Department for International Development
DPG	Development Partners Group
DRI	Disability Rights International
ELN	Ejército de Liberacion Nacional
*EmOC	emergency obstetric care

*ESC	economic, social, and cultural
EZLN	Ejército Zapatista de Liberación Nacional (Zapatista Army of National Liberation)
FARC	Fuerzas Armadas Revolucionarias de Colombia
FCGH	Framework Convention on Global Health
FGM	female genital mutilation
HRBA	human rights–based approach
*HRC	Human Rights Council
ICCPR	International Covenant on Civil and Political Rights
*ICESCR	International Covenant on Economic, Social and Cultural Rights
*ICPD	International Conference on Population and Development
IFP	Inkatha Freedom Party
IMF	International Monetary Fund
IPV	intimate partner violence
ITNs	insecticide treated bed nets
IWW	International Workers of the World
LGBT	lesbian, gay, bisexual, and transgender
LRA	Lord's Resistance Army
MCH	maternal child health
*MDGs	Millennium Development Goals
MoHSW	Ministry of Health and Social Welfare
MMR	maternal mortality ratio
MSM	men who have sex with men
NAFTA	North American Free Trade Agreement
NALSA	National Legal Services Authority
NGO	nongovernmental organization
NHRI	national human rights institution
*ODA	official development assistance
OHCHR	UN Office of the High Commissioner for Human Rights
PEPFAR	U.S. President's Emergency Program for AIDS Relief
PHR	Physicians for Human Rights
PHU	primary health unit
PJF	Policia Judicial Federal (Federal Judicial Police of Mexico)
PLWAs	persons living with HIV/AIDS
PMA	Pharmaceutical Manufacturers Association
PMTCT	prevention of mother-to-child transmission
PPP	public-private partnership

PTSD	Post-traumatic Stress Disorder
*QALYs	quality-adjusted life years
SAM	social accountability monitoring
*SBA	skilled birth attendant
*SDGs	Sustainable Development Goals
SRH	sexual and reproductive health
SRHR	sexual and reproductive health and rights
TBA	traditional birth attendants
UDHR	Universal Declaration of Human Rights
UHC	universal health coverage
UNDP	United Nations Development Programme
UNICEF	United Nations Children's Fund
WHO	World Health Organization

Introduction
How Do We Understand Suffering?

We humans can tolerate suffering: we cannot tolerate
meaninglessness.
—Desmond Tutu, *Believe: The Words and Inspiration of Desmond Tutu*

Human rights are being violated on every continent. . . . Human
suffering anywhere concerns men and women everywhere.
—Elie Wiesel, Nobel Peace Prize Acceptance Speech,
December 10, 1986

Before I had my two children, I had a miscarriage. I was living in New York City at the time and medically it was not a major event. I required surgery, but I was admitted to the hospital very early in the morning and by that same evening I was released and at home. Of course, emotionally it was deeply, deeply painful. Earlier, I had been invited to go on a human rights fact-finding delegation to the state of Chiapas in southern Mexico that was scheduled for the week after my unexpected miscarriage. I had lived in Mexico for years and been to Chiapas many times before, and the political events that prompted the delegation felt very immediate to me. And, undoubtedly to escape the emotional pain I felt and to stop feeling sorry for myself, the very next week I did indeed go.

Chiapas is the state where the Zapatista Army of National Liberation (EZLN, according to its Spanish acronym) had launched its revolt on the day that the North American Free Trade Agreement (NAFTA) went into effect on January 1, 1994. The EZLN was protesting economic and political policies that left indigenous people systematically marginalized and impoverished. Its goals included achieving basic citizenship rights, indigenous control over resources (especially land), and demilitarization of indigenous areas.[1] In December 1997, when I was there on this occasion, paramilitary violence was at its height in Chiapas. The Mexican government was exploiting religious and political fault lines in these impoverished indigenous communities and arming paramilitary groups with Orwellian names, such as "Peace and Justice," in order to terrorize potential Zapatista sympathizers. On December 22, 1997, thirty-six women and children were killed in Chenalhó, a community in *los Altos*, the "mountainous region," of Chiapas.[2] In the weeks preceding the Acteal massacre, as it came to be called, an upswing in violence had already exacerbated the displacement of Zapatista-sympathizing communities.

It was in one of those communities of internally displaced persons that I encountered a woman who was hemorrhaging as a result of a miscarriage. She was just about at the same stage of pregnancy as I had been the week before. However, in her case the hemorrhage was a life-or-death situation. She was weak from the loss of blood and obviously terrified. Her husband and the elders in the community had decided that it would be better for her to "die with dignity" than to be taken to the nearest hospital because they viewed the public health facilities as an arm of the government counterinsurgency.[3]

I was immediately gripped by the sense of, "there but for the grace of God go I." After all, I could easily have been in the same situation. I dropped the neutral human rights investigator role and the delegation arranged for this woman to be accompanied to the hospital in San Cristóbal de las Casas by a representative of a local nongovernmental organization (NGO) who the community elders accepted. The NGO representative made sure that the woman would not have to answer any political questions—which was a common tactic that government facilities at the time were using to intimidate Zapatista sympathizers—and that she was treated appropriately by the health providers. Afterward, the woman—alive and healing—was transported back to her community by the same NGO representative.

In retrospect, however, it was *not* "but for the grace of God" that she was in a life-or-death situation—and that I, the previous week, was not. It was because of very human choices about laws and policies about women's education and the use of health facilities; it was because I was a white, middle-class woman with good health insurance living in a city with excellent health care; and it was because I was able to make decisions about my own body, and my own life—whereas she was not.

I cannot count how many times during the years I have been engaged in this work that I have heard that the "will of God" led to the death or suffering of a woman, a child, or a family. And often "God's will" has seemed to be tinged with a good dose of misogyny. I remember Lidia, for example, who had a protracted labor and was unable to stop her own body from crushing the skull of her unborn child and then she expired herself, because allegedly she would not confess to an adulterous act. And there was Carolina, married to a loutish drunk, who even as she exsanguinated from an overdose of misoprostol, spent her final hours soaking her own blood up in rags, in a desperate attempt to prevent her children from finding her in a pool of blood upon returning home from school. Her suffering was apparently "deserved" because she had tried to have an abortion, fearing the prospect of having to support another child with her abusive, alcoholic husband.

Men are not always part of the problem, of course. In Ethiopia, I met Mahmoud, whose wife had died a few years before we spoke. He told me how he continued to dream of her every night and when he awoke, gripped by the reality that he was alive and she was not, he would feel deeply depressed, wishing for his children's sake that he had died instead. Indeed, I could see that the children were not doing well, and one of them had been recently hospitalized for kwashiorkor, a condition of acute malnutrition. Mahmoud told me that he knew that there must have been something he had done to make his wife die and for him and his family to suffer so awfully, but he could not tell what. And he went on to say through tears—very unusual for a man from Ethiopia to share in front of a foreign woman—that he believed that part of his transgression was precisely not knowing what deep wrong he had committed. Mahmoud was consigned to his own private Hell for eternity, wondering what he had done to bring the wrath of an unforgiving God on his family. It was unthinkable for him to believe that indeed he had committed no great sin and that in fact his wife had died because of a profound injustice—an injustice for which humans, and not God, were responsible.

Health and Suffering as Reflections of Social (In)justice

It is impossible to do health and human rights work for very long and still cling to the notion that our own sadness, our own pain, is somehow special. The late Nigerian author Chinua Achebe captured this in *Things Fall Apart*: "You think you are the greatest sufferer in the world? . . . Do you know that men sometimes lose all their yams and even their children? . . . Do you know how many children I have buried . . . ? . . . If you think you are the greatest sufferer in the world ask my daughter . . . how many twins she has thrown away."[4] The truth is that all of us eventually live broken lives. The question is how we make sense of the fragments.

I argue in this book that applying a human rights framework to health forces us to think about how we understand our own suffering and that of others, and the fundamental causes of that suffering. What is our agency—our power to act—as human subjects? What is the agency of other humans in decisions that affect our health, and how is the line drawn between what are mutable human policies and decisions and what we may see as "natural"? Richard Horton, editor of the *Lancet*, has argued, human rights are important in relation to health "because they bring a moral dimension to our discussions about the suffering of others and because of the duties they impose on each of us."[5]

In this book, I seek to contribute to an understanding of how we construct narratives about suffering, in moral but also in legal terms, and of the connection between conceptions of power relations and state responsibility that those narratives entail. I argue that, ultimately, applying a human rights framework to health should also cause us to act differently because treating with indifference the too-often unjust suffering of others, whether on our street or across the globe, denies the importance of the lives of others and, in turn, undermines all human dignity in this increasingly interconnected world.

Of course, not all suffering and ill-health are a matter of human rights violations. Plenty of suffering and illness in this world can be blamed on the genetic lottery, poor choices that lead us to wreck our own lives and those of the people we say we care about, bad luck, and our human penchant for selfish and brutish behavior. And pain and suffering are part of the essential fragility of our existence, part of the texture of our lives. But there is also injustice, which stems from arbitrariness—the arbitrariness of the color of our skin, the genitalia attached to our bodies, and the place in the world in which we were born, for example. There is the injustice of miasmas of corruption and massive indifference to the misery of fellow human beings and of laws and policies and practices that embed ideological, religious, and cultural prejudices in our daily lives and rob certain people of the ability to live with dignity and well-being. That is the suffering I am concerned with in this book.

In 1948, the United Nations General Assembly adopted the Universal Declaration of Human Rights (UDHR), with no dissenting votes. Article 28 of the Universal Declaration calls for "a social and international order in which the rights and freedoms" in the UDHR can be fully realized.[6] I believe that if we took that call seriously, the landscape of global health and justice would be dramatically different. For example, we could no longer tolerate the fact that in some countries a girl has a greater chance of dying in childbirth than graduating from primary school. Nor would we be able to simply lament that nearly seven million children under the age of five die every year from preventable diseases of poverty while in the United States and elsewhere, middle- and upper-class children and their parents find distraction in incessant materialistic accumulation.[7] Rather, something about this egregious imbalance, and the fact that so many of us can live our lives of privilege with such long shadows of suffering emanating from them, would strike us as fundamentally wrong—as a "manifest injustice" in Amartya Sen's words, which demands not just charity but breaking out of our passivity to create fundamental change.[8]

In the last twenty years, so-called human rights–based approaches (HRBAs) to health and development have proliferated among NGOs as well as international agencies.[9] In 2003, the United Nations issued a "Common Understanding" of what an HRBA requires in development programs.[10] Moreover, human rights advocacy organizations, courts, and quasi-judicial international bodies, among others, have increasingly been engaged in interpreting and applying human rights norms in health contexts, from HIV/AIDS to maternal health, and there has been tremendous clarification of norms relating to the right to health itself. As the UN "Common Understanding" on HRBAs states, common themes can be identified across these efforts, including emphasis on nondiscrimination and equality, participation, accountability, and the rule of law.[11] What it means to apply these HRBAs in theory and practice, and to elements of human rights frameworks more broadly, and how applying these HRBAs challenges conventional public health and development approaches, are the subjects of much of the rest of this book.

I argue throughout this book that the core of applying a human rights framework to health involves understanding that patterns of health and suffering reflect power relations as much as they do biological or behavioral factors. If HRBAs, or human rights frameworks generally, are to be meaningful to the people on whose behalf we purport to work, they must strive not just to analyze but to remedy what Paul Farmer calls the "pathologies of power" that produce gross inequities within and between our societies.[12] When we begin to rethink power relations and to question the root causes for our own and others' suffering, it "de-naturalizes" both the biological individualism of the medical and health fields and many of the societal arrangements that perpetuate poverty, inequality, and violations of human rights; we see that these forces do not "just happen"; that they are neither "natural" nor inevitable acts of God. Thus we can begin to reexamine what it means to say that something *causes* someone's illness or condition, and also look at what produces certain distributions of power and privilege in society. We can begin to question prevalent narratives for thinking about poverty, inequality, human rights, and health that we often take for granted.

Many of these questions have no easy answers. No area of human rights more acutely poses queries about what is required of society for individuals to live lives of dignity than health. Think, for example, of the baby born very prematurely, who is kept "alive"—in some very limited meaning of that word—in a hospital in the economic North at inordinate expense to the public's coffers, or of the person with terminal cancer in a middle-income country whose "few more months" may cost more than what it would to immunize the majority of children in a rural community. Where do the boundaries of social and state responsibility lie? These are some of the questions of life and death with which we need to wrestle honestly and sincerely, and without empty sloganeering, if we care about applying human rights frameworks to health.

Further, we need to be willing to follow the implications of the conclusions about what justice in health would require, which I argue often demands that we rethink our approaches to both global health and human rights. For example, I believe we should all feel outrage at how arbitrary it is that the woman in Chiapas could have easily died (and all too many women do) while my own miscarriage meant simply a minor medical procedure. If we share that visceral indignation, even when the suffering is across borders— "out there"—we first need to understand what factors underlie that arbitrary difference in life chances; what makes it injustice rather than tragedy; and what opportunity structures exist, for different actors, to change those circumstances. And then, we need to act. This book is a call to begin to remake our institutions, and social and legal arrangements, at national and global levels, as a matter of what we owe to one another as full human beings with equal dignity.

Much of this book discusses women's and children's health, both because they have been the focus of my own work and because they are particularly sensitive reflections of patterns of justice and injustice. Poverty and inequality are inscribed in the malnourished, and too often stunted, bodies of children. Show me a profoundly malnourished child and I will show you factors of social and gender injustice within the family; in the community; in access to information, health care, and education; and in the food-security policies, budgeting priorities, and legal and policy frameworks of the country.

Or take maternal mortality. As I have often emphasized, maternal mortality is not principally a medical problem; it is primarily a social problem and a problem of political will at both the national and international levels. Hundreds of thousands of women and girls are still dying every year in the global South not because we do not know how to save them—we do, and we have for well over half a century—but because their lives are not valued, because their voices are not listened to, and because they are discriminated against and excluded in their homes and communities and by health-care systems that do not prioritize their needs.[13] Those are issues of fundamental human rights and social justice, and rights therefore need to be at the center of responses.

Amazing advances have been made not only in the conceptual clarification of HRBAs to health and development in recent years but also in the evolution of the right to health itself. A flurry of recent books on the right to health in international law and in regional perspective attests to the intensity of activity, as well as to scholarly attention.[14] Yet an enormous gap exists between theoretical discourses and practice. Human rights frameworks and HRBAs remain marginal in mainstream development as well as in health policy and programming across much of the world. Not only is the enjoyment of the right to health a very distant dream for most of the world's inhabitants, but even the *idea* of an enforceable entitlement relating to health care and public health protections seems disturbingly irrelevant to most discussions about health and development that take place at national and global levels.

Now that we have a clearer idea of the concepts and principles that characterize an HRBA to health, I believe that we need to translate that knowledge for development economists and governmental policy makers, for health practitioners, and most of all for the people whose lives and well-being are affected. We need to make human rights frameworks relevant for them by making explicit assumptions regarding how social change happens and how applying a human rights framework to health would make a difference in practice.

Human rights are all too often thought about by health professionals and the public as abstract principles or as relating only to laws and policies. On the contrary, as I make explicit throughout this book, applying HRBAs should change decision making, and in turn opportunity structures, in specific ways at multiple levels of government and throughout the stages of the policy cycle. One aim of this book is to illustrate how human rights frameworks are relevant to the decisions that policy makers, providers, programmers, activists, and judges face in their daily work and in turn how human rights strategies can be deployed to produce changes in normative recognition, policy processes, and social mobilization, which ultimately have the potential to create social transformation.

Addressing the "So What" Questions

In addition to showing *how* human rights frameworks can be operational-ized in practice, we also need to address the "so what" questions in a broader sense—Why should people care about applying human rights to health? Why do these frameworks matter? I believe that to answer these questions ade-quately requires the development of an empirical evidence base with respect to their impacts. Human rights frameworks and HRBAs are still reasonably new, but now that we have a better sense of common elements of what they include, we need to move beyond hortatory invocations of their importance to establishing what difference they can make in diverse people's lives. I ar-gue throughout this book that establishing and measuring impact must go far beyond merely pasting some indicators that might be easy to grasp—such as "respectful care"—onto traditional public health programs. Developing such an evidence base also requires new methodologies to capture the full impacts and, more broadly, lessons of applying human rights frameworks, which go beyond standard public health outcome and process measures.[15]

Trying to point to *value added* of human rights in conventional health programs is enticing, as we want national governments to adopt HRBAs; yet I fear it will ultimately be self-defeating because applying human rights prin-ciples will not necessarily accelerate progress in conventional measures. In addition, doing so reduces human rights to a purely instrumental value. Throughout these pages, I argue that a meaningful HRBA cannot merely re-package a conventional public health program. On the contrary, applying an empowering human rights framework to health transforms the evalua-tive space—the outcomes of interest as well as the process. For example, as discussed in later chapters, if we take seriously that human rights require shifting power dynamics, as I suggest, then we need metrics to assess political and institutional changes, shifts in public perceptions, and changes in outcomes.

What we measure reflects what we care about. Therefore, answering the "so what" question also necessarily calls for engaging in a dialogue with people outside the human rights field about normative questions—about how things *should* be, about what we *should* care about. The "so what" question inevitably leads to discussions about the purpose of health policies and programming in particular and of social and economic development more generally—and even about the nature of power and justice. In applying a human rights framework to health, in the context of maternal health, for example, we do not care simply about averting deaths. Rather, from a human rights perspective, women and girls have the right to live lives of dignity, which includes enjoyment of their sexual and reproductive health and rights (SRHR) as well as other human rights. As part of enabling them to do so, we should ensure that they have the conditions to go through pregnancy and childbirth safely. But applying a human rights framework also requires giving them meaningful choices throughout their lives, which go far beyond the health sector.

The great majority of women who die from pregnancy-related complications have lived lives marked by poverty, deprivation, and discrimination. From the moment of their births, these girls and women often face a funnel of narrowing choices whereby they are unable to exercise meaningful agency with respect to what they will do with their lives, how they will express their sexuality, how much they will be educated, with whom they will partner, when they will have sex, whether they will use contraception, and finally—as in the case of the woman in Chiapas who was suffering a miscarriage—what care they will get when they are pregnant or delivering, even when their lives hang in the balance. Applying a human rights framework to health in the context of maternal health, demands opening spaces, by shifting the opportunity structures—the resources and barriers—different actors face—to enable these women to live with dignity.[16] Answering the "so what" question requires fundamentally rethinking the nature of the problem, as well as the solution.

I also argue throughout this book that to effect transformative social change we need to shift thinking not merely in relation to health, as large a challenge as that is, but in relation to the demands of human rights. Part of the distressing disconnect between the normative development of human rights law relating to health and what public opinion and public policy in many countries reflect, relates to narrow conceptions of human rights—as civil and political rights only—and the consequent limited demands of social justice. Much of this book, therefore, explores the implications not just of different paradigms of health but also of conceptions of state responsibility and the ways in which we understand how power is exercised to limit people's abilities to enjoy their health rights and live lives of dignity. This book does not seek to proselytize for human rights or HRBAs; applying human rights frameworks to health is only meaningful insofar, and if and when, it leads to greater social justice.

This book is not directed especially at international human rights scholars, although I do include some discussion of evolving norms of international law and the need for further evolution. I believe that if we want to transform the world we cannot continue to talk among the converted; we need to reach people in other disciplines who come from different perspectives. We also need to reach the future leaders in law, development, and public health. This book is therefore an attempt to contribute to widening the circle and showing students, as well as practitioners from other fields who might not be immersed in human rights, why applying a human rights framework to health can matter.

Personal Stories: A Personal Voice

I am convinced that the reasons that human rights matter are often best understood within the context of individuals' lives. Statistics are, of course, necessary to illustrate trends and probabilities, and to place individual stories in context. However, by sharing stories of real people (whose names have been changed to preserve their privacy unless their names are within the public domain) and places throughout this book, I hope that the dilemmas and issues faced in the field will feel more immediate for many readers. Humans are, as Jonathan Gottschall argues, naturally storytelling animals; we make sense of our lives through narratives, narratives derived from religion, from national founding myths, and from family lore passed on from generation to generation, among other things.[17] And because we understand our own lives in the form of narratives that we live out, the form of narrative can also help us understand the lives of others.[18]

As emphasized in many anthropological studies, rights exist as lived experiences, not as abstract concepts in international instruments, and the ways in which rights are made meaningful are often through social relations and interactions.[19] I hope, therefore, that by capturing some elements of the particularistic through personal narratives, I will also be able to convey the universal commonality of humanness, as well as of human rights.

In addition, much of this book deals with the inexorably normative world we live in; throughout, I emphasize that the law and narrative are inseparable. The legal opinions discussed and the interpretations of human rights law are located in specific narratives about power, individuals, and the state, which in turn have an enormous impact on the social meaning of rights, as well as on our personal subjectivities.

As the stories collected here trace the work I have done in my professional life, they are in a sense my story as well. My mother's family is from Argentina and I grew up bicultural and bilingual. I originally became a human rights lawyer largely because the horrors of the Dirty War in that country loomed large in my childhood consciousness, as did later my outrage at the role of the U.S. government in many of the dictatorships and dirty wars across Latin America.[20]

I have had the privilege of living half of my adult life outside the United States. Living and working within countries, even when living in situations of tremendous relative comfort, is vastly different from parachuting in to conduct studies or field visits. No course or long-distance project supervision can as effectively reveal the true nature of the challenges of global health and development initiatives as can living and working in another culture for extended and formative periods. My perspectives on different places described here are deeply subjective and have been shaped not only by the sometimes dramatic political events that occurred during the times I was working in a certain place but also by the people I got to know.

However, the fact that nearly all of the stories in this book are from around the world in no way implies that I fail to see the gross inequities in the United States and the U.S. health system. Far from it. My father's father was a member of the IWW (International Workers of the World) and a lifelong union activist who transmitted to me his conviction that a truly inclusive democracy in the United States would require much greater substantive equality. As inequalities have continued to grow in the United States since my youth, I hope that some of the reflections in this book can encourage people in the United States to consider the way we might treat health and health care within the United States differently if we were to apply a human rights framework to some of the enormous social challenges we face.

I also want to highlight the role that the United States plays in shaping possibilities for enjoying health and related rights throughout the world. For example, in 2014, I was in Argentina when it again defaulted on its debt because of a small group of holdout creditors—vulture funds—and a U.S. court applied its parochial vision of what the "rule of law" required without any consideration of the equity effects of such a ruling or the perverse narrative it was creating regarding sovereign debt accumulation and payment.[21] The Human Rights Council condemned the activities of the vulture funds and called for a multilateral framework for sovereign debt restructuring.[22] Perhaps because I could easily have grown up in Argentina instead of the United States, the prevalent U.S. discourse around the events—that those were "the rules of the game" to get access to U.S. equity markets and "otherwise Argentina could go elsewhere and pay higher prices"—was a particularly acute illustration of how privilege justifies itself through the narratives we create about ourselves, not just at individual levels but also at societal levels, and that the two are inextricably intertwined, as I discuss throughout these pages.

The Structure of This Book

The rest of this book is divided into two main sections and a conclusion. In Part I, "Starting Points," I suggest that a transformative engagement between health and human rights requires rethinking conventional approaches to human rights, as well as to health. I came to public health not from the perspective of healing, as many others do, but from a traditional lawyer's training in human rights and with a profound concern for social justice. At the time, in the early 1990s, the human rights movement was almost exclusively focused on civil and political rights violations. But as some others did, I grew to feel that if the movement did not address social injustice, it would remain a marginal discourse for social emancipation.

In Chapter 1, beginning with a description of one of the first cases of torture that I ever worked on in Mexico, I set out thoughts about what torture does to us as human beings—the nature of suffering it inflicts and how it strips away the possibility of self-government, agency, and therefore human dignity. The concept of the equal dignity of all human beings, of the need to see other people as ends in and of themselves rather than as instruments for the advancement of our own or others' aims, is the core of a rights framework. And that simple concept—of according all people equal dignity—has enormous implications for the way our societies and world are organized.

I go on to explore the links among human rights, dignity, and health, beginning with a three-pronged paradigm that Jonathan Mann and colleagues set out in the early 1990s, at the beginning of what has become known as the health and human rights movement. There are serious health consequences to torture, and unfortunately the historical involvement of health professionals in torture and other abuses is all too common. Indeed, some forms of abuse in the health sector rise to the level of torture or cruel, inhuman, and degrading treatment.

However, most violence that affects women's and children's health is in the home or in private spaces close to home. Therefore, as human rights law, and domestic law in many countries, has recognized, to address the kinds of violence and suffering that women and children face, regulation of power must extend beyond the public sphere and into the private sphere of the home. Yet the way the public continues to think about human rights often continues to be too limited. If torture shatters the worlds that people construct, these abuses of children, especially girls and sexual minorities, sometimes disabled, often prevent the victims from ever fully developing a sense of themselves as full subjects of rights.

Chapter 2 begins with another example from my early days of human rights advocacy work in Mexico. During the course of investigating an atrocity by the Mexican military in a remote region of Chihuahua state, I found myself watching an infant die. Stunned by the mother's lack of indignation over her child's death, I argue that extreme poverty cannot be seen as a "background condition" but should be understood as just as much a violation of human rights as acts directly committed by state agents. The powerlessness wrought by extreme poverty is as devastating as that inflicted through torture, and the effects are the foreseeable result of human decisions about policies and programs at multiple levels. Yet even when there are obvious health consequences, we still too often fail to appreciate the human causality and state responsibility that lie behind these deprivations of dignity.

International law has advanced significantly in terms of eroding unhelpful distinctions between civil and political (CP) rights and economic, social, and cultural (ESC) rights, as has the jurisprudence of various national courts. Indeed, in both international and some national law there is now a concept of minimum essential levels of ESC rights necessary to life with dignity, as well as implications for leveling the playing field. However, just as with reframing state obligations regarding the private sphere, there is still a long way to go to change public understanding of ESC rights so that they are seen as *real* rights. I argue that to do so requires examining our assumptions about prevailing neoliberal economic paradigms and state responsibilities, as well as about the ways in which power prevents people from exercising freedom in practice and the consequent implications for how we think about justice.

In Chapter 3, I argue that conventional approaches to medicine and public health also require rethinking. Describing an incident that occurred early in my public health career in Haryana, India, I illustrate the limitations to empowering people through conventional public health approaches that treat social determinants—such as caste, gender, and racial hierarchies—as "distal," or background, factors, as opposed to the proximate behavioral causes on which most interventions as well as research focus.

Applying a human rights framework does not and cannot mean ignoring the need for access to biomedical advances. As Paul Farmer argues, the right to health must include the "right to sutures"—and blood, essential medications, and other supplies.[23] At the same time, a meaningful HRBA also calls for contextually grounded strategies to chip away at the power structures that perpetuate patterns of illness and suffering. These are all too often relegated to background conditions that cannot be touched in the short term in public health planning and policies; as a result, they never get addressed. After distinguishing between a right to health and the application of an HRBA or a human rights framework to health, which includes these social determinants that relate to other rights, I explore how such an approach, which builds on work in social medicine and social epidemiology, demands a fundamental shift in the way that health is generally understood in mainstream medical and public health practice.

In Chapter 4, starting with a story from the remote jungle "department" (state) of El Chocó in Colombia, I emphasize the significance of health systems within an HRBA to health. Health is largely a result of social determinants that go beyond the health sector. However, health systems reflect the patterns of discrimination and inequalities found in the overall society; alternatively, they can also help to facilitate greater substantive democracy. Health systems lie at the core of the realization of the right to health, as well as of HRBAs to health. In a rights framework, a health system is understood as a core social institution—"akin to the justice system or a fair political system"—rather than a delivery apparatus for goods and services.[24] So, for example, a society in which rich and poor alike feel that the health system is fairly prioritizing their needs is a more just society than one in which rich and poor are treated in different institutions with different standards of care—simply because of access to money.

A fundamental distinction of an HRBA to health systems is a focus on accountability. Arguing that an HRBA requires a "circle of accountability," Chapter 4 describes how such an approach would differentiate it from a conventional approach at each stage of the policy cycle, from the initial situational analysis through planning and budgeting processes to program implementation and monitoring and review mechanisms to remedies.[25] Returning throughout the chapter to the context of Colombia, I outline a systemic judgment by the Colombian Constitutional Court in 2008, which called for restructuring the health system along rights principles. I highlight the importance of that historic judgment, especially to the extent that it arguably destabilized entrenched assumptions and interests in the Colombian health sector and triggered a chain of varied effects. Throughout the book, I emphasize that applying a human rights framework in a transformative way aims to change dynamics of relationships between the public and the state to a relationship of entitlement and obligation and to dis-entrench patterns of power and privilege, which systematically deprive some people of their health and other rights. At the same time, I note challenges for meaningful change that continue to exist in the Colombian context.

In Part II, "Applying Human Rights Frameworks to Health," I examine specific aspects of HRBAs to health, and human rights frameworks more broadly, and I make more explicit how human rights frameworks can be applied by different actors to produce social transformation, providing examples throughout. As Part II develops human rights concepts introduced in Part I, readers may find these chapters somewhat more academic than those in Part I. However, it is precisely my intent that the explanation and application to the stories I introduce will make these legal concepts more accessible to nonlawyers. Human rights–based approaches require a broad, multidisciplinary response that depends on all of us, whether we are legal, development, or public health practitioners; professionals as well as ordinary citizens.

A fundamental part of the argument I make in these pages is that the divide between theory and practice is deeply fallacious; how we think about global health problems shapes what we do about them. It is useful to analyze specific conceptual elements of HRBAs to unpack what they imply in practice and to determine where both the theoretical and practical dilemmas lie. In showing how human rights tools and strategies to health have been deployed in concrete contexts by different actors, I note that many examples are partial, effecting only incremental changes. Yet that need not be discouraging, as changes in certain choice situations and relationships of power can trigger a cascade of changes, which in turn create meaningful improvements in the enjoyment of health and other rights by many other people.

Chapter 5 begins with a story of a maternal death in Sierra Leone, one of the poorest countries on earth and which was ravaged by a brutal civil war for many years and most recently has been decimated by Ebola. In what may seem a somewhat unlikely context, I return to the importance and meaning of accountability within a human rights framework. Perhaps what a human rights framework uniquely adds to other work in public health that is focused on social determinants lies precisely in the definition of relationships between rights-holders and duty-bearers. This identification of duty-bearers, in turn, permits the creation of a framework for accountability, including judicial recourse.

I stress, however, that accountability cannot mean adding remedies to broken systems. Real accountability calls for changes not only at multiple levels of decision making regarding health or, as described earlier, the establishment of a circle of accountability across the policy cycle but also across different relationships of entitlement and obligation: providers and patients; programmers and policy makers; policy makers and parliamentarians; elected governments and citizens. Further, in this chapter I explore not just different mechanisms but also different aspects of state obligations for taking positive measures in human rights; that is, *for what* is the state accountable? *How much* effort is the state expending? And *how* it is going about the process?

In Chapter 6, I return to Latin America. Through a story of rural health promoters from Puno, Peru, I explore the complex and challenging subject of participation in health. A fundamental aspect of a human rights framework is that people are not treated as passive recipients of goods and services but as participants in decisions that affect their well-being. I argue in this chapter that to understand meaningful participation in a human rights framework requires understanding where power resides and how power operates to keep people from challenging inequity, even when their health and well-being are at stake.

Active participation depends on the conditions for pluralistic democracy in a liberal state, including transparency and access to information. It is important to remember that participation also includes the voice of health professionals who are themselves often silenced within hierarchical and punitive health systems. However, I argue that effective participation that leads to mobilization for transformational change also requires going beyond liberal understandings of power to challenge how discourses and agendas, as well as boundaries for participation, are defined. Indeed, human agency and dignity are constrained in many ways that are invisible, and setting health and other priorities based on people's subjective assessments of their own suffering, as is done in conventional public health, may in fact entrench unfair background conditions that reduce people's own expectations for their lives. Ultimately, enabling people to participate in ways that challenge their own internalized subordination calls for the development of critical consciousness.

In Chapter 7, based on a discussion of a young, disabled woman who died of pregnancy-related complications in KwaZulu-Natal, South Africa, I examine the implications of a rights framework's demands that equality and non-discrimination be placed at the center of a public health and development agenda. The South African context illustrates sharply how intersecting forms of discrimination, based on race, disability, gender, and other axes of identity, conspire against diverse people living in poverty to deprive them of life choices.

A focus on equality has dramatic implications for public health and mainstream development. Conventional public health all too often remains in the thrall of health maximization, which measures "success" using averages and aggregate statistics, often based on achieving the "biggest bang for the buck." From a human rights perspective, national averages are not sufficient in measuring impact; disparities among populations can be more revealing of the obstacles underlying the achievement of well-being for certain historically disadvantaged groups in society.

This chapter further explains that the principle of "equality" in human rights has different faces. Formal equality requires equal treatment for similarly situated people and is closely related to demands for universalization of services. However, substantive equality acknowledges that in fact all people do not have equal starting points, and therefore different measures are required to achieve equal enjoyment of health and other rights. Conventionally, the human rights community has been overly reticent about taking stands regarding social inequality, which is a profound social determinant of population health. Not only is there increasing empirical evidence that social inequality is bad for our health, but I argue that the equal concern and respect for people, which meaningful substantive equality requires, demands as a normative matter certain degrees of economic equality and the macroeconomic policies that achieving such conditions would entail.

Yet fairness in health is not simply a matter of addressing income inequality or social exclusion, as it might be in relation to other rights; it also depends on considering other factors, such as the severity of a person's illness. After all, we have some notion that very sick people should be given priority in terms of resources over people who are suffering from relatively trivial conditions. Similarly, we consider comparative effectiveness of different interventions because to ignore efficiency considerations entirely has not just economic consequences but also equity consequences in terms of how many people end up suffering. Because even reasonable people will disagree on the relative weight of these different factors, addressing inequality in health requires a process that enables meaningful deliberation among those affected.

Chapter 8 examines human rights obligations beyond borders and begins with the story of a woman's death in a district hospital in Tanzania, a highly aid-dependent country. So many of the causes of people's poverty and ill-health in the global South are a result of global institutional arrangements and decisions taken beyond their national borders—in Washington, D.C.; New York; London; and even Seattle, Washington. Human rights law generally considers the relationship between people and national governments, which by itself can obscure the important actors and forces that have influence that cuts across national borders and boundaries. But this has begun to change.

This chapter explores differing concepts of global accountability and health governance, as well as a variety of emerging efforts to hold donor states responsible for extraterritorial obligations, in order to make advances with regard to the health of the poor in the global South. I discuss not only traditional forms of international aid cooperation but also the role that unjust institutional arrangements play in systematically putting some countries at a disadvantage in relation to others. I close the chapter by returning to a fundamental theme of the book: What is at stake in competing narratives of "sustainable development," which will be the future development agenda?

Finally, in the Conclusion, I reflect on what it can mean to apply a human rights framework to health—as opposed to other frameworks for social change—and why people who are concerned with social justice should care. Through the story of a boy I met in a psychiatric hospital in Argentina, I come back to the main message of this book: With the concerted efforts of people around the globe, another world is possible.

There is no recipe or magic bullet for the realization of human rights to health for all people. Throughout this book, I emphasize that progress can be and has been made. But meaningful human rights frameworks and HRBAs are about social transformation, which demands struggles for power and not "pleas to have human rights conferred" by the state.[26] Those struggles are inherently political, messy, and complex. Transformative change does not follow a linear path. Indeed, the ever-increasing array of toolkits to "show people how to apply HRBAs" will end up being counterproductive if they imply that to do so is akin to following a generic, technocratic formula. As I suggest in the later chapters, versions of human rights already coexist far too comfortably with neoliberal economic paradigms and are easily palatable to those who benefit from the status quo. If HRBAs to health, and human rights frameworks more generally, are to fulfill their promise in changing the systems that perpetuate inequality and injustice, they must subvert entrenched and insulated institutions and what have become virtually hegemonic views of the world. If rights are to be useful, they should play a role in destabilizing both norms and practices that deny certain people equal respect and concern. This book is not a manual on HRBAs to health; it is, on the contrary, a call to hold onto the radical possibilities of applying human rights frameworks to health.

When I began my work on health and human rights, an eminent international expert dismissively informed me that to spend my time promoting a legally claimable *right to health*—and maternal health in particular—was as useful as dedicating my life to knitting coats out of butterfly wings. As we see in these pages, a lot has changed in the twenty years since that moment. But there is still an enormous amount of work to do. If we collectively hold onto the emancipatory potential of using a human rights paradigm to promote social justice, I am convinced that we can transform, albeit incrementally and with inevitable setbacks, the landscape of global health and rights.

Concluding Reflections

My mother never failed to say "there but for the grace of God go I" whenever we passed a homeless person on the street in New York City. I only came to realize much later that, in her case, it was not a way of eliding the social and economic policies that distinguished her—our—fortune from theirs. Rather, it was a practice of mindfulness, an acknowledgment of the human being in front of her, and a reminder to be compassionate on a daily basis.

In the 1980s, when then-President Ronald Reagan's deinstitutionalization of patients in psychiatric hospitals, coupled with cuts in social services, resulted in approximately 140,000 mentally ill people living on the streets in cities across the United States, my mother's reflective comments took on a special significance.[27] My brother had long struggled with mental illness, moving in and out of private institutions. In looking into many of the faces of the people who found themselves suddenly living on the street, it was impossible for me not to reflect on the arbitrary twists of fate that led to the possibility of a life of dignity for my brother compared to a life of squalor, hopelessness, and degradation faced by so many others. It was impossible to maintain the pretense that there was anything essentially different about my brother—or about us as a family—that justified the difference in outcomes, or conferred protection from the fear and loathing with which people with mental illness are routinely regarded in the United States, as well as in other places around the globe.

I argue throughout the rest of this book that defining health as a question of human rights forces us to examine how we make sense of and respond not only to our own suffering or that of our close family and friends but also to that of others, including those living very far away. As humans, we instinctively try to give meaning to our losses as well as to our fulfillment, to create narratives about what has happened to us. Too often we use a kind of self-interested, albeit un–self-conscious, logic about when suffering is "bad luck," when there is some "implication that God was a party to the outcome," or when tragedy is simply inevitable because that is the way things are "in those places" or "those cultures."[28] I want us to question that logic.

For example, when U.S. missionary Dr. Kent Brantly came back from Liberia with Ebola in 2014 and was cured at Emory University Medical Center, he gave a news conference thanking God for his survival.[29] Undoubtedly inadvertently, the implication was that God may not care so much about the thousands of Liberians and West Africans who did not survive. But God did not cure Dr. Brantly; what cured Dr. Brantly was excellent medical care, coupled with probably an already stronger immune system than many undernourished people in West Africa had.

And I want us to question when narratives are created and too often embedded in laws, around whose suffering matters. For example, a thirteen-year-old girl is sexually assaulted by her uncle, but for her to choose to have a life plan that does not include the fetus she was forced to carry is "evil and selfish," imposing suffering on the innocent "child." And isn't it possible that a sex worker—female, male, or trans—also suffers when raped and has a right to bodily integrity, as well as labor protections?

But I also want to be very clear: I do not believe that human rights are fundamentally at odds with all religious traditions. There is no question that pain, sorrow, and suffering are part of this life, or a cycle of lives. I do not reject the notion that there can indeed be a value in suffering.[30] Any parent knows that it is a mistake to try to protect a child from all disappointment and pain. After all, resiliency is crucial to our development as human beings. The needless suffering caused by unfairness in our societies and our world is the subject of this book. And unlike the "glad tidings of great joy" promised in the Bible or other blessings and enlightenment that entice people in an afterlife, a human rights framework emphasizes a universal claim to dignity in this world. It is not redemption but justice that I argue a human rights framework offers.

At the same time, taking seriously the ways in which power structures suffering within and between countries requires rethinking narrow human rights frameworks as relating only to a small slice of civil and political issues, a view that continues to prevail in much of the world. Taking suffering seriously calls for us to challenge what those conceptions of human rights say about our understanding of the role of the state, the demands of justice, and, ultimately, our ways of being together in this broken world.

PART I

Starting Points

Chapter 1

Dignity and Suffering: Why Human Rights Matter

We accord a person dignity by assuming . . . they share the same
human qualities we ascribe to ourselves.
  —Nelson Mandela, speech, Cape Town, South Africa, May 10, 2004

Where, after all, do universal human rights begin? In small places,
close to home—so close and so small that they cannot be seen on
any map of the world. Yet they are the world of the individual
person: the neighborhood he lives in; the school or college he
attends; the factory, farm or office where he works. Such are the
places where every man, woman and child seeks equal justice, equal
opportunity, equal dignity without discrimination. Unless these
rights have meaning there, they have little meaning anywhere.
Without concerted citizen action to uphold them close to home,
we shall look in vain for progress in the larger world.
          —Eleanor Roosevelt, speech, United Nations, New York,
                                                  March 27, 1958

I graduated from law school with an Echoing Green Foundation Fellowship
to bring human rights cases from Mexico to international tribunals and treaty
monitoring bodies.[1] One of the first cases I worked on involved the annihilation of nearly an entire family. Francisco Quijano Santoyo was allegedly
engaged in drug trafficking and was involved in a shootout that resulted in

the death of a police officer. The next day, antinarcotics agents from the Federal Judicial Police (PJF, according to the acronym in Spanish), the Mexican equivalent of the FBI, surrounded the family's house in Mexico City and exterminated two of three other brothers: Jaime and Erik. In human rights language, that kind of murder by state agents is referred to as "extrajudicial execution," a rather technical term for the bloodbath that occurred in this case.

Another brother, Héctor, was injured and detained after the shootings and eventually tortured to death. It was a particularly brutal torture; the PJF agents cut out Hector's tongue with a small knife and attached electrodes to various parts of his body. Eventually he died of cardiac arrest. But what made Héctor's torture almost unimaginably horrendous to me was that the PJF forced his mother and sister to listen to and watch parts of it, which is of course a torture in and of itself.

Six months afterward, Héctor's father, Francisco Quijano Garcia, who had been campaigning publicly for an investigation into the deaths of his sons, was himself disappeared; his body was found months later at the bottom of an unused well. The police accused an associate of Mr. Quijano Garcia, but the man, who was convicted of homicide in the case, stated he had confessed under police coercion.[2]

I got to know Héctor's sister, Rosa, quite well. We were about the same age. We'd both just gotten married. I felt like my adult life and career were just beginning. Her life as she knew it had just ended; her world had been shattered.

I learned from Rosa something that I have heard repeated by torture victims too many times to count in the intervening years: the most awful thing about torture is not the physical pain, as intense and unbearable as that can be; the most awful thing about torture is that it destroys a person's sense of herself and her world.

Elaine Scarry has described the "unmaking of the world" that occurs through torture.[3] Focused on the effects of the physical pain, Scarry explains that "as in dying and death, so in serious pain the claims of the body utterly nullify the claims of the physical world."[4] Anyone who has experienced it knows that intense pain makes us small; rather than feeling our bodies in space, space and time are limited by our bodies. The physical pain experienced by torture victims destroys the world they project as well as the one they know. "This unseen sense of self-betrayal in pain, objectified in forced confession is also objectified in forced exercises that make the prisoner's body an *active* agent, an actual cause of his pain."[5] Pain, as Scarry writes, is a central part of that destruction of one's world.

But, as I learned from Rosa, personally experiencing physical pain is not always a prerequisite. Seeing a loved one being tortured and being impotent to stop the pain can also unmake one's world. In *Prisoner Without a Name, Cell Without a Number*, Jacobo Timerman relates his own experiences as a prisoner in a clandestine prison during the Argentine Dirty War. He speaks particularly to the experience Rosa had in Mexico:

> Nothing can compare to those family groups who were tortured often together, sometimes separately but in view of one another, or in different cells, while one was aware of the other being tortured. The entire affective world, constructed over the years with utmost difficulty, collapses with a kick in the father's genitals, a smack on the mother's face, an obscene insult to the sister, or the sexual violation of a daughter. Suddenly an entire culture based on familial love, devotion, the capacity for mutual sacrifice collapses. Nothing is possible in such a universe, and that is precisely what the torturers know.[6]

Torture destroys any possibility of human agency in the victim through its physical effects; but it also destroys the narrative we construct to make sense of ourselves emotionally and psychologically.[7] It is this shattering of human agency—and, in turn, of human dignity—that lies at the core of torture and makes it the quintessential abuse of human rights.

In this chapter, I discuss understandings of human dignity, the link between health and human rights, and why human rights matter. The equal dignity of all people is the basis for the notion of universal human rights. Dignity requires the conditions that enable one to govern one's self and exercise ethical as well as physical independence within a specific social context; it also requires us to respect the humanity in others.

There is an important link between torture—the classic violation of human rights and dignity, defined in more detail later in this chapter—and health, in terms of both the severe physical and psychological impacts on victims as well as the frequent use of specialized knowledge by health professionals in carrying it out. Moreover, some abuses in health care—through the manner in which services are inflicted and through the denial of treatment—rise to the level of what is considered "torture or cruel, inhuman, and degrading treatment" under international law. The common thread among these different facets of torture and inhuman treatment is that they stem from, and result in, a denial of the full humanity of the victim.

I go on to argue, however, that confining our focus on torture to the actions of state agents, whether police or health personnel, reflects an inadequate conception of human rights and state responsibilities—especially if we are concerned about the health of women and children. Women and children overwhelmingly face abuse in the private sphere, and applying a human rights framework to health must enable us to redress that suffering. The annihilation of self that occurs when an adult is tortured by strangers is only one kind of assault on dignity; it can be just as awful when children are raised to internalize a sense of themselves as inferior or defective—a sense of themselves as less than fully human or even deserving of abuse—before they are able to acquire any degree of autonomy. Thus, human rights frameworks need to be empowering, as well as protective, of agency across multiple spheres.

Human Dignity: A Universal Concept with Varying Conceptions and Implications

Recognition of the dignity inherent in all human beings is the basis for human rights.[8] Across countless cultures and philosophical as well as religious traditions, there is a concern for the "equal dignity of the human person," which is set out in the Universal Declaration of Human Rights and in many other international documents. Dignity has been assailed as meaning different things to different people. As the late legal philosopher Ronald Dworkin argues, dignity has fallen into "flaccid overuse." Yet, at its core, the principle of dignity is most often explained in terms of requiring that people be treated as ends and not mere means. Thus, torture is the ultimate example of reducing victims to being means—means to obtaining information, exacting revenge, or expressing discrimination toward or contempt for a certain group.

The liberal philosopher Immanuel Kant was a leading articulator of this meaning of human dignity: "Everything has either a price or a dignity. Whatever has a price can be replaced by something else as its equivalent; on the other hand, whatever is above all price, and therefore admits of no equivalent, has a dignity. But that which constitutes the condition under which alone something can be an end in itself does not have mere relative worth, i.e., price, but an intrinsic worth, i.e., a dignity."[9] Kant's insight has implications for how we relate to others as well as to our own lives. That is, if life has objective, intrinsic value, then it follows that both your own life and the lives of others have that value. It is not just you who can possess dignity while other human beings are slaves. Out of respect for your own dignity, you must treat yourself as an "end"—or an independent subject. At the same time, out of respect for the dignity of others, you must treat them as ends in and of themselves, and not as means for your own benefit. Kant's notion that we should be able to universalize how we wish to be treated implies that achieving dignity in one's own life requires respect for humanity itself, which is fundamental to the concept of universal human rights.

Many scholars have pointed out a conceptual dilemma here: if dignity is intrinsic, it should not need protection through laws and policies.[10] Yet violations of human rights, such as torture, clearly constitute affronts to dignity, and the purpose of reflecting human rights in law both at the national and international levels is to protect people's dignity. Despite this theoretical dilemma, I believe that, on a commonsense level, the notion that every human being possesses an intrinsic worth and that this worth should be recognized by other human beings and enshrined in our laws and social arrangements can be compatible with the idea that, sadly, too often it is undermined in practice.

Much has been written critiquing the Westernized individualism of modern human rights, sometimes with ample justification. However, this concept—the fundamental dignity of all human beings and the prescription to treat people as ends and not means—is not just a Western philosophical concept. Kant's proposition that we cannot adequately respect our own humanity unless we respect the humanity in others has strong resonances with a number of religious and cultural traditions. The Bible's "Golden Rule," for example, calls on people to treat others as they would want to be treated. Similar notions regarding seeing others as full human beings can be found in the beliefs of Jewish thinkers, such as Martin Buber, as well as in Sufi and Hindu traditions. Buber writes about the distinction between relationships grounded in treating others as "*Its*" or objects—and fuller "encounters" with others as subjects or "*Thous*."[11] In a similar vein, the rule of dharma in Hinduism basically states, "One should never do that to another which one regards as injurious to one's own self."[12] "*Namaste*," the common Indian salutation, is a humbling acknowledgment of being on equal standing with the person greeted.

In African traditions, there is the notion of "*Ubuntu*," which can be roughly translated as "I am because we are."[13] *Ubuntu* is found in diverse forms in many societies throughout Africa; among the languages of East, Central, and Southern Africa, the concept of *Ubuntu* captures a world view about what it means to be human.[14] Desmond Tutu, the South African archbishop emeritus and Nobel Peace Prize laureate, explains that, on an interpersonal level, *Ubuntu* means that every person's humanity is bound up in each other.[15] For his part, the scholar Kwame Anthony Appiah, who has West African—Ghanaian—roots, associates his attachment to the idea of dignity with his father, "who grew up in Asante, at a time when the independence of its moral climate from that of European Enlightenment was extremely obvious."[16] Appiah goes on to note that those Asante conceptions depended on a sense of one's own dignity being connected to the dignity of one's fellow citizens.[17]

In stressing universality, I do not want to overstate the claims to uniformity: the essential human qualities that support a claim of worth, dignity, and shared humanity vary across philosophical and religious traditions. In some, there may be a concern for the sentience and the capacity of fellow humans to suffer (and in some philosophers' arguments this would extend rights to animals as well);[18] in some religious traditions, there may be a focus on the quality of having a soul. In a modern human rights framework, dignity is reflected in the human capacity for agency, or self-government, which enables a person to make (and take responsibility for) choices and decisions about one's self and the course of one's life.

The kind of self-government necessary for human dignity need not—and, in my view, should not—be understood as autonomy in a vacuum, isolated from societal context. This book is not a philosophical treatise on the nature of our constitutive attachments to others or the voluntariness of our relation to our own ends, which are deeply contested among different philosophical traditions. I believe that both extremes—excessively individualized rights schemes and the kind of cultural relativism that rejects the plasticity of human social arrangements and dignity as a value—are overly rigid.

On the one hand, neither communities nor cultures are stable and monolithic. Reified assertions of unchanging cultural norms empty them of their political content and disconnect them from the realities of how they are used to prop up all sorts of inequitable social norms and power hierarchies.[19] We must recognize not only that communal ideals shift over time but also that the notion of a community as a closed circle of group harmony is also false and disregards the multiple identities that we each carry within ourselves.

I am the product of two different religions, national and class backgrounds, and ethnicities, and therefore it may be particularly easy for me to see the false necessity of ascribing one particular identity to any given individual. More generally, however, rigid notions of identity—of gender identity, for example—disregard the multiplicity of meanings that a particular identity (such as gender) has for diverse people. Indeed, the construction of collective identities, based on gender, as well as ethnicity, religion, and race, for example, is a continual and ongoing process, not one definitive event with constant flux stemming from the inherent conflicts within each group.[20] As Kant proposed, we humans have the capacity and duty to examine our conscience, which unites out thoughts and feelings, and that capacity can allow us to resist dominant moral codes and create the possibility for reform.[21] If we believe in human dignity and the capacity of human beings for choice and agency, it follows then, as I discuss in later chapters, that we cannot accept that identities and roles imposed on people are immutable. In the decades of my doing this work, there have been many times in the most "traditional cultures"—from deep in the Amazon to remote African villages—that I have witnessed transformations in self-understanding about the role of women, which in turn produced changes in behavior with spouses, children, and others, and eventually led to modifications of expectations and group practices. Or sometimes it is judicial decisions, such as the *Atala* decision by the Inter-American Court of Human Rights, that can destabilize social narratives of identity even in a devoutly Catholic context such as Chile regarding the assumption that the "best interests of the child" means a lesbian cannot have custody.[22]

On the other hand, I also recognize that true self-government requires the power to make meaningful decisions for one's self within the thick networks of relationships in which we actually live. This requires a conception of being human that acknowledges that we are all embedded in social contexts, and exercising ethical independence in our lives requires navigating the relations in those contexts. As philosopher Charles Taylor argues: "Discovering my own identity doesn't mean that I work it out in isolation, but that I negotiate it through dialogue, partly overt, partly internal with others."[23] A dynamic relationship and mutual dependence exists between an individual and the conditions as well as between an individual and other people—children, sexual partners, community members, and so on—that allow an individual to develop into a full person.[24]

Throughout the rest of this book, I argue that a human rights framework based on a notion of dignity as including a respect for the humanity in others contains within it an understanding of our inescapable interconnectedness as members of multiple communities and societies. That interconnectedness, in practice, is shaped by different power relations that affect the possibilities for some people to live with dignity, and in our invariably gendered, racial-ized, class relations, our identities are enacted and reenacted continually in ways that can reinforce or can transform the status quo. Therefore, experiencing dignity is inextricably linked with participating in (re)shaping the conditions of our society, and with who gets to count as a full and equal member.

The narrow liberal idea of rights based on atomistic autonomy is, as we discuss in this and later chapters, connected to an idea of the liberal state. In the nineteenth century, traditional liberal state, male, property-owning, adult citizens were conceived of as free and equal. The role of the state was seen principally in terms of preserving their autonomous liberty, through po-lice, military, and judicial protections. A more modern conception of the state as a welfare state, or a "social state of law" (*estado social de derecho*), recognizes that the diverse citizens in a society cannot exercise their liberties freely, or participate fully in society, without some background equality in distribution of resources and opportunities. No subject more than health rights illustrates the need to adapt traditional rights analyses, as former South African Constitutional Court Justice Albie Sachs stated: "Health care rights by their very nature have to be considered not only in a traditional legal con-text structured around the ideas of human autonomy but in a new analytical framework based upon the notion of human interdependence. A healthy life depends upon social interdependence: the quality of air, water, and sanitation which the state maintains for the public good; the quality of one's caring rela-tionships, which are highly correlated to health; as well as the quality of health care and support furnished officially by medical institutions."[25]

This is the challenge of developing emancipatory rights frameworks con-cerned with dignity: they must navigate an understanding of our identities as socially constituted and yet also allow for individual agency; they must strike a balance between recognizing that identities are not preassigned, essentialist, and immutable, yet also not so fluid as to be readily changeable; and people must be protected by the institutions of the state, yet also must be empowered materially by the state and enabled to express different aspects of themselves freely.

Violations of Dignity and Rights: When Do We Stop Treating People as Fully Human?

Torture, as Dworkin writes, "is designed to extinguish that power [to make decisions], to reduce its victim to an animal for whom decision is no longer possible. That is the most profound insult to his dignity . . . it is the most profound insult to his human rights."[26] That is precisely what happened to Héctor Quijano.

Conversely, it is impossible to torture someone whom one sees as a fully human being. It is not the case, as some people think, that torture is generally committed by sociopaths, untethered by conscience, but rather that humans have a seemingly infinite capacity to justify inhuman actions to ourselves. Sociologists and psychologists have studied the different conditions, at societal, institutional, and individual levels, under which certain people can be dehumanized by others to the extent that it leads to torture. For example, Erving Goffman writes about the "mortification of self" and breakdown of normal social behavioral expectations that occur in "closed institutions" such as military boot camps, prisons, or psychiatric hospitals.[27] Other scholars have pointed to the existence of a tendency to blame the victim, or what Ervin Staub calls a "just-world view"—the belief that the person being tortured must have done something terrible to deserve what is happening to him or her.[28] This was true of the atrocities committed by the military dictatorship in Argentina and the abuse committed by the police in Mexico, as well as the "enhanced interrogations" conducted by the U.S. government in Iraq, Afghanistan and elsewhere. It is not just evil people and psychopaths who torture other human beings; structural factors foster the dehumanization of a certain group of individuals and allow perpetrators to stop seeing the victims as fellow human beings. Genocide is the ultimate expression of the denial of humanity of an entire group or population.

Torture, although perhaps the quintessential violation of an individual's human rights, is of course far from the only deprivation of civil and political rights that denies dignity and people's ability to carry out life plans. When we lack the freedom to elect our government or the freedoms of association, information, and movement, or if we face detention without due process, our ability to govern our lives—and in turn our dignity—is deeply affected.

Historically, people have been treated as less than human on the basis of differentiation with respect to particular aspects of their identity, which is why nondiscrimination is a central tenet in human rights law. For example, the U.S. Constitution originally accorded slaves the status of three-fifths of a person.[29] And to this day, racial discrimination permeates U.S. society, police, and the criminal justice systems, as well as every point in the U.S. health care system.[30] To be born black in the United States, according to critical race theorist Patricia Williams, writing in the 1980s, is to "embody" an otherness in relation to being born as the white self, and it is a threatening otherness that must be controlled or repressed. To this day, we have examples in the media all the time of how being especially a young black male in America is still a marker of dangerousness to be contained, from Florida to Ferguson, Missouri. For "blacks"—as Williams deliberately referred to a set of social actors—rights are a "magic wand of visibility and invisibility, of inclusion and exclusion, of power and no-power. The concept of rights, both positive and negative, is the marker of our citizenship, our participatoriness, our relation to others."[31]

In the Spanish colonies, there were theological debates about whether just the black slaves brought from Africa or both they and the indigenous people of Latin America lacked souls, because the possession of a soul was thought to define "humanness."[32] Historically, a narrative of femininity in parts of Latin America is deeply tied to a vision of *criolla* women of European heritage as "clean and modern" as opposed to indigenous women who were thought to be dirty and animal-like.[33]

Women generally have historically been—and still often are—treated as less than fully human, as chattel or children or even on a par with animals.[34] Women in many countries are still denied the right to inherit land and are required to obtain consent from men for certain medical procedures. And throughout the world, cultural norms and practices regularly define women not in terms of their humanity but in terms of their sexuality, which is to be managed and controlled. Women are the objects of both desire and misogyny, and in seemingly equal measure seem to need to be protected or repressed, rather than treated as subjects with rights, including to sexual pleasure.

One principal way in which women's ethical and legal subjectivity is diminished is through laws and practices that reduce them to mere means for reproduction and childrearing. As Betty Friedan said, "There is no . . . full human dignity and personhood possible for women until we assert and demand the control of our own bodies, over our own reproductive processes. . . . The real sexual revolution is the emergence of women from passivity, from *thingness*, to full self-determination and dignity."[35] Among other courts, the Colombian Constitutional Court has explicitly used a "dignity" argument to strike down draconian abortion restrictions. In 2006, the court reasoned that to not leave any exceptions for the life and health of the mother, or for rape or incest, reduces the woman to being "a womb without conscience."[36] The Argentine Supreme Court was even clearer in striking down restrictions on abortion in the case of sexual assault: "From the notion of human dignity comes the principle that establishes [women] as an end in an of themselves and not merely a means or instrument of reproduction."[37]

People with various disabilities have also been denied full human status by discriminatory laws as well as by social norms throughout history that dictate certain physical standards for humanness as well as define "normal" behaviors.[38] Indeed, it is only in the last twenty to thirty years that the international human rights movement has begun to take seriously the violations of dignity faced by people with disabilities, including mental disabilities. Laws reducing "imbeciles" and "lunatics" to some less-than-human status, depriving them of control over basic decisions in their lives, including reproduction, were more the norm than the exception historically, and they continue to be in force in too many countries.

Historically, laws enshrined distinctions between citizens and others of lesser status based on property ownership as well—and across much of the world today, we still consign vast swaths of humanity to being less than fully human in practice, if not law, merely because they are poor. Stop at virtually any traffic light in Dar es Salaam or Freetown or Mumbai or Lima—or a hundred other cities across the globe—and there will be an immediate assault of beggars parading their misery in exchange for a handout. We, the well-off, who walk along or drive by in cars with the windows rolled up, tend to look right through the beggars, avoiding their eyes. However, the destitute and ill—trapped by their seemingly inexorable invisibility as human beings— often go to lengths to make themselves seem more pitiful and deserving of charity than the rest. Societies in which we tolerate these manifestations of tremendous inequality and extreme poverty structure this relationship between the well-off and the very poor, fostering systematic dehumanization that makes dignity impossible. Confronted endlessly with this visual barrage of deformities and desperation, the people in the cars or rushing by on the streets invariably stop seeing the extremely poor as fully human but rather as objects that inspire compassion at times and undoubtedly contempt and loathing at others.

And one step removed from the street—on the web, on our TV screens, and in our newspapers—the masses of people displaced by war or earthquakes, starving to death, or stricken with terrible diseases, which should have been preventable, are paraded before us; CNN, Al Jazeera, and the BBC are constantly feeding us some new atrocity or humanitarian crisis, as our ability to empathize and see the people on the screen as equal human beings grows ever more tenuous.

In human rights we used to believe that simply drawing attention to a horror would be enough to make people take action. Yet, the spectacles of misery all too often fail to focus our attention on the ways in which our social and economic arrangements systematically create the situations in which some people are treated as means rather than ends—with grave effects on their health, as well as on their dignity. As Susan Sontag writes, "The imaginary proximity to the suffering inflicted on others that is granted by [these] images suggests a link between the far away sufferers and the privileged viewer that is simply untrue, that is yet one more mystification of our real relations to power."[39]

But in this inexorably interconnected world, we are not innocent spectators of suffering in our own countries or across the globe. For example, what if wages in a country are too low for laborers to exercise choice about their life plans while the wealthy live in palaces? And what if people in the United States or Europe are relying on the cheap labor provided in Guatemala to harvest sugar or in Bangladesh to make clothing—under conditions that make it impossible for them to live with dignity? Do we not owe those strangers the treatment that we would wish for ourselves, and shouldn't we insist that our governments apply appropriate trade and labor regulations in the countries from which we import products? What level of concern for "the other" is feasible, or required by respect for human dignity, in our globalized world?[40] My intention in these pages is to encourage readers not just to have a knee-jerk reaction of sympathy, which as Sontag notes, "proclaims our innocence as well as our impotence,"[41] but to explore how a rights framework might make us rethink what we owe each other as full human beings, through the laws and institutional arrangements we devise at national and global levels.

Dignity, Health, and Human Rights

Dignity, health, and human rights are intimately connected. In a classic 1994 article, Jonathan Mann and colleagues described three dimensions of connections between health and human rights. The first dimension relates to the health impacts that result from human rights violations—especially, in their discussion, civil rights violations such as torture. The second dimension involves the impact of health policies, programs, and practices on human rights—again in their original conception, with a focus in particular on civil rights. The final dimension, and one that I discuss at length throughout this book, involves the recognition that health and human rights are integral dimensions of, and can be complementary approaches to advancing human dignity and well-being.[42]

Let's start with the recognition that human rights abuses, such as torture, are not only violations of human dignity but also quite evidently bad for people's health, as is clear from the Quijano case. As director of research and investigations for Physicians for Human Rights (PHR) in the 2000s, I supervised PHR's investigation into the health effects of the so-called "enhanced interrogation techniques" that the George W. Bush administration was using on detainees in the "war on terror." In 2006, the Bush administration was claiming that these techniques did not constitute torture because they did not meet the threshold of pain and suffering required under the UN Convention against Torture, which the United States had ratified and implemented through domestic legislation.

In day-to-day conversation, we often use the word "torture" quite loosely. In international law, Article 1 of the UN Convention against Torture sets out four essential elements of the definition of torture: (1) *intentional* infliction; (2) of *severe* pain and suffering (physical or mental); (3) for a specific purpose (that is, *to obtain information, intimidate, punish, or discriminate*); and (4) *with* the involvement, instigation, consent, or acquiescence of a state official or person acting in an official capacity.[43] The severity of pain and suffering must pass a certain threshold level. However, judging whether a specific action meets that threshold depends on all circumstances of case, including duration; intensity; physical and mental effects of the action; and gender, age, and state of health of the victim. The PHR investigation, based in part on in-depth interviews with former detainees, clearly demonstrated that the techniques used did constitute torture.[44]

The investigation into these so-called enhanced interrogation techniques reinforced that, given the right circumstances, normal individuals have a seemingly infinite capacity for the basest of cruelties, often believing that such behavior is directed at achieving some higher objective—in this case, information about the "war on terror." Moreover, medical professionals, despite having professional duties of loyalty to patients, are not immune from succumbing to instrumentalizing people to achieve some "higher" goal set out by the state.[45] Additional investigations by PHR demonstrated the extent to which health professionals—psychologists, in particular—had been involved in the development and application of the enhanced interrogation techniques.[46]

The second dimension of Mann and colleagues' paradigm involves the effects of health policies, programs, and practices on human rights. Quarantine, "shelter in place," and isolation policies can certainly violate civil liberties and create discrimination and stigmatization, if not carefully tailored, which became all too apparent at different points in the Ebola outbreak that began to spread quickly in 2014 in West Africa. International law recognizes exceptions for public health and public order, and the Siracusa Principles and other international documents have been developed to provide criteria to reduce inadvertent discrimination and disproportionate restrictions on civil rights during public health emergencies.[47]

For now, I want to focus on the centrality of not reducing people to means in a human rights framework, as we are concerned with people's dignity. Syphilis experiments, for example, were systematically carried out for forty years on African Americans in the United States.[48] The Tuskegee Syphilis Study, conducted from 1932 to 1972, was a research study on the outcome of untreated syphilis on hundreds of African American men in Georgia. The study participants were essentially on a decades-long deathwatch, as the study officers did not treat their advancing and deadly syphilis. A fundamental distinction between a human rights approach to health and a conventional utilitarian approach is that whatever the objective may be—a cure for syphilis or the promise of some other medical breakthrough—it can never justify treating fellow human beings as mere means to that end.

Again and again, in health as well as more broadly, we see that the most egregious abuses are committed in the name of some higher purpose. Mann felt that inadvertent discrimination was so common in public health that it should be assumed, and need to be disproven.[49] Moreover, it is not coincidental that, as in the case of the syphilis study, research abuses commonly affect populations that are discriminated against, marginalized, or vulnerable.

It is important to note that the Tuskegee study represented an appalling breach of a number of ethical standards in public health, in addition to the human rights violations it entailed. And in the aftermath of the scandal it caused when the public realized what had been going on for decades, the United States adopted practices and institutions to manage the use of human subjects in research.[50] Almost all countries in the world now have some institutions that conduct ethics review of medical, public health, and social science research involving other human beings.

Torture and Cruel, Inhuman, and Degrading Treatment (and Other Abuses) in Health Care

The manner of provision of health care, as well the failure to provide health care, can result in practices that rise to the level of torture, or cruel, inhuman, and degrading treatment, as they are defined in international law. In the context of health care, steep asymmetries of power are inherent—consequently, massive suffering and dehumanization are all too easily accepted and even normalized. For example, labor-and-delivery wards across the world have distinctly veterinary qualities to the care women are being provided, where basic issues of privacy, respect, and common consideration for human dignity are too often lacking.

Also in the reproductive health care context, forced sterilization has been found to constitute torture.[51] The UN Committee on the Elimination of Discrimination Against Women (CEDAW Committee), for example, has noted that decisions about one's body and reproductive capacity are essential to being able to live the life one chooses, and depriving a woman of these capacities strips her of essential dignity.[52] And again, it is no coincidence that discriminated against populations, such as the Roma in Slovakia and the indigenous women in Peru, who are already treated by society as less than fully human, can end up being targeted for sterilization by the health system.

Denial of access to treatment can also deny women of fundamental choices over their lives and has been found to constitute torture when such denial produces severe pain and suffering. For example, in the case of *KL v. Peru*, a young Peruvian girl was forced to carry an anencephalic fetus to term because of the interpretation of restrictive abortion laws.[53] After giving birth to a baby that had no brain, KL was forced to breastfeed the baby during the four days it lived. KL was later diagnosed with severe depression that required psychiatric treatment.[54] The UN Human Rights Committee found that Peru had subjected KL to "cruel and inhuman treatment" and reasoned that in preventing KL from having a therapeutic abortion, KL's severe suffering was entirely foreseeable.[55]

Denial of care can be direct, as in the case of KL, where it emerged as an open conflict between her petition and the decision of the hospital. But denial of care that rises to the level of "inhuman and degrading treatment" can also be achieved through laws, policies, and regulations in which there may be no open conflict between the patient and facility. For example, the denial of access to pain relief, if it causes severe pain and suffering, can be considered "cruel, inhuman or degrading treatment" under international law.[56] But there is a gap between international norms and national regulations, as well as between public and political attitudes. That millions of people around the world continue to die of cancer and HIV/AIDS and other conditions, in excruciating pain every year, is related to how we understand the cause of that suffering and the state's responsibility for taking measures to redress it.

Let me give an example of what the denial of pain medication means to an individual person. When I was living in Peru I got to know Dolores, a young woman who lived in the Cono Norte section of Lima. Before any gentrification began, the Cono Norte was a large slum area far removed from the picturesque poverty that tourists like to snap photos of in rural villages. The area Dolores lived in was filled with bleak cement structures, half constructed and chaotically set out on unnamed, unpaved streets, made more gray by the perpetual foggy mist, or *garrua*,[57] that blankets Lima. It was a long time after she got sick before we knew Dolores had cancer. She coughed, her throat hurt, her glands were swollen. She saw doctor after doctor but was unable to get an accurate diagnosis—the doctors took her money and prescribed ineffectual cough syrups and antibiotics, and when these failed to work they told her it was a manifestation of psychological repression. She was told she would be cured if she could only learn to voice her anger. It got worse, she lost her voice, and it hurt so much to swallow that she stopped eating solids. Finally, she was diagnosed with esophageal cancer. By this time, it had metastasized; chemotherapy was ineffective. But even when she knew that she was dying, the health system still failed to provide her with the pain medication that might have allowed her to die with some dignity.

Dolores died in agonizing pain; having lost her voice, her face, disfigured by the agony, wore the perpetual expression she felt, frozen for weeks in a "howl" and reminiscent of the Norwegian artist's famous painting.[58] Her parents had set up a bed for her in the room next to the living room. Although she had previously taken care of everyone else in the family, family members now took turns feeding Dolores through a tube, cleaning her bedpan, and washing her body so that it would not get sores. Dolores spent her last months unable to sleep and wracked by anxiety and depression, as well as physical pain. I visited Dolores multiple times as she deteriorated and witnessed the center of this family's home become transformed into a site of grief and anguish. It was unbearable for me, let alone her parents and the rest of her family, to see her suffer so much—and to be completely impotent to alleviate any of her misery.

The intensity of Dolores's pain, and that of many terminally ill patients like her, is as world-destroying as that inflicted in some forms of torture. Yet it need not be this way. Most of this book, like most of my work, is concerned with the conditions under which people are born and live, but dignity has everything to do with how people end their personal narratives as well. Palliative care is part of allowing people to die with dignity, as is the choice of euthanasia under some circumstances.

Even from a purely utilitarian perspective, dying in unbearable pain should not happen to anyone in the twenty-first century. Morphine is an inexpensive drug and although palliative care would not be prioritized by conventional cost-effectiveness measures, as the dying do not recover, health economists are beginning to rethink those metrics in relation to pain relief.

But some might argue that the state is not responsible for Dolores's suffering in the same way that a state agent is when torturing, as in the Quijano case, because the source of the pain is internal to the person and not caused by the health care system. Yet it was completely foreseeable that Dolores would end up in such pain, and morphine is an economical medication that easily could have been administered to allow Dolores to die with dignity and with little or no pain. We expect the state to undertake a wide array of actions to prevent what are the predictable consequences of not providing pain medication. Consider, for example, that we call for our governments to provide traffic signals because the resulting motor-vehicle accidents and injuries in the case of not doing so are entirely foreseeable. Similarly, the omission of providing pain medication can be considered *an affirmative act*, an act for which the state should be accountable through administrative and legal mechanisms. Dying patients do not get access to pain medication because health care workers are not trained in pain management or because regulations on controlled substances prevent their prescription and accessibility in the health system.

How we understand the reason for people's suffering is crucial to enabling us to apply transformative human rights frameworks to health. If morphine and other pain medications are cheap and effective and if the failure to make those medications available and accessible results in the suffering of millions of terminally ill and other patients every year, we need not accept that suffering as "natural" or inevitable. Once we see how this inhuman treatment is *caused by* human decisions it follows that the laws, policies, and regulations that fail to take account of the claims to dignity that people in immense pain are forced to endure must be changed as a matter of justice, not just compassion.[59] Under international human rights law, states have the obligation to *prevent* as well as punish and redress torture and cruel, inhuman, and degrading treatment.

Human rights groups have campaigned successfully to change laws and regulations regarding access to palliative care across multiple countries.[60] When Human Rights Watch and other organizations have done so, they have argued that first, it is reasonable to expect that a state will not interfere with the delivery of palliative care to a patient; that is, they will not create undue barriers, through regulations or otherwise, to access. Second, the state has an obligation to ensure the availability of essential medicines, of which morphine is one recognized by the World Health Organization. Third, all states should implement a national public health strategy and plan of action; even if they cannot provide pain medication to everyone immediately, palliative pain relief should be part of that strategy and plan of action. And fourth, states are obligated to train their health personnel in pain management, which is part of making the medications accessible in practice. If these steps were instituted across the world, millions of people would be saved immeasurable suffering.

Torture and Suffering in the Private Sphere

One way to expand the domain of rights is to reinterpret both what it means to act and how we understand causal responsibility. Inaction by the state should be seen as action when, as in Dolores's case, the effects of such inaction are entirely predictable and preventable and we can identify reasonable measures for the state and other duty-bearers to take. Another way to expand rights and the responsibility of the state is to expand our consideration of assaults on dignity experienced in the so-called private sphere.

As I mentioned, in a narrowly circumscribed liberal paradigm of rights, freedom is seemingly exercised in a vacuum. Individuals in the liberal state are assumed to be "free" so long as the state does not force them to do something against their will. This is how we have traditionally thought about the right to be free from torture—as a shield from police (as in the Quijano case), as well as other state agents, including those in the health sector. Rights are conceived, in Roberto Unger's words, as "a loaded gun that the right holder may shoot at will in his corner of town." This view of rights in terms of isolated autonomy largely construes society and community as artificial constructs—rather than as processes through which our full identities emerge as individual human beings, as I suggested earlier.[61]

The idea implicit in such a view, that "every man's home is his castle"— that rights only protect from infringements in the rigidly defined "public sphere"—is particularly inapposite for women and children who suffer the most direct violations of their rights within the "private sphere" of the home. For decades, feminists have pointed out that it is impossible to establish a true democracy in a society if each home is a dictatorship within which women have no rights. The "personal is political"—the "private sphere" is porous, and abuses of power exercised in the private sphere do not allow certain people to be genuinely free in any sphere of their lives. The same is true for how we raise children. The realization of children's rights requires many public and societal changes. But it also fundamentally requires changing relationships within families so that decisions taken in children's names or on their behalf are justified to them, and justifiable in terms of their "best interests."[62]

Taking seriously the suffering of women, children, sexual minorities, and others requires a shift in the conception of rights and ensuing state obligations from the way in which they were set out in theories of the traditional liberal state. For example, both women and children are far more likely to face cruel, inhuman, and degrading treatment from domestic abuse than from police officers. In Tanzania, for example, three-quarters of children are subjected to physical or emotional abuse by the age of eighteen.[63] Nearly a third of girls are subjected to sexual abuse,[64] and not just in resource-poor settings, or the "developing world." In the United States, in 2014, when it came to light that pro-football star Adrian Peterson had inflicted a "good old-fashioned whoopin'" on his four-year-old son, many rose to his defense as merely standing up for traditional authority, despite the sequelae of that punishment resulting in the child's treatment in the emergency room.[65] This kind of torture is often every bit as brutal as that suffered at the hands of state agents and, more often than not, children are witnesses to the violent abuse of their mothers or siblings—just as in the Quijano case, as Héctor's mother and sister were forced to be. But in "private" settings—schools, homes, churches—the victims are often forced to see or even to live with the perpetrators, day in and day out.

International law, as well as domestic law in many countries, has evolved to address the obligations of states to protect people from abuses within the private sphere. For example, the UN Convention on the Elimination of All Forms of Discrimination Against Women (CEDAW), promulgated in 1979, and the Convention on the Rights of the Child, which was promulgated a decade later and as of 2014 has been ratified by every country except for the United States, South Sudan, and Somalia, transcend this rather artificial public-private divide and call for states to take responsibility for changing social practices that affect women and children, respectively.[66] Subsequent normative development takes this evolution further, including extending obligations of nonstate (that is, private) actors.[67] Moreover, in most countries there are national laws against domestic violence, at least against women if not children; and in some there are criminal prosecutions of perpetrators, and NGOs and agencies dedicated to helping survivors.

An enormous gap remains, however, between what the laws say and the pervasiveness of these forms of torture and abuse in practice.[68] Just as with other forms of torture and inhuman treatment, the health impacts of intimate partner violence (IPV) are pervasive and irrefutable. Physical impacts of IPV include high rates of arthritis, chronic neck or back pain, chronic pelvic pain, stomach ulcers, hypertension, and frequent headaches.[69] Some of the mental health effects include higher rates of depression, anxiety, posttraumatic stress disorder (PTSD), suicidal ideation, and substance abuse.[70]

Perhaps even worse, women and children who suffer from domestic violence too often believe they deserve the torture to which they are continually subjected. For example, in a global survey conducted in 2005, approximately two-thirds of women who had been subjected to domestic violence believed that it was appropriate for their husbands to hit or beat them for reasons that included not completing housework, disobeying their husband, refusing sex, and actual or suspected infidelity. A husband's most common justification was suspecting a wife of being unfaithful.[71] Further, women who are subject to abuse have little or no control over household resources, and little education.[72] Therefore, their opportunity structures severely limit their ability to exert agency.

In the case of domestic violence against children, it is often not that the torture shatters an already formed world or a fully constructed sense of identity; rather, emotional, physical, and sexual abuse prevents them from forming a sense of themselves as full human beings in the first place. Sometimes such abuse relates to condemning or castigating a child's expression of sexuality or gender identity as he or she is just beginning to have a sense of how that fits into his or her personhood. As I have stressed, we human beings construct the meaning of our lives every day through the small interactions we have with the people around us.[73] When people or society mirror a confining or contemptible picture of themselves, it ends up, as British sociologist Steven Lukes notes, "imprisoning them in a 'false, distorted and reduced mode of being.'"[74]

This process of internalizing domination is what leads so many girls—and members of sexual minorities and other marginalized groups—to see themselves as less than full human beings, with no claim to equal dignity. These are often the girls who then tend to believe they "deserve" to be beaten or neglected or abused in other ways as women; these are the members of sexual minorities who end up living under a cloak of shame and self-loathing. Recognizing this process of internalized domination, and its enormous health consequences, demands that our rights frameworks not only provide protection from abuse and access to entitlements, but also rethink the resources necessary to overcome internalized barriers and thereby create new opportunity structures for people to claim their dignity.

Changing laws and institutional practices is an important part of changing the common script through which we create our material and social realities as is ensuring equal access to endowments such as education and employment. But part of applying an empowering human rights framework to health and promoting a human rights culture must also entail changing the mirror that is held up to our private worlds, as those mirrors also create narratives for our lives and the conditions for developing our identities. Transforming our societies so that everyone can be accorded dignity requires actively working through both education systems and campaigns targeting popular culture to change how we see and relate to one another within those "small places"—close to and within our homes—"where human rights begin."

Concluding Reflections

The Quijano case as it developed was just the tip of an iceberg, which allowed me, together with Mexican colleagues, to bring a case in which we documented how PJF agents were involved in repeated instances of torture and other abuses of fundamental human rights. Yet, rather than being investigated or prosecuted, the perpetrators were transferred around the country, and even sometimes sent to serve on UN peacekeeping missions. The case created a scandal when the revelations were made public to a U.S. congressional committee holding hearings on the possibility of the signing of NAFTA and to the UN Committee Against Torture, which subsequently issued a scathing finding.[75] Other outrages also surfaced around the same time with respect to the PJF. Eventually, the then–attorney general of the country, Ignacio Morales Lechuga, stepped down and was replaced by the then-director of the National Human Rights Commission, Jorge Carpizo MacGregor. The PJF agents named in the report were suspended or fired, if not fully investigated or sanctioned for the abuses they had committed. In terms of broader reform, the National Human Rights Commission instituted a policy of tracking all agents allegedly involved in human rights abuses, which it continues to do to this day.[76] Of course, torture and abuse by the PJF did not stop there; indeed, over the years with increasing drug-related activity in Mexico, it may have increased. But that is the constant challenge of human rights work, and it does not mean that holding some officials to account and changing policies is meaningless. Far from it; it shows us that incremental changes are possible—and, as I argue throughout this book, these incremental advances can trigger further changes and open different spaces that lead to new struggles, often with different sets of actors, but also can lead to greater transformation.

During the years I lived in Mexico, Rosa slowly began to piece together fragments of her broken world. She and her husband moved out of Mexico City to a resort community. They opened a business renting jet skis and diving equipment to tourists. She got pregnant and had a child. Nothing would ever be the same again, but she managed to reestablish a kind of equilibrium. If someone met her in later years, it might not even occur to them that Rosa had not always been this woman who engaged in easy pleasantries with her tourist clients, that there was a time when she had been a very different woman, with different dreams for her life. If anything, understanding what had happened to her family as an injustice and having it recognized and acknowledged publicly as a flagrant violation of fundamental human rights enabled Rosa to make meaning out of the horror, and in turn to move on.

I got to know another family who was denied even that level of emotional closure. My husband and I lived in Mixcoac—a working-class neighborhood of Mexico City, a block away from the Lucha Libre, the professional wrestling ring. It turned out to be the perfect neighborhood for a human rights lawyer. When PJF agents sat outside our door day and night, knocked out the streetlights and wiretapped the corner pay phone as well as our house phone (this was before cell phones), we acquired a certain status among the neighbors, all of whom had their own problems with the universally hated Mexican police. There were no washing machines at the time, and Gabriela came to Mixcoac to do our laundry once a week with her three-year-old daughter, Josefina, in tow.

Gabriela and her sister, Patricia, had had a tough life, growing up in an impoverished household often without enough food. Becoming domestic workers is often the only option for girls who grow up in the circumstances of Patricia and Gabriela. Armies of young girls across Latin America—and much of the rest of the world—work in conditions with almost no labor protections in practice. If they are fortunate enough not to be abused physically or emotionally, they can easily still end up being oppressed by their own insignificance in cruelly indifferent societies, as happened to Gabriela.

As we got to know each other, Gabriela increasingly confided in me about her abusive husband. Sometimes she would ask for a little extra money if she had to pay for a place for her and her daughter to sleep away from him for a night or two, and sometimes the results of an "argument" would be visible on her body. I urged her to move out on more than one occasion, but the reality was Gabriela could not afford to leave; she had no other options.

One week Gabriela failed to show up for work. Patricia called that night; she wanted to know if her sister had shown up. Patricia was worried. She said Gabriela had called her the day before saying that she was scared for her life; her husband had beaten her terribly and threatened to kill her. This was not the first time he had made such threats, and I tried to reassure her that Gabriela had likely taken Josefina away for a few days.

But Patricia's worst fears proved to be correct. A few days later Gabriela's body was found, having been beaten badly. Josefina was missing. Although we were told that there was physical as well as circumstantial evidence that pointed to him, Gabriela's husband was never charged, an omission that seemed directly related to his being friends with the police in the district. Josefina was never located.

We stayed in touch, albeit sporadically, with Patricia and her daughter. I knew Patricia would never recover from the murder of the sister with whom she shared everything or from the disappearance of her niece. The years passed and Patricia dedicated herself entirely to her daughter, and she was as proud as any mother could be. But in some important way, the impunity in Gabriela's murder and Josefina's disappearance, and Patricia's sense of powerlessness, had taken her life from her too; there was a background of grief that made her into someone she would otherwise not have become.

When I lived in Mexico, the impunity of the police and military for torture and other abuses, including homicides, was shocking. The security forces not only were not serving the protective functions they were supposed to fulfill in a democratic state but also had become predatory; it was largely the poor like Gabriela and others in the working-class neighborhoods such as Mixcoac, who suffered the toll of their abuses. Nevertheless, there is even greater impunity and, too often, public acceptance of poor people being mistreated in health facilities, and deprived of essential care. And despite tremendous advances, far too many women and children are subjected to abuse and neglect of all forms within homes—across not only Mexico but the world.

Applying a meaningful human rights framework to health requires transforming our narratives of people's suffering, as well as transforming the ways in which power is exercised to deprive people of power and dignity, whether through acts or omissions and whether in public or private. In turn, as I discuss at length in later chapters, it requires identifying the contours of the state and societal responsibilities needed to transform those conditions, and the social, political and legal opportunity structures for different actors to do so.

The Powerlessness of Extreme Poverty: Human Rights and Social Justice

Like slavery and apartheid, poverty is not natural. It is man-made, and it can be overcome and eradicated by the actions of human beings. And overcoming poverty is not a gesture of charity. It is an act of justice. It is the protection of a fundamental human right, the right to dignity and a decent life.
—Nelson Mandela, BBC News, February 3, 2005

People used to say that it is awful, regrettable, or troubling that so many children go to bed hungry. . . . Today . . . we can now picture the poor not as shrunken wretches begging for our help, but as persons with dignity who are claiming what is theirs by right.
—Thomas Pogge, *Freedom from Poverty as a Human Right*

Around the world, it is the poor who suffer the vast majority of civil and political rights violations, including torture, in both public and private spheres. In the years I lived in Mexico, far more of the clients I worked with were like Gabriela, with limited choices and struggling to make ends meet—and not like Rosa, who was decidedly middle class. There was the teenager who was playing soccer with friends, who must have irritated the wrong police officer on the wrong day because he ended up tortured to death in a local jail for simply urinating in public. Or the campesino (peasant farmer) who was mercilessly harassed and finally murdered with impunity by drug traffickers when he wouldn't relinquish the land his family had received from "The Great One"—Lázaro Cárdenas—after the Mexican Revolution.[1] Or the young woman who got caught up in helping a drug dealer for money, was subjected to a Kafkaesque trial, and was then sexually assaulted by a guard in prison. Or a dozen other people for whom severe poverty itself was a prison of despair.

Profound poverty makes people hostages to their fates, and entire futures dissolve because of petty bureaucratic decisions or arbitrary abuses of power. In *Behind the Beautiful Forevers*, Katherine Boo writes of Annawadi, a slum in Mumbai, India, saying that for the very poor, good fortune "derived not just from what people did, or how well they did it, but from the accidents and catastrophes they dodged. A decent life was the train that hadn't hit you, the slumlord you hadn't offended, the malaria you hadn't caught."[2] People who are not just of modest means but who live in extreme poverty are constantly faced with "Sophie's choices" about which child goes to school, which will get health care, who will get to eat that day.[3] When poverty takes away such basic power over one's life, it makes self-governance and therefore dignity impossible, and it represents violations of a series of human rights, including health and other economic and social rights, under international law.

I was still doing conventional civil and political rights work in Mexico when I participated in a fact-finding delegation to Baborigame, a small village in the southern part of the Sierra Tarahumara in the state of Chihuahua. Baborigame would be a short flight to Tucson, Arizona, where some of the most sophisticated medical care in the world is available. But the Sierra Tarahumara is a mountainous area, and in the early 1990s it had extremely poor infrastructure. The terrain and difficulty of access made the Sierra Tarahumara ideal for cultivating opium poppies, and drug lords forced many of the indigenous campesinos who owned small tracts of land in the area to do just that. As I have described elsewhere, in 1992, the Mexican military burned down much of the village of Baborigame, took away men to torture them, stole and killed livestock, and displaced the entire population.[4] Allegedly the military was eradicating opium poppies, but it is entirely possible that the eradication merely reflected a transfer of control between the cartels, on whose payrolls were many of the Mexican officials engaged in the so-called "drug war."

Along with a small group that included both Mexican and international human rights activists, I went to investigate the events that had occurred in Baborigame.[5] One morning, the helicopter going to survey the eradicated crops from the air was full and I stayed behind with the missionary nuns, who did what they could to attend to the impoverished Tepehuac community in this isolated area of northern Mexico. The Tepehuac community, like the vast majority of indigenous groups in Mexico, was disproportionately represented among the most severely impoverished in the country. At the time, the government was providing almost no water, sanitation, or health services to this remote area. The small group of nuns provided basic primary care and did whatever they could for patients who required more complicated attention, such as a man with leprosy who had lost some of his limb function.

I had no idea that I was going to watch a child die that day. By the time his mother, Pilar, brought him in, the infant was so dehydrated and weak that he was incapable of crying. Given the nuns' meager supplies, there was nothing to do but pray and watch as life faded from his tiny body. Pilar held his body and cried softly. We all cried. The commonly accepted narrative that the destitute or those in certain "other" cultures experience less grief over the loss of a child because it is so common is simply not true. But it may allow the privileged to distance themselves from the implications of having to address the immense suffering of fellow human beings, whether in the slum across the street or across the world.

Apart from the images of the last minutes of the child's life, what I recall most vividly from that day more than twenty years ago was that his mother did not express the rage, in addition to sadness, which I felt so acutely—rage that her community lived without adequate water, sanitation, and food; rage that there was no accessible health care when her son did fall ill as a result; rage that her son had died an entirely preventable death because of these deprivations and the systematic discrimination against indigenous populations in Mexico. Pilar understood the military's arbitrary detentions, tortures, theft of livestock, and wanton destruction of property as human rights violations. Indeed, denouncing those abuses to my delegation is what had brought her and her neighbors down the mountain. Nevertheless, her anger did not appear to extend to her living conditions, which were the underlying cause of her son's death. What was striking on that cold morning in 1992 was the absence of the mother's sense of the terrible injustice implicit in her son's suffering and death. To her, as with so many mothers and families I have met before and after her, the death of her son was simply "the will of God."[6]

I have no doubt that the impotence Pilar felt—and her actual powerlessness—was just as profound as that which Rosa experienced as she watched her brother being tortured. Indeed, when the World Bank published the groundbreaking *Voices of the Poor* study in 2000, which attempts to understand people's experiences of poverty through discussions with tens of thousands of poor people around the globe, what came across was that "again and again, powerlessness seems to be at the core of the bad life."[7] The very poor are at the mercy of fate, as well as the capricious whims of those in power; when poverty is combined with other axes of identity, such as ethnicity in this case, or gender, race, or caste, the disempowering effects can increase exponentially. Moreover, as the World Bank study showed, being extremely poor not only means going without food or shelter or education, it also often means being treated badly by institutions, such as the health and justice systems, and excluded from voice in those institutions as well as in the larger society.

Yet the human decisions and human actions that lay behind the death of Pilar's son seem more obscure, more invisible, than what happened to Héctor Quijano. Once again, how we understand causation and the boundaries of human responsibility lie at the heart of how we respond to different forms of suffering. That is, if we understand Pilar's son's death as misfortune or personal tragedy, it elicits a very different response than if we understand it as injustice, for which the ground was laid by human decisions and actions, not by divine will. Although the first perhaps creates sympathy, the second calls on us to translate compassion into political, social, and legal action.

Philosopher Thomas Pogge writes that extreme poverty—and the suffering and human rights violations that it creates—are intimately connected to our social arrangements at national and global levels: "Severe poverty today, while no less horrific than that experienced by the early American settlers, is fundamentally different in context and causation. Its persistence is not forced on us by natural contingencies of soil, seeds, or climate. Rather, its persistence is driven by the ways that economic interactions are structured: by interlocking national and international institutional arrangements. . . . We can avoid it . . . by restructuring national and global legal systems so that everyone has real opportunities to escape and avoid severe poverty."[8] It was through experiences such as the one in Baborigame, that I came to feel at a visceral level that for human rights frameworks to be relevant to the struggles for dignity of the great majority of the world, these frameworks needed to provide useful approaches to restructuring those national and global systems.

In this chapter, I first set out the interconnectedness of all human rights—economic, social, cultural, civil, and political. I go on to explore what it would mean to conceive of issues relating to social and economic conditions—and to health, in particular—as rights, and how doing so is directly related to our understanding of the importance of dignity and has consequences for how we address lack of access to the most basic conditions of public health and health care. I then describe how modern human rights law has evolved, including eroding the differential treatment of categories of rights. But I also note challenges presented by prevailing neoliberal economic paradigms and their relationship to narrow conceptions of rights. I argue that traditional arguments against health and other ESC rights are misplaced, and reveal certain limited assumptions about society, the obligations of the state, and the demands of justice. It is only when we question those narratives that we can develop empowering approaches to human rights—and development—which can better address the root causes of poverty and advance the health and dignity of the most disadvantaged among us.

Interdependence and Indivisibility of Human Rights: The Right to Health as Set Out Under International Law

As discussed in Chapter 1, the deprivation of civil rights—through torture or the arbitrary detentions by the military in Baborigame, for example—have severe health consequences. Indeed, health is both the result of the enjoyment of a wide array of different human rights, as well as a precondition to be able to participate fully as an equal citizen in society and to live a life of dignity. It illustrates vividly the importance of thinking about the realization, as well as the violation, of human rights in terms of their interdependence and indivisibility.

The Universal Declaration of Human Rights, which was promulgated by the United Nations General Assembly in 1948, reaffirmed member states' "faith in fundamental human rights, in the dignity and worth of the human person and in the equal rights of men and women and [their determination] to promote social progress and better standards of life in larger freedom." The Declaration includes both CP rights and ESC rights, including the right to a decent standard of living.[9]

The recognition of all human rights as being inextricably intertwined makes intuitive sense. We cannot think about an active citizenry participating in public affairs if those citizens are uneducated. Conversely, we cannot imagine a meaningful right to work without freedoms of association and information for workers. Further, as in Baborigame, much of poverty is inextricably linked with discrimination along gender, religious, racial, ethnic, or other lines. And it is often a noxious combination of intersecting discriminations, as well as stigma, that entrenches people in poverty and limits their ability to exercise agency.

In 2014, a long way from Baborigame, I met Paula, whose life story illustrated exactly how these different kinds of rights deprivations combine to limit life choices. Paula was one of the plaintiffs in a court case being brought on behalf of a group of Kenyan women who had been involuntarily sterilized because of their HIV status. She was in her 40s when I met her, with a tenacity that must have helped her through the many hardships and the constant discomfort she suffered as a result of a poorly performed bilateral tubal ligation (BTL). Paula had been born into abject poverty in a village in western Kenya, had been forced to drop out of school after completing primary school, had gotten pregnant multiple times against her will because the successive men in her life had not allowed her to use contraception, and had been infected with both syphilis and HIV. None of Paula's partners had provided for her after her children were born and she often had to support not only herself and her children but also these men, as well as her grown brothers. She had been subjected to emotional and physical abuse by nearly all the men in her life and, finally, by the health system, which coerced her into having a BTL by threatening to withhold the infant formula and antiretroviral (ARV) medications vital to both her and her child's survival. Paula's experience of the funnel of narrowing choices over her life was inextricably shaped by the interactions between her economic exclusion and the brutal gender discrimination she faced which led to lack of education and abuse, as well as the stigma and ignorance surrounding HIV. In real people's lives, autonomy and entitlements, and different kinds of rights that enable living with human dignity, are inseparable.

Nevertheless, during the Cold War, CP rights (such as rights to bodily integrity and freedom from torture) and ESC rights (such as rights to work, education, and health) were divided into twin covenants, in which the obligations had very different status under the law. The right to health was treated as an ESC right under international law and was included in the International Covenant on Economic, Social and Cultural Rights (ICESCR), which was promulgated in 1966. Because of the manner in which obligations are worded in the ICESCR, much of the right to health was not immediately enforceable, in contrast, for example, to civil rights, such as the right to be free from torture or cruel, inhuman, and degrading treatment. Rather, it was subject to "progressive realization" in accordance with a state's "maximum available resources."[10]

Article 12(1) of the ICESCR, which is the core formulation of the right to health under international law, sets out the right of everyone to the "highest attainable standard of physical and mental health." Article 12(2) announces steps states should take toward its progressive realization: "reduction of the stillbirth-rate and of infant mortality and [provision] for the healthy development of the child; improvement of environmental and industrial hygiene; prevention, treatment and control of epidemic, endemic, occupational and other diseases; and the creation of conditions which would assure to all medical service and medical attention in the event of sickness."[11]

The distinction between the way CP and ESC rights were treated in the twin covenants reflected and affected interpretation, discourse, and practice under international law. Health and other ESC rights were largely relegated to being merely "programmatic" rights, rather than "real" legal rights subject to judicial enforcement. One of the staunchest supporters of this view in international circles, the United States, stated at the former UN Commission on Human Rights: "The realization of economic, social and cultural rights is progressive and aspirational. We do not view them as entitlements that require correlated legal duties and obligations."[12]

At first glance, the right not to be tortured is intuitively universal; it is ostensibly a "negative" right, requiring only restraint from the government. However, the right to the highest attainable standard of health may seem to be different; it may appear to be a "positive" right, requiring affirmative actions and spending. Yet these distinctions are misleading. In practice, ESC rights require forbearance on the part of the state—such as refraining from engaging in forced evictions—and CP rights require affirmative actions and expenditures.

For example, vast resources are poured into meeting minimum standards for "fair and free" electoral processes in impoverished countries, which require massive international assistance. According to a 2006 United Nations Development Programme (UNDP) report, the cost of one vote in one election averaged USD 1 to USD 3 in the United States and Western Europe; USD 4 to USD 8 in "consolidating democracies," such as Lesotho; and up to USD 45 in post-conflict situations.[13] In India, the general elections that began in

April 2014 were projected to cost a staggering USD 5 billion,[14] which is equivalent to more than 90 percent of what the country allocated for health in that fiscal year.[15] High costs are also a price we pay for adhering to the right to a fair trial, including the costs of public defenders. Yet the cost of CP rights, such as fair and free elections and the right to due process, is largely hidden through general taxation, and we do not in general question the responsibility of the state to provide these fundamentals to human dignity.

In practice, no rights can be implemented from one day to the next; all require "progressive realization." Think of achieving the right to be free of torture and cruel, inhuman, or degrading treatment. If we think only about acts committed by police and military, such as in the Quijano case or in Baborigame, we would still require long-term investments in legal reforms, as well as institutional reform with respect to the security forces as well as judiciary. And, as discussed in Chapter 1, when we expand our conception of torture to include omissions as well as actions in health care settings, and domestic abuse, the actions for which the state is responsible extend to a far broader range of initiatives aimed at prevention, at educational and attitudinal change, in addition to legal, regulatory, and policy reform.

Since the Cold War thawed, international law has evolved considerably to some extent dissolving these unhelpful distinctions. The Vienna Declaration, the outcome document stemming from the Vienna Conference on Human Rights in 1993, contributed enormously by stating that, "all human rights are universal, indivisible and interdependent and interrelated" and that the states must promote and protect all human rights and fundamental freedoms.[16]

All human rights (civil, political, economic, social, and cultural) are now understood at the international level to give rise to three dimensions of governmental obligations: the duties to respect, to protect, and to fulfill.[17] The duty to respect requires refraining from direct interference; the duty to protect requires guarding from the interference by others (for example, through regulating private actors, as discussed in Chapter 1); and the duty to fulfill requires affirmative actions aimed at promoting the realization of the right, including access to care in the case of health.[18]

What Does It Mean to Treat Economic and Social Issues, Such as Health, as Rights?

In development and social policy, health has conventionally been construed in terms other than "as a right," so it is worth exploring the question of what it would mean for Pilar and her child in Baborigame or Paula in Kenya—or anyone—to claim health as a right. If extreme poverty means that the world controls our lives in ways that leave us bereft of ethical independence, then the assertion of rights to economic and social entitlements, such as health, is a claim on the responsibilities of the state to ensure the conditions under which people can exercise meaningful agency. That claim, in turn, requires shifts in both the resources people have and the barriers they face that shape their ability to exercise choices; in other words, it requires shifting their "opportunity structures."

But why should justice or fairness call for the state to take steps to equalize access to such entitlements with respect to health and health care when it does not in other areas? Indeed, "fairness" often means "getting what you pay for." For example, we would not expect to pay USD 50 and be able to purchase the latest smartphone or expect to buy a Ferrari if we only have USD 10,000 to put toward a car. If we buy an economy-class ticket on an airline, we do not expect to get the same service as we would business class. To suggest otherwise seems far-fetched. Why should health, including health care, be different?

Philosopher Amartya Sen provides a useful way of thinking about this. Sen argues that to assert that health (or any other social issue, such as education or housing) is an issue of human rights implies that (1) it is of special importance and (2) it is subject to social influence.[19] That health is of special importance has been persuasively argued on both normative and empirical grounds.

Our intuition that health is of special importance is related to the distinction Kant draws between that which has a price and that which is fundamental to dignity, as I mentioned in Chapter 1. As we discussed in that chapter, within a rights framework, to live with dignity requires being able to pursue a life plan. That, in turn requires preserving a normal range of opportunities in life or, using Sen's terms, certain "capabilities." There is abundant evidence that health is critically important for people to be able to maintain productive work and to have the capacity for physical as well as ethical independence in their lives.[20] Health is a precondition to exercising basic self-government, and it is inextricably connected to the capacity to live with dignity. Therefore, health, including health care, cannot be treated as just another commodity to be allocated by the market, such as an airplane ticket or a car.[21]

As an empirical matter, it has often been pointed out that in almost every culture there are greetings, sayings, and rituals that highlight the special significance people place on health. For example, as Jonathan Mann noted in the mid-1990s, in virtually every language, toasts are commonly raised "to your health," and expressions exist equivalent to my own grandmother's constant refrain, "So long as you have your health."[22]

The second requirement Sen sets out for thinking about health as a right is that it be subject to social influence. We cannot claim a right to beauty, grace, or musical aptitude because they are largely matters of genetics, fate, or personal effort. Consider, for example, Yo-Yo Ma's ability to play the cello, Francisco de Goya's creative genius, Lionel Messi's soccer talent, Serena Williams's tennis skills, or Wislawa Szymborska's poetic voice. We don't have rights to those talents, and indeed they are commonly called *gifts* or *giftedness*. Rights can only be achieved through social arrangements, which shows that such arrangements are not optional but necessary for us to enjoy our dignity fully. Think of the right to a fair trial or the right to fair and free elections, for example. These are matters of social institutions and arrangements—they cannot be achieved through personal effort or talent; they are subject to external social forces and they require public commitments. The same applies to a right to health.

Some people would say that it is silly to talk about a right to health, as so much of good health is indeed a matter of genetics, personal behavior, or simply luck. That is true—and it is precisely for this reason that there is no human right to be healthy under international or any national law. And in many countries, including the United States, there is still no acknowledgment of a right to health at all. But under international law, the right to health is phrased as the right to "the highest attainable standard of physical and mental health," which as noted earlier presumes both individual differences and societal differentiation based on resource availability.[23]

However, as noted, the "right to health" under international law, as set out in the ICESCR and elsewhere, does extend beyond health care. Often when we think of obligations relating to health, we think of medical care. But in fact, the reasons people are able to be healthy are generally much more related to public health interventions—such as clean water, sanitation, nutritional measures, and control of occupational hazards—than to care received at a hospital or local health clinic. As was evident in Baborigame, this is particularly true for children. Unsafe drinking water, inadequate availability of water for hygiene, and a lack of access to sanitation contribute to about 1.5 million child deaths each year and account for almost 90 percent of deaths from diarrhea.[24] These conditions also contribute to the spread of infectious disease, and of the more than seven and a half million children who died before their fifth birthday in 2010 almost two-thirds died of preventable infectious causes.[25]

These public health interventions are frequently invisible compared to medical interventions—unless you are in a country or place, such as Baborigame in the early 1990s, that does not have them, when that becomes painfully apparent. Just as with medical care, these public health interventions require institutional arrangements and societal commitments. They cannot be achieved by individuals acting alone. Consequently, it makes sense that these "preconditions to health" or "underlying determinants" are part of the right to health.

Leveling the Playing Field and a Minimum Threshold Level

As in Baborigame, extreme poverty frequently manifests itself as lack of access to the most basic preconditions of health, as well as access to care. The consequences of considering health and other ESC issues as rights are that the state then has a duty to "level the playing field" in terms of access to basic preconditions of health and care. These are not simply conditions that can be left to the market. A right to health does not call for equalization of all outcomes, or all incomes, though, and in Chapter 7 we discuss in much greater depth the extent to which applying human rights frameworks to health demands substantive equality.

In addition to a commitment toward equalizing access and entitlements, however, there is also an obligation on the part of the state to provide certain minimum standards to the entire population. The duty to provide such a minimum threshold level is not subject to progressive realization under international law or certain national jurisprudence; it is an immediate obligation that stems from what is necessary to protect the dignity of the most disadvantaged members of society.

The concept of an "existential minimum" or "vital minimum," including access to food, housing, and social assistance, as well as to health care, for the worst off was set out early in the jurisprudence of the German constitutional court, and is tied to the concept of human dignity. It has subsequently been adopted by constitutional courts in a number of South American and European countries. As in Germany, which linked the notion of a "vital minimum" to the purposes of the state, in Colombian constitutional jurisprudence, the notion of a "vital minimum" (*mínimo vital*) has also been explicitly tied to the political formulation of Colombia as a "social state of law" (*estado social de derecho)* under the 1991 constitution, and the protection of human dignity. Thus, through social protection systems and otherwise, these states have a legal, not just moral, obligation to ensure a minimum threshold, which is necessary to enable human dignity.

In international human rights law, the UN Committee on Economic, Social and Cultural Rights (CESCR) has also adopted the notion of a minimum core content as being both essential to enabling individuals to live with dignity as well as for the appropriate understanding of ESC rights as real rights.[26] The CESCR has articulated the minimum core in different ways over the years. In its third General Comment, in 1990, deprivations of a significant number of citizens of "minimum essential levels" of ESC rights under the ICESCR, including essential foodstuffs, essential primary health care, basic shelter and housing, and the most basic forms of education, would be a presumptive violation of state obligations. In CESCR's General Comment 14, issued in 2000, the "basic obligations" of states' parties to the ICESCR with respect to the right to health in particular are far more extensive and also include measures relating to equitable distribution of health facilities, goods and services, and national plans of action with respect to health.[27]

The concept as well as the application of a minimum core content in international human rights has received scholarly critique for, among other things, its lack of ambition and clarity.[28] Nevertheless, a legal obligation to provide a vital minimum as a matter of right is essential if we hope to begin to transform conceptions of prerequisites for dignity as well as the duties of the welfare state or "social state of law."

Advances in Rethinking ESC Rights, Especially Health Rights

Accepting a threshold minimum is only part of a larger reconceptualization of state obligations to ensure ESC rights, including the right to health. The twenty-plus years since Vienna have witnessed astounding progress in the evolution and elucidation of international norms relating to the right to health in particular, as well as to ESC rights more generally. According to the World Health Organization (WHO), every country in the world has now ratified at least one treaty containing health-related rights.[29] Treaty-monitoring bodies have issued important interpretations of norms relating to health rights, including Article 12 of the ICESCR, which are clarificatory, if not binding.[30]

The groundbreaking UN Convention on the Rights of Persons with Disabilities, together with significant Additional Protocols to the American Convention on Human Rights and the African Charter on Human and People's Rights, have entered into force. Further optional protocols to various treaties, including the ICESCR, now permit quasi-judicial petitions to challenge violations of health and other ESC rights in cases where domestic remedies are inadequate. Conference declarations and other official outcome documents, resolutions from the Human Rights Council, and reports of UN Special Rapporteurs (or independent experts) have also elucidated standards relating to aspects of health and other ESC rights, even though they are not "hard law."[31]

Institutional commitment to HRBAs to health and development has also greatly expanded among agencies. Intergovernmental agencies, including UNICEF, UNDP, and the WHO, now have units devoted to rights-based analysis, policies, and programming. Some donors, as well as NGOs and national governments, have explicitly adopted HRBAs with respect to issues varying from sexual and reproductive health to water and sanitation. And in 2013, the WHO published a monograph collecting evidence regarding the effects of HRBAs on women's and children's health.[32]

At the domestic level, many recently enacted or reformed constitutions, such as Kenya's 2010 constitution, explicitly include the right to health. Further, in Nepal and elsewhere governments are enacting health policies that refer explicitly to rights principles; and where there are gaps, courts are enforcing access to entitlements. In cases from South Africa to India, and Costa Rica to Colombia,[33] we have increasing examples of the enforceability of health and related rights. Beyond enforcing individual entitlements to care and preconditions, courts are transforming health policies—whether in relation to HIV/AIDS medications in South Africa, maternal-child health programming and food policy in India, or the structure of the health system in Colombia.[34] These judgments are having impacts both material and symbolic on real people's lives. Coupled with social action and political mobilization, judicial rulings are permitting members of marginalized groups—from persons living with HIV/AIDS (PLWAs) to transgender people—to conceive of themselves as fully human subjects whose demands are underpinned by notions of legal, as well as political, entitlement.

Further, health rights advocacy has not been limited to formal legal forums. In addition to pressing for international and domestic law reform
and judicial advances, many human rights NGOs—especially in the global
South—have been increasingly active in educational and political mobilizing campaigns around health and other ESC rights in their countries. Issues
ranging from water privatization to the impacts of trade agreements on access to medicines are now being fought by NGOs as human rights issues,
when in the past they would have been mere "policy issues."

Moreover, coalitions that include both health and development groups,
along with more traditional human rights advocacy organizations, have
placed health and other social concerns on the democratization agenda in
countries from South Africa to Peru in the last twenty-five years.[35] National
human rights institutions have forcefully investigated such issues as involuntary sterilization as fundamental rights concerns and conducted inquiries
with respect to abuses of sexual and reproductive health, bringing about
sweeping policy changes as a result.[36]

Increasing efforts to promote social accountability at local and national
levels are being enhanced through the Internet and social media, which have
permitted international and regional networks of advocacy organizations to
easily share information about rights-based strategies relating to health care,
food, housing policies, trade agreements, and other issues that affect poor
people's health. Programs to map violations geospatially and cell phones that
permit crowdsourcing, together with other increasingly cheap technologies,
will undoubtedly enable innovations in accountability for health and other
social rights in the near future that are unimaginable today.

Rethinking Rights: Challenges

Nevertheless, these developments must be seen within the larger political and
economic context, which is overwhelmingly dominated by neoliberal economic policies and narrow liberal conceptions of rights, including those related to health and health care, and ensuing state responsibilities. Neoliberal
economic policies, in general, seek to transfer control of the economy from
the public to the private sector, reducing the obligations of the state and leaving in effect market forces with respect to access to health and other social
rights. All too often, the result of such policies has been to consign large
populations to being "externalities" of growth or austerity policies—means
to achieving larger societal ends. The needs of people who live at the edges of

society in extreme poverty are often disregarded in a political and economic focus on abstract economic development goals. As a result, those affected by such policies too often find their humanity and dignity shunted aside, as they are relegated to the gutters on the road to modernity.

Despite advances in international law and at the domestic level, public policy and media discussions, as well as many legal frameworks, continue to distinguish between CP rights and ESC rights. For example, in 2007 the *Economist* magazine ran an editorial that typifies this widely held view. It attacked the tendency to "dilute" traditional CP rights by "mixing in a new category of what people now call social and economic rights." The article argued that "no useful purpose is served by calling [food, housing, and so on] 'rights.' When a government locks someone up without a fair trial, the victim, perpetrator, and remedy are pretty clear. This clarity seldom applies to social and economic 'rights.' It is hard enough to determine whether such a right has been infringed, let alone who should provide a remedy, or how."[37] As noted, the editorial's argument that ESC rights are fuzzy "programmatic" rights that elude judicial remedy ignores the last two decades of jurisprudence and legal and constitutional reforms in many countries, as I discuss further in later chapters.

However, perhaps even more important for our purposes now, the concept of human rights that the *Economist* editorial advocates—one that is widely understood in public discussions—limits human rights to a very palliative role in the regulation of power. The narrow liberal approach to human rights set out in the *Economist*—identifying a violation, a perpetrator, and a remedy—assumes an underlying state of equilibrium in a society in which all citizens are free and equal, as discussed in Chapter 1.[38] The violation upsets the equilibrium; the remedy restores it. Think of the Quijano torture case, in which bringing the perpetrators to justice theoretically restores the equilibrium. Of course, far more is required in practice, and the Quijano case illustrates how the institution of the PJF had to be reformed, and indeed still needs to be. This paradigm, which has been widely used in the human rights movement—of identifying a violation, perpetrator, and remedy—is thus not really appropriate for creating or describing the sustained systemic change needed with regard to CP rights.

But in the case of health and other ESC rights, we are definitely not seeking to return to a status quo ante in a fixed society, with fixed rules about income and how resources are allocated. Think back to Article 28 of the UDHR, discussed in the Introduction, which sets out a right to "a social and international order in which the rights and freedoms set forth" in the Declaration can be fully realized.[39] Such a social (and international) order requires that progressively realizing the right to the highest attainable standard of health for diverse individuals and groups will necessarily involve evolving claims about what we owe each other as different, but fully equal, human beings. The responsibility of the state to meet these demands of distributive justice suggests not only flux but also contestation, which requires legitimate, democratic processes to resolve. In this conception, rights cannot be understood as immutable constraints on government action, as they are in a narrow liberal construction; rather, rights constitute social practices that create spaces for vital social deliberation on how to arrange social institutions to meet population needs, especially of the most disadvantaged.

Examining Assumptions About the State, Society, and Justice

In the aftermath of the global recession that began in 2008, austerity policies and state retraction from social services has become the norm—even in social democracies across Europe, where certain entitlements to social welfare had seemed unquestionable. National courts and international human rights treaty-monitoring committees are increasingly being asked to assess whether policies that appear to imply retrogression, or backsliding, with respect to social entitlements, have been implemented in reasonable and proportionate ways, with adequate protections for the most disadvantaged.[40]

In some cases, politicians seem to reflexively accept the politics of scarcity and austerity because of a failure of imagination, while in others there is a glorification of the "minimal" or laissez-faire state as being the ideal. The latter generally argue that using the power of the state to redistribute wealth through fiscal powers and regulation is not only inefficient but also unjust because it interferes with peoples' liberties. Thus, again, neoliberal economic positions are closely aligned with a libertarian, or at least narrow liberal, version of rights and the state.

The problem with this argument is that there is no "natural" or neutral distribution of wealth in a society; what a person ends up with in terms of resources will always depend on a combination of personal talents, parental heritage, luck, and the laws in the country in which he or she lives.[41] I believe it is a mistake for human rights advocates to argue for redistribution of wealth through taxation as though it were a form of humanizing the underlying economically rational situation. This always puts ESC advocacy in a remedial or "defensive" posture. On the contrary, the distribution of wealth and privileges within a society and across societies is the result of socially created customs, laws, and regulations that permit and entrench those distributions, including ones that favor market expansion and limit social protections, including for people living in extreme poverty. Friends in Nordic countries have told me that they in no way feel that high rates of taxation are "taking something" from them; they had no "right" to that wealth to begin with.

Compare, for example, how much wealth is inherited in the United States—and elsewhere. The rate at which estate taxes are set and what the loopholes are determine a great deal of inter-generational wealth—and, in turn, of prospects for the future. Yet in the United States and across many societies, legal rules and social norms foster the belief that a child of someone who has become very wealthy during his or her lifetime has some inherent claim to that wealth as a matter of right. Many children of inherited wealth tend to internalize some degree of superiority, as though the world were theirs and they were entitled to more from life than the poor. Children who grow up in severe poverty, in turn, tend all too often to believe the converse. But that need not be the case.

Indeed, in a human rights framework that establishes obligations to respect the equal dignity of all people, it should not be. As the late legal philosopher Ronald Dworkin wrote: "A laissez-faire political economy leaves unchanged the consequences of a free market in which people buy and sell their product and labor as they wish and can. That does not show equal concern for everyone. Anyone impoverished through that system is entitled to ask: 'There are other more regulatory and redistributive sets of laws that would put me in a better position. How can government claim that this system shows equal concern for me?'"[42] Moreover, as Cass Sunstein points out: "Those who denounce state intervention are the ones who most frequently and successfully invoke it. The cry of laissez faire mainly goes up from those who, if really 'let alone,' would instantly lose their wealth-absorbing power."[43] All politics are coercive, and it is most often the powerful who benefit from the way in which a given state is choosing to exert its regulatory power.

This need not be our understanding of the conditions necessary to exercise rights and live with dignity. For example, the Colombian Constitutional Court has articulated that the "social state of law" (*estado social de derecho*) set out in its 1991 constitution was formulated as it became clear "the extent to which human beings are not really free or equal due to natural and social limitations, among which the economic ones stand out. The realization of freedom and equality require measures, actions, entitlements and services that a person by herself cannot achieve. The democratic state thus evolved from a liberal democratic state to a social democratic state, animated by the purpose of ensuring that the material prerequisites of freedom and equality are effectively guaranteed."[44] Similarly, the South African Constitutional Court, writing of the commitments undertaken through its visionary 1994 constitution, stated: "Millions of people are living in deplorable conditions and great poverty. . . . These conditions already existed when the Constitution was adopted and a commitment to address them and to transform our society into one in which there will be human dignity, freedom and equality, lies at the heart of our new constitutional order. For as long as these conditions continue to exist that aspiration will have a hollow ring."[45] And as early as the 1970s, the Indian Supreme Court stated, "The mandate of the Constitution is to build a welfare society in which justice—social, economic and political—shall inform all institutions of our national life. The hopes and aspirations aroused by the Constitution will be belied if the minimum needs of the lowest of our citizens are not met."[46] Thus, the narrative of rights, and of dignity, in these countries, allows courts to assess laws and policies in ways that ensure attention is provided to the most disadvantaged.[47]

As noted, the United States, by contrast, has been among the staunchest of opponents to recognizing ESC rights at the federal level.[48] Although at the state level, the right to education has been advanced through courts and social movements, the United States notably does not recognize a right to health care or health, and it famously frames specific entitlements to health care in terms of an abstract right to "privacy."[49] For example, in the United States, a woman's right to an abortion is based on protecting her "personal dignity and autonomy" considered in a vacuum, divorced from the wider social and economic conditions of a woman's life.[50] If a poor woman cannot afford to pay for an abortion, the U.S. Supreme Court has held that the government has no obligation to subsidize it. Further, not a penny of the Affordable Care Act can be allocated to abortion services. And the preclusion of federal funding to subsidize poor women's abortions is probably one of the single greatest barriers to care and contributors to late-term abortions by poor, adolescent, and marginalized women.[51]

The narrative of abortion as a private decision based on personal, "intimate suffering" also illustrates how the framing of rights issues has implications for public health responses. When rights frameworks fail to recognize the real differences in power that poverty and other social conditions impose on people's autonomy to make choices about their well-being, health issues become, as Lynn Freedman writes, "Strictly individual problems conceived of as 'risk factors' to be treated with education in strategies of avoidance. Thus as the legal language imposes deeper and deeper constrictions on our expectations of entitlement and our understanding of justice, the corresponding health debate becomes more and more impoverished as well."[52]

Reframing Global Poverty and Development from a Rights Perspective

If a rights perspective changes the calculus of what we—and the state—owe the most disadvantaged within our own societies, it also changes how we think about what we owe fellow human beings at the global level. As I discuss at length in Chapter 8, a great deal of extreme poverty in the world and deprivations of economic and social rights more generally are determined by decisions taken beyond national borders. Just as it is arbitrary that institutional arrangements within a country systematically favor certain classes over others, it is also arbitrary—if historically determined—that global institutional arrangements systematically deprive populations in certain countries of basic human rights. Thomas Pogge argues, "Severe poverty should be classified as a human rights violation" because "it is a foreseeable and avoidable effect of how the world economy is currently structured [which] foreseeably produces avoidable human rights deficits on a massive scale.[53] Development is generally thought of as an affirmative act of "giving aid." But Pogge asks us to rethink our view of causation to see how the rules of the global game systematically disadvantage some countries and the poorest people within those countries, with foreseeable health consequences.

In classic development thinking, poverty has been understood in terms of income poverty, as a generic shortage of income. Generally it has been defined as less than USD 2 a day (according to purchasing power); and extreme poverty as less than USD 1 a day, although more recently as less than USD 1.25 a day. According to these measures, approximately a billion people live in extreme poverty around the world. And recent studies have shown that 72 percent of the "bottom billion" now live in middle-income countries, notably in India and China.[54]

As the traditional view of poverty did not consider context or ability to convert income into access to food, education, housing, and health care, the formula was simple: increase jobs and income, and it will be better for the country—and poverty will be reduced. However, over the last fifty years, some schools of economics have focused on the global system and the relationship of "peripheral" to "central" economies, which historically established a perpetual cycle of dependency.[55] And the path out of such cycles goes far beyond merely creating jobs, as these will pay wages that allow for increasingly less purchasing power within their countries; rather, the structures of dependency, including financial transaction regulations, need to be fundamentally altered.

In recent decades, development thought and practice have come to focus on poverty reduction in new ways, including "human development" and HRBAs. Amartya Sen, the philosopher who is the father of human capabilities theory, first introduced the idea of human development, and of poverty as a series of "unfreedoms." Severe poverty, as discussed at the beginning of this chapter, means a lack of freedom to make choices over one's life, and extreme poverty is an accumulation of unfreedoms that translates into an inability for self-government and ethical independence. In turn, human development is usually defined as the expansion of capabilities and freedoms, or the increase of the ability to "be and do" what one wishes.[56] Income, in this view, is not an end in itself but a means to expanding choices, and only one of several. The UNDP issues annual human development reports which define human development as enlarging people's choices and set out the most critical requirements for expansion of choices as living a long and healthy life, being educated, and having access to resources needed for a decent standard of living.

An HRBA to development is consistent with a human-development approach in terms of the goal of expanding choices or agency. However, in a rights framework, lack of access to basic health facilities, education, or housing are understood as violations of obligations to ensure minimum essential levels of different rights, for which states should be held accountable as duty-bearers. Just as there is an essential minimum in domestic contexts, in the context of international development policies, including antipoverty strategies, CESCR has stated that the core obligations for ESC rights "establish an international minimum threshold that all development policies should be designed to respect."[57]

The dynamic of duty-bearer and claims-holder in a rights framework underscores how extreme poverty and the attendant violations of rights are relational. As I discuss throughout this book, those relations are based on discrimination, exclusion and stigma, as well as access to certain endowments, that perpetuate people's deprivation and their lack of control over their lives. And the opportunity structures that they create vary. For example, Paula in Kenya faced different limitations on her choices than Gabriela did in Mexico, which in turn was different from the ways in which Redit's choices were restricted in rural Ethiopia after her mother died.

The UN General Assembly adopted the Millennium Declaration in September 2000, which attempted to unify the global development agenda around the idea of "people-centered development" and the eradication of extreme poverty. The next year, the UN Secretary General released the "Road Map," a plan for implementing the Millennium Declaration that included the Millennium Development Goals (MDGs), which subsequently became the blueprint for global development for the next fourteen years.

The MDGs provided a narrative to the aid system and a frame for thinking about development progress. But arguably, they only painted a thin patina of concern for true people-centered "human development" onto what remained a neoliberal global institutional framework.[58] Indeed, although initially hailed as a tremendous global commitment to poverty eradication, by focusing on narrow technical approaches to achieve specific outcomes, the MDGs arguably went backward to a 1980s concept of development as fulfilling "basic needs" rather than as a process for empowering individuals to have greater choices and control over their lives.[59] As we will come back to throughout this book, if we recognize people as having dignity and agency, they are not merely passive beneficiaries of development programs. In Chapter 8, we return to how an HRBA would demand a shift in approach to promote "sustainable development" and Sustainable Development Goals (SDGs) in the post-2015 world, aimed at change in the structural relations that underpin patterns of severe deprivation and underdevelopment.[60]

Concluding Reflections

Since I was in Baborigame in 1993, a lot has changed there. In the intervening years, the Mexican government adopted a national insurance scheme, Seguro Popular, and extended health care across its territory, even in remote areas such as the Sierra Tarahumara.[61] It also adopted a conditional cash-transfer scheme called Oportunidades to try to address some cross-cutting barriers faced by people in poverty.[62] In explaining the basis for Seguro Popular, the plan's architect and then-Minister of Health Julio Frenk argued it was centrally based on rights: "Whereas Mexico had made strides in the exercise of political and civil rights as a result of its democratization process, it was clear that the next great challenge was to ameliorate social inequality by assuring the universal exercise of the right to health care. . . . This was the over-riding ethical framework in which the reform was presented."[63] Moreover, between 2009 and 2011, Mexico's constitution was reformed and, subsequently, the law of protection writs (*amparos*) was reformed to enable people to pursue legal redress in collective cases of ESC violations. Critics will claim, rightly, that the conquest of rights, and health rights in particular, is incomplete in Mexico, and severe poverty and inequality persist. Yet these advances were unthinkable in Baborigame in 1993, and they show that remarkable progress in paradigms as well as practice is indeed possible in a relatively short span of time.

However, in a remote part of southern Malawi—Neno—the conditions were not unlike what I had seen twenty years earlier in Baborigame. In 2013, I met a woman named Happiness, whose life had been anything but happy. She had given birth to twelve children, three of whom had died. Two had died of AIDS-related causes, the third of maternal causes, although that child also had HIV. Happiness recounted to me the story of her own life, as well as that of the daughter who died in childbirth. At the age of 64, Happiness was now caring for nine orphaned grandchildren and lived in absolute destitution. Her husband was nearly blind because of cataracts and could no longer help with the small farm they depended on to eke out their existence. Her life was a series of strokes of fate, very few of which she had any control over.

I have come to see that gradations of abject poverty are meaningfully measured not in currency but in food—in the infrequency of a person's access to any kind of meat or protein and in how small the quantity of food that ends up on each plate. It is measured in whether children are attending school, whether they have untreated diarrhea and skin rashes, whether they sleep on mats or directly on dirt floors, and whether they have ever worn shoes. It is measured in how far you have to walk from your home to the borehole that is your only source of water and in how many families share it; it is measured in whether you have access to even the simplest of shared pit latrines or whether everyone is defecating in the open. It is fundamentally measured in whether you have any choice about these issues. By any of these measures, Happiness and her family would count among the poorest of the poor.

She and I talked for hours that day, peeling through layers of past and present, laughing and crying together under an enormous baobab tree. From the time Happiness was a small child, so much of her life had been shaped by gendered social norms, and later by governmental neglect of her and her children's basic rights: lack of access to water and sanitation, to education, to basic health care; the cruelty and abuse without any recourse that her daughter had suffered at the hands of her son-in-law; lack of sexual and reproductive autonomy; and entrenched gender-based discrimination. In more human terms, as we talked I tried to imagine what it would be like to wake up with her sorrows every day. Happiness conceded to me that she had considered suicide at times, but she had thought about where that would leave her grandchildren. As we talked, a scrawny cat crawled in and out of Happiness's lap, and I marveled at how this woman summoned the kindness and energy to keep gently stroking it.

Happiness struck me as an extraordinary woman, unmarred by the bitterness that would deform so many in her situation, and managing to maintain purpose in a life blighted by extreme hardship. She eagerly offered to share with me the meager amount of food the family had, saying that I "looked hungry." I was awed by her generosity and warmth, as well as her openness to sharing her story with me. It occurred to me then, as it has at other times, that for those who face the kind of brutal deprivation and tragedy that Happiness did, there is simply no time to grieve all the sorrows in life. She told me she had never had the chance to cry over all of the things she recounted to me, and was obviously grateful for the space to do so. For people who nobody bothers to record by means of birth documents or identity cards, for people who live in perpetual invisibility, the opportunity to construct the narrative of their lives and tell their story to someone who takes the time to ask them what the details have meant to them can provide some measure of solace. Yet, it seemed far too little to be able to offer in this case.

I was left thinking that although much has changed in human rights law and activism regarding the suffering of people living in extreme poverty and in the entitlements of people on the ground in many places, these changes "elsewhere" still mean nothing to Happiness and millions of others around the globe, who through no fault of their own were born in places that have yet to benefit from these shifts.

We have a long way to go in shifting the global and national narratives of what causes severe poverty and what it means in people's lives, as well as the responsibilities of states, individually and collectively in development, to address it. The tragedy of poverty is precisely that it remains so naturalized. Those who are trapped in it accept it too often as fate, Divine will, or just "the way things are." Happiness, just as Pilar in Baborigame twenty years earlier, understood her suffering not as injustice but as the lot she had been dealt by God. And those who can distance themselves generally do.

At the global level, Susan Sontag argued that globalizing poverty may "spur people to think that they should care more," but it also may "invite them to feel that the sufferings and misfortune are too vast, too irrevocable, too epic to be much changed by any local political intervention."[64] Applying a meaningful human rights framework to health and development not only demands more than handouts for the poor, which may alleviate guilt but does nothing to change the underlying causes of their suffering, it also requires challenging this apathy through concrete steps, including law and policy reform, programs, litigation, and social mobilization as I discuss throughout this book.

However, the meanings of "rights" are contested. In this chapter, I have argued that consigning human rights to a narrow range of political issues is not justifiable conceptually and condemns the human rights framework to wither in irrelevance because it fails to address the pressing priorities of the vast majority of people in the world. Until we—poor and wealthy, global North and South alike—begin to grasp fully the magnitude of the injustice of extreme poverty in terms of violations of fundamental rights and dignity, we will be unable to pursue the implications of that understanding through concrete, if iterative, actions, to transform the way we organize our societies and our world.

Chapter 3

Redefining Health: Challenging Power Relations

> Where systematic differences in health are judged to be avoidable by reasonable action they are, quite simply, unfair. . . . Putting right these inequities—the huge and remediable differences in health between and within countries—is a matter of social justice. . . . Social injustice is killing people on a grand scale.
> —WHO Commission on the Social Determinants of Health, 2008

> The fact that holders of such power may relinquish it with reluctance must not deter us from pursuing what is just.
> —Sir Michael Marmot, Chair of the WHO Commission on Social Determinants of Health, 2009

Before I decided definitively to pursue a career linking global health with human rights, I spent some months working and living at a small, privately funded health-care center in Haryana, India, a small state that borders Punjab. Delhi's explosive growth since the 1990s has made the area I was in significantly less rural today. But back then, it took several hours, on several buses, to get to the health center from Delhi, and it was a different world. Indeed, Kabliji Hospital was founded as a rural health center, with the specific goal of providing free care to the poor and of the same quality that they could receive in urban areas.[1] The health center was surrounded by acres of mustard fields. It was possible to walk for hours between villages. Electricity and running water were scarce and unreliable; telephone landlines did not reach very far outside the city (and mobile phones were not yet common); and the night sky still had that profound blackness punctuated by the magical iridescent radiance of stars, which is unimaginable in areas with dense populations and heavy electrical usage.

Kabliji had a small outpatient clinic in the village of Ghamroj, where I would accompany the local nurses and doctors. Ghamroj has since been transformed, but at the time it looked the perfect portrait of a typical, north-Indian village. Dotting the unpaved streets were neatly thatched mud huts and brightly colored saris hanging out to dry, all against a backdrop of buffalo languidly roaming the seemingly endless fields.

The most common complaint at the tiny outpatient clinic was from mothers who were bringing their children in for treatment of diarrheal disease. Some of the young doctors simply prescribed antibiotics; some provided the women with oral rehydration salts and advised them on the preparation of oral rehydration therapy. Some of us noted that these women were retrieving water from a large pond very close to the outpatient clinic, where buffalo and cows could be seen bathing, drinking, and defecating throughout the day. But why would these women use this water and risk making their children sick when there was a well in the middle of the village?

The young doctors and I assumed—in just the way that most conventional public health planning does—that the women must have been ignorant about the effects of dirty water on their children's health and that they therefore required health education. And so we set about to educate them about the importance of clean water, emphasizing the links between diarrheal dehydration and malnutrition, and encouraging them to go the small extra distance to the well in the center of town. And, as in most conventional public health programming, our efforts to reshape knowledge, attitudes, and practices were targeted at mothers, not asking them about their needs but treating them as primarily instrumental, as caretakers for their children.

It was some weeks after we had embarked on this endeavor that we discovered why the women were using the pond. The women's behavior was not because of a lack of education or out of laziness—as some of the urban-based doctors who were doing their rural service had claimed. It was because most of the women who we saw repeatedly bringing their sick children in for treatment were Muslims who lived near the tiny outpatient clinic. Muslims face discrimination in India, and there is a painful history of inter-religious violence in the country. But that was not the whole story.

Ghamroj was dominated by a particular Hindu warrior caste, and these families had converted to Islam from Hinduism because they were Dalits, or "untouchables," who fall at the bottom of the Hindu caste system. This is the case for many Muslims in India, who descend from low-caste Hindus and convert to Islam to escape their Dalit status.[2] However, as is often the case in India, the rest of the Hindu community in Ghamroj did not recognize their conversion and continued to treat them as Dalits. Although by law discrimination and segregation against Dalits is proscribed, they continue to be discriminated against and excluded from much of society.[3] Female Dalits face a double burden of discrimination based on both caste and gender, and Haryana is particularly known for conservative gender roles and exceptionally high rates of violence against women.

As a result, the women faced great violence and possible death if they attempted to use the well in the center of town. The next nearest well was more than two miles away, at the health center itself, which would have required the women to carry the heavy buckets back and forth every day. The decision to use the pond water was entirely rational, given their constrained circumstances.

The lesson was a simple but powerful one for me, one too often forgotten or ignored in public health. We so frequently focus on biological or behavioral factors that we can easily overlook the social, political, economic, and cultural factors that shape the resources and barriers—the opportunity structures—that people have to take account of with respect to their health. Yet evidence suggests that these determinants are often the most critical to the patterns of health and disease in a given society.

In this chapter, I examine how looking at health through a human rights lens can fundamentally transform our understanding of health issues and what to do about them. I begin with the WHO definition of health and describe how from a human rights perspective health and suffering are produced, experienced, and need to be understood in the contexts in which we live. I argue that a rights paradigm challenges both the widely entrenched biomedical approach to health, as well as the conventional public health approaches that focus on biological and behavioral determinants of health, abstracted from the ways in which power is exercised to shape our well-being. Just as in Chapter 2, I suggested that extreme poverty is unnatural, patterns of health and ill-health are caused largely by "social determinants," which are products of human choices that get encoded in laws, policies, and budgets, not natural phenomena. Understanding the causes of ill-health—the causes of our suffering—is key to being able to claim rights to health, as well as to other social entitlements. I illustrate the shift in thinking that applying a rights framework has meant over the last twenty years, with respect to sexual and reproductive health and rights, but I also underscore how contested narratives of rights can be.

Defining Health, a Right to Health, and Human Rights–Based Approaches to Health

That social conditions profoundly affect a broad range of health outcomes has been abundantly demonstrated in an ever-growing literature from social epidemiology, as well as from earlier work in social medicine and medical sociology.[4] Rudolf Virchow, the father of social medicine, famously argued that in order to heal individuals, one must treat the sick society.[5] In recent years, the field of social epidemiology has brought attention to the overarching importance of social determinants to population health—relating patterns of disease with the way society is organized in terms of, for example, class and racial inequalities, as well as employment, educational, and housing patterns.[6] "Social determinants" are far broader than the "underlying determinants," or preconditions, such as water and sanitation, referred to in Chapter 2 as a part of the right to health. The WHO Commission on Social Determinants of Health, which released its groundbreaking report in 2008, defines social determinants as the conditions in which people are "born, grow, live, work, and age," and which shape their health status.[7]

This understanding of the importance of social factors is central to construing health as a right, even if all social determinants are not part of the right to health per se. Indeed, it was at the core of the definition of health set out in the preamble to the newly formed WHO's constitution in 1946, which first proclaimed, "The enjoyment of the highest attainable standard of health is one of the fundamental rights of every human being without distinction of race, religion, political belief, economic or social condition."[8] The WHO constitution also noted, "Health is a state of complete physical, mental and social well-being, and not merely the absence of disease or infirmity."[9]

It is easy to dismiss this definition as utopian. Other than sexual ecstasy or perhaps the infant attached to its mother's breast, when does anyone ever feel a complete state of physical, mental, and social well-being? And this definition of health has indeed been controversial. In part because of these debates, the core formulation of a right to health in international law did not adopt the WHO language, although the concept has played an important role in the international instruments and declarations.

As noted in Chapter 2, those who shaped the wording of the ICESCR chose the phrasing, now in ICESCR Article 12 (1): "The right to the highest attainable standard of physical and mental health." They recognized that the ability of any state to guarantee its people such a right will inevitably be constrained by resources and by other factors. There is no right to *be healthy* under international or national law. Although we may wish that the state could guarantee "complete physical, mental and social well-being" for every woman, man, and child, those who formulated binding international rights law acknowledged that a state can at best be held legally accountable for establishing standards and for providing access to preconditions of health, as well as care.

From a rights perspective, there are serious problems with the definition of health in the preamble to the WHO constitution. Such a wide definition makes it impossible to carve out an enforceable legal entitlement relating to a right to health. Rights are building blocks to live lives of dignity, not complete end-states in and of themselves. There are many other values besides health within a life of dignity. Some of them are other, distinct human rights, such as freedom of information and equal protection of the law and political participation, and some of them are not, such as love. It would be a mistake both conceptually and strategically to attempt to have a *right to health* subsume all rights relating to any social determinants.[10]

However, a human rights framework explicitly acknowledges the interdependence of all rights, CP rights and ESC rights, and therefore a HRBA requires multisectoral approaches to health. A human rights framework is inherently concerned with the social relations—and power relations—that structure possibilities for health. What the 1946 definition in the preamble to the WHO constitution did—more than sixty years before the WHO Commission on Social Determinants issued its report—was to very clearly suggest that health is not just a matter of biological or behavioral factors. Think, for example, of how caste, gender, and religion manifested themselves in the Haryana example at the beginning of this chapter. The diarrhea and disease that those children suffered from were not an inevitable product of "natural" biological phenomena. Their suffering was the result of deeply discriminatory social relations, which in turn affected their parents' (and because of gender roles, their mothers') ability to exercise agency and choice over basic decisions, such as where to gather water to be able to keep their children from falling ill.

It is often easier to see how unjust social arrangements affect health in societies other than our own. Indeed, outside certain parts of South Asia, the differentials in life prospects stemming from caste seem entirely arbitrary and repulsively discriminatory. Yet, in our own societies, those same kinds of injustices too often become invisible. We retreat into accepting the status quo and focusing on individual behaviors rather than identifying and acting on social injustice and political failures.

For example, in the United States, there is overwhelming evidence that racial and ethnic disparities affect every aspect of our health system and reflect entrenched racial inequalities and discrimination in the larger society. It must be noted that race, which involves historically constructed power relations, is a concept that shifts and is used for multiple (and sometimes malign ideological) purposes. Yet "race" identifies a cluster of institutionalized practices that reinforce domination of some over others. And just as Dalit women in Haryana, India, face dual discrimination, women of color in the United States do as well. For example, they are three times more likely to die of maternal causes than are white women. These women of color have less education, live in segregated neighborhoods, have fewer employment prospects with poorer insurance coverage, and, especially in the case of undocumented women, are less likely to seek help in a timely manner.[11]

It is clear that race discrimination is a "fundamental cause" of disease in the United States, in the sense that associations between race and health are robust and transcend specific diseases or conditions. In the mid-1990s, Bruce Link and Jo Phelan demonstrated that the disparity in mortality from tuberculosis between white men and African American men at the beginning of the twentieth century was replicated at the end of the twentieth century in the disparity between the two groups in mortality from cardiovascular disease.[12] Subsequent work on racial disparities has only reconfirmed the importance of adopting systematic approaches to addressing the underlying causes of poorer diagnosis, treatment, and outcomes among people of color across a range of conditions. Yet media and public discourse invariably focus on individual behavior, choice, and habits, isolated from the social contexts in which people live, when explaining poor outcomes from maladies such as diabetes or cancer. When surveyed, providers often focus on noncompliance of patients to explain differing results.[13] Personal responsibility rather than social accountability are inevitably emphasized.[14]

For this reason, the 1946 WHO definition of health, despite its apparent idealism, continues to be so important today. Changing approaches to health to prioritize social determinants will require enormous changes in public consciousness about what causes ill-health in the United States, just as it will in India and elsewhere. But more than sixty years ago—long before people were even discussing the phrase "social determinants"—this WHO definition took a step toward denaturalizing the suffering produced by social causes. And in this sense it was a tectonic shift in perspective from the traditional medical and scientific approach to health that prevailed at the time in the West, and continues to do so to this day despite the many advances in social medicine and social epidemiology.

Challenges to the "Biomedical Paradigm"

This WHO definition of health, further developed in later conference declarations and other documents, represented a dramatic expansion of the so-called biomedical paradigm, in which health is in fact construed as *the absence of* disease or infirmity or, slightly more broadly, the absence of pathology.[15] Consider for a moment how health is treated when you are at the doctor's office. The "normal" on the cholesterol test or blood pressure test is evidence of *health*. This "biomedical" approach to health is so entrenched in both research and training of health professionals, as well as in public discourse about health in the West, that it is widely taken for granted.[16] The WHO conceptualization of health as a positive state, embedded in social contexts, challenges a number of key aspects of this paradigm.

First, in the biomedical paradigm, states of ill-health are abstracted as "conditions" distinct from the person suffering from them. In the West, we have become used to thinking this way, but that was not always the case. For instance, Greek *humoralism*, which prevailed as an explanatory framework until the nineteenth century, tailored diagnosis and treatment to individual cases, associating individual health with internal balances as well as factors such as air, weather, and social dynamics. This perspective continues to shape many other cultures today; Eastern medicine also tailors remedies to the physical and emotional expressions seen in individual patients.

And take, for example, schizophrenia and bipolar disease, two widespread sources of "psychiatric disability" in the West. These are not treated as abstract conditions in many non-Western societies. Rather, the observable episodes of mania, catatonia, or paranoia are treated as the afflictions because they force the person to withdraw from his or her social roles. However, when the person is not suffering an episode, that person is treated as "normal" and not defined, as in the West, as "a schizophrenic."[17]

Second, modern Western medicine draws a distinction between physical and mental health. The abortion context demonstrates that, just as our concepts of rights can narrow public health discussions and responses, so too can our conceptions of health affect the scope of entitlements women enjoy. In a number of countries where exceptions to the criminalization of abortion are based on "threats to the life or health of the mother," it has been contested whether "health" includes mental health as well as physical health. Staunchly antichoice advocates have argued that opening up the concept of "health" in such a way would allow women to claim they were "depressed" merely because of becoming pregnant.

Furthermore, these separate categories are simply not the way people think of health and ill-health in many other cultures. For example, when I conducted interviews with family members of women who died in pregnancy and childbirth in eastern and southern Africa, informants would almost invariably refer to feelings of "profound pain" (e.g. "uchungo" in Swahili). The pain they described had both physical and psychological manifestations, including muscle weakness, chest pain, and headaches, as well as pain associated with what in the West might be called depression, such as lethargy, uncontrollable sadness, and fatigue. It also had social manifestations, such as the inability to attend to work and withdrawal from social interactions. It would be incomprehensible to most of the people I interviewed to attempt to put labels that insisted on differentiating between their physical and psychological symptomatology, and to abstract those from their social situation.

Similarly, in the cosmology of the Quechua-speaking descendants of the Incas in Peru, physical, mental, and spiritual well-being are all inextricably connected. An indigenous *curandero* (healer) in the southern Peruvian highlands is most likely to begin a diagnosis with a reading of the patient's coca leaves. Whatever views Westerners might hold toward such practices, the knowledge and ability to interpret the meaning of symptoms that the *curandero*, or other traditional healers have, is firmly rooted in their ability to link the physical complaints a person might have to their emotional state and their interpersonal relations. And that ability depends on a deep knowledge of a specific context.

In sharp contrast, the biomedical model fundamentally abstracts our understanding of health from social and cultural context, to define it as some variant of "species normal functioning." Just as with the narrow liberal state, individuals are construed as floating free of their social environments, which are seen as rather thin constructs, rather than pivotal to the understanding of our selves and our well-being.

Yet, as early as the 1970s, Arthur Kleinman was distinguishing between "disease" as a maladaptation or malfunctioning of biological or psychological processes and "illness," which comprises the personal, interpersonal, and culturally determined reactions to disease.[18] In a human rights framework, our understanding of health and ill-health has to encompass both the biological and the socially constructed dimensions of the experience.

By contrast in the biomedical paradigm, health and pathology are not only defined in isolation from the broader setting in which people live but also treated as objectively ascertainable by scientific experts (medical researchers or clinicians). Moreover, the judgments prescribed by those experts (diagnoses) are often assumed to be a truth that is beyond question either by individual patients or by the public in general.[19]

Since the mid-twentieth century, in the United States and elsewhere, critiques from bioethics have attempted to increase the autonomy and authority of patients in patient-doctor interactions, chipping away at the traditionally unfettered paternalism of physicians to decide what is in the best interests of the patient.[20] So, for example, the nature and amount of information a physician might have to share with a patient or her family when discussing various courses of action has dramatically changed over the years. Yet, the promotion of increased autonomy for patients and "shared decision-making for improved outcomes" in bioethics has stopped short of questioning the inherent exercise of power in the ability to define disease and deviance from some abstract idea of "normal."[21]

Let me be clear, however: A human rights approach to health is not an anticlinical or antiscientific stance. Health has *both* biological and social dimensions. As I discuss further with respect to the state's accountability for adopting appropriate measures in Chapter 5, human rights strategies must be based on solid scientific evidence. Religion, ideology, and other forms of hatred wrapped up as tradition are responsible for vast suffering across countries of differing development levels.

In addition, the astounding pace of progress in biomedicine makes it even more urgent to address the inequities in the enjoyment of those advances. While living in Tanzania, I watched helplessly as my then-ten-year-old son became very ill very quickly. Wracked with coughs that left him blue and gasping for air and vomiting, we were medically evacuated to South Africa for urgent care. There is nothing like seeing your desperately sick child recuperate to make you appreciate the benefits of scientific progress and modern medicine. And there is nothing like living in a country that does not have an adequately functioning health system to make you appreciate the enormity of the privilege of being able to seek care in another country, when the overwhelming majority of people cannot.

In short, rights frameworks absolutely need to be grounded in the best evidence we have from public health, as well as concerned with the equitable distribution of the fruits of scientific advances. At the same time, however, thinking about health in terms of rights makes us critically question the implications of defining health and ill-health in isolation from what it means to diverse people in their lives.

How We Understand Suffering and What It Says About a Claim for a Right to Health

How we understand health and ill-health is dialectically related to how we understand the reasons for our suffering and that of others. How we make sense of the conditions that befall us and our loved ones has everything to do with whether we can see it as injustice and, as a result, claim *rights* to health.

For example, the Peruvian woman I described in Chapter 1, Dolores, died an excruciating death from esophageal cancer. She and her family, who were all deeply religious, wracked their brains for the sin that this poor young woman must have committed to bring upon herself such suffering. She had not smoked, she did not drink, and she was even entirely chaste. Encouraged by the quacks they attended, they concluded in the end that she had literally swallowed her anger and resentments and that, in place of the gratitude to God that she was meant to feel, these had built up in a giant mass that eventually closed off her throat.

In more than twenty years of interviewing families of women who have died of pregnancy-related causes, I have heard all kinds of explanations—from having been hit on the head by a mango during pregnancy (Sierra Leone) to not wearing a hat and letting the sun steal her unborn baby's soul (Peru). In many places, the notion of witchcraft is very strong. This may be especially true in parts of sub-Saharan Africa, but the idea that people put curses on one another is widespread throughout much of the world. In many places from

Turkey to the Middle East to Latin America, it is often the "evil eye" (or *mal de ojo* in Spanish) from which people need to be protected by talismans or cured through "ritual cleansings" (or *limpias* in Spanish). In Latin America, these cleansings are often performed with items such as eggs or animals, such as *cuy* (guinea pigs, in the Peruvian Andes). In much of the world, I think it would be difficult to find even highly educated people who did not at least privately credit *mal de ojo*, or other forms of cures or spells, with some power.

These explanations often coexist with what is objectively verifiable. In Malawi, for example, one family understood the reason for a young woman's death in delivery not simply as a mistaken failure to get to a health facility quickly when she was going into labor but as the result of a curse placed on her by a neighbor who wanted her land. It was the family's view the curse incapacitated her from making the decision to seek care in a timely way.

At other times, the idea of these curses is developed as a response to colonialism or official regulation of behavior. In some cases, the "cure" for the suffering induced by the curse is a traditional practice, which itself creates suffering. The evolution of female genital mutilation (FGM), or cutting, in Tanzania, as documented by Chiku Ali and Agnete Strom, is a powerful example of this. Traditionally FGM was generally performed as a coming-of-age ritual, as a way of maintaining girls' chastity. But Ali and Strom note: "Cutting of babies as young as one year of age started in the early 1970s. The natives sent a loud message to the outside world: circumcising babies was necessary in order to cure a mystic spell placed on them by the ancestors. This curse was now called *lawalawa*, a local synonym for the Swahili word *peremende*, meaning candy."[22] *Lawalawa* was described by natives as swelling and itching in a child's genitals and vagina. According to Ali and Strom, "The phenomenon of *lawalawa* did not exist before the authorities decided that FGM must be banned immediately. . . . It seems that the natives invented *lawalawa* to legitimate FGM, even though the performance had to lose some of its meaning."[23]

Mystic spells from ancestors may seem alien or primitive to many readers, and for elders to use *lawalawa* as an excuse to mutilate young girls' genitalia is indeed a horrific abuse of power. But the notion of illness as punishment for transgression of social norms and communally ascribed virtues is common throughout the world.

Consider, for example, public health messages in the United States regarding abstinence from overeating and smoking, getting enough physical exercise, and reducing stress. We are constantly being told by the media what we should do to be able to maintain our health. Of course scientific evidence shows that such behavior *is* good for us. This is very different from the example of *lawalawa*, you may say. And that is true.

Nevertheless, these behaviors come to be defined as "virtuous," and we come to associate enjoyment of health with virtue and suffering with transgression, individual insufficiency and personal failure. At a friend's funeral that I attended a few years ago, a man who had been her officemate spoke about her life. My friend had died far too young of lung cancer—very advanced when it was detected—although she had never smoked or worked with chemicals. Her officemate recounted how he ate bags of artificially orange-colored Cheetos, while she ate carrot slices for lunch; he never exercised, whereas she was an avid yoga and exercise enthusiast; he was quite overweight and she was not. He commented ruefully on the irony of all of this, and most people in the audience no doubt felt, as I surely did, that it was deeply *unfair*, that somehow someone "who does everything right" should not be stricken down early, while someone else lives a slothful, hedonistic life with impunity—as though illness and health were matters of punishment or worth.

Whether it is a magical curse, divine punishment, or some other variant of individual responsibility, when we think about the reasons for our suffering—and that of others—in these terms, it obscures the societal and political responsibilities for patterns of health and ill-health. It is in the hazy gray area, where the boundaries of individual responsibility and social determinants meet, that the scope of the right to health—and the ensuing obligations of states—are defined. These are profound questions of moral philosophy, culture, and religion. And, as discussed later in this chapter, there may be no area where narratives of "sin" and "transgression" are more clearly embedded in policies and laws than sexual and reproductive health. But regardless of the topic, invariably the boundaries of individual and societal responsibility become encoded in how societies legally treat entitlements to health and health care.

For example, Richard Epstein expressed the still widely held view in the United States some decades ago that individuals will take more responsibility for their health if forced to pay the full costs of their own health care. At the "margins," as economists like to say, people may overeat or smoke or take other risks that are bad for their health: "Noble intentions quickly lead to an endless tangle of hidden subsidies [and] perverse incentives which in the long-run often backfire on its intended beneficiaries."[24] Thus, the essence of the argument in Epstein's widely influential book, *Mortal Peril*, was about the dangers of the government subsidizing universal health care—an argument that surfaced again in discussions on the Affordable Care Act.

The notion that people need to *earn* health-care access, or preconditions to health—as if it is something we can do all by ourselves outside of social factors and determinants—is inconsistent with the concept of a *right to health*. In some cases, people convicted of serious crimes are deemed to have forfeited their right to vote because they breached the values of the community. Nevertheless, in general we do not need to *earn* fundamental rights necessary to live with dignity and participate fully in our communities and society. This is true of civil rights, such as due process or freedoms of expression or religion, and it has generally come to be accepted about some ESC rights as well, such as basic education. Similarly, if we believe that people have rights to health, the state bears some responsibility for providing access to preconditions as well as care. Access to care and the preconditions of health is not matter of desert, but of universal entitlement.

Nevertheless, the question of *to what extent* the state bears responsibility for preventing and mitigating suffering and how much must be left to the responsibility, or fate, of the individual will be disputed across societies. All rights are sites for contestation as well as tools of struggle. And we shall see throughout this book that—given constant technological innovations and medical discoveries, demographic and environmental shifts, and evolving social and cultural norms—this is acutely apparent when we think of defining the ever-changing boundaries of an enforceable right to health that includes care.

Challenges to Mainstream Public Health

If the biomedical approach to health tends to focus on technical interventions to treat physiological conditions, as Jonathan Mann wrote, the traditional framing of the public health question as " 'We have a cancer problem, now what do we do about it, within the existing social system?' inevitably leads to a focus on individual behavior." The question is largely construed as a matter of personal volition in mainstream public health.[25] This is exactly what happened in the example I set out at the beginning of this chapter; we moved from treating the diarrheal disease as a purely biological issue of bacteria in the children to be treated with medicine to seeing it as a public health issue, and then attempting to change mothers' behavior.

However, the dynamics of power at work in structuring health outcomes remain largely invisible if analysis focuses on the independent effects of individual behavior or individual biological risk factors. Focusing on individuals precludes fundamental challenges to the status quo. Thus, as long as we were focusing on educating mothers about hygiene and sanitation, we failed to see that the caste and gender relations in the village, and not a lack of knowledge, were determining the parameters for their behavior.

In a rights framework, a core public function of epidemiology—the study of the distribution and determinants of disease—is precisely to make the connections among impoverishment, discrimination and inequality, and health, visible. This requires challenging deeply held assumptions about why people, and certain people, end up suffering from certain afflictions. Thus when we ask what makes women die of pregnancy and childbirth complications, the answer is not simply hemorrhage or eclampsia. That is *how* they die. Nor is it individual choices and care-seeking on the part of women; those are the result of specific opportunity structures. Rather, to really understand *why* women die, we need to understand the roles that poverty, gender, inequality, and social exclusion and the political failure to address them play as causal factors.

This, in turn, requires contextual, multilevel analyses. As a result, a rights framework calls on us to jump between "levels" of causation. Conventional public health generally distinguishes between so-called proximate and distal causal factors. Issues relating to poverty or social norms are generally considered to be distal factors, which are consigned to the background, and public health efforts concentrate on more proximate factors. These proximate "population-level risk factors"—such as obesity rates—are often taught in separate courses in schools of public health and focus on targeting behavioral change. Not surprisingly then, distal factors are often forgotten when it comes time to design and fund interventions and, in turn, the status quo does not get transformed. In a rights framework, by contrast, those distal factors are more meaningfully understood to be *fundamental* or *determining* factors. Nancy Krieger writes in a similar vein: "Driving health inequalities are how power—both power over and power to do, including constraints on and possibilities for exercising each type—structures people's engagements with the world and their exposures to material and psychosocial health hazards. Notably, neither type of power readily maps onto a metric of proximate or distal."[26]

Take another example: lead paint exposure in children, which for generations was a major problem in the United States. It is now well documented that exposure to lead "down to the lowest blood lead concentrations yet studied" is associated with a wide range of toxicity and can affect almost every organ system in the body.[27] Perhaps the very first "health rights" case that I ever worked on, while still a law student in the late 1980s, involved a child-care center in Chelsea, Massachusetts, a low-income city in the Boston area. This child-care center, largely serving minority children and particularly the Latino community, was almost directly underneath the bridge that spans the Mystic River. The Maurice J. Tobin Memorial Bridge, the largest bridge in New England, was at the time being repainted. The lead paint that had been on the bridge was being removed and much of it was flaking down onto the yard of this child-care center. Unfortunately, lead paint has a sweet flavor and is attractive to children. In this case, the Massachusetts Public Interest Research Group (MassPIRG) was able to negotiate with the Massachusetts Bay Transportation Authority to construct a dome over the child-care center to prevent the lead paint flakes from falling into the yard during the de-leading of the bridge.

But when we looked into litigation around Section 8 housing in Boston—Section 8 authorizes the payment of assistance to private landlords in the United States for rental housing, which by law was supposed to be free of lead paint—we realized that bringing a claim might mean that some of these families would lose their only source of shelter.[28] These children were exposed to the risks of lead paint consumption for the same reasons that their housing was so precarious: they were poor minorities whose parents had very constrained opportunity structures, just as the women in Haryana had. Given very limited language, education, financial and other resources, and sometimes lack of immigration status, they faced enormous barriers, and had few choices about where to live, work, and send their children to child care or school. Separating out these social determinants as "background factors" and reducing the public health issues to individual behavior might solve some basic needs. But it cannot allow us to address the multivalent needs of real human beings who find themselves facing a confluence of factors limiting their ability to exercise choices, including in relation to protecting their children's health.

In its groundbreaking 2008 report, the WHO Commission on Social Determinants of Health attempted to reframe public as well as scientific understanding of the importance of social determinants in causing ill-health. That report stated,

> The poor health of the poor, the social gradient in health within countries, and the marked health inequities between countries are caused by the unequal distribution of power, income, goods, and services, globally and nationally, the consequent unfairness in the immediate, visible circumstances of people's lives—their access to health care, schools, and education, their conditions of work and leisure, their homes, communities, towns, or cities—and their chances of leading a flourishing life. This unequal distribution of health-damaging experiences is not in any sense a "natural" phenomenon but is the result of a toxic combination of poor social policies and programmes, unfair economic arrangements, and bad politics.[29]

The WHO Commission's report drew on hundreds of studies that had been done showing the significance of social determinants, and even more work has appeared subsequently on connections between specific social determinants such as socioeconomic status gradients and health.

For example, Steven Woolf and colleagues examined whether correcting the social conditions that account for excess deaths among individuals with inadequate education might save more lives than medical advances in the United States.[30] The authors concluded, "Spending large sums of money on such advances at the expense of social change may be jeopardizing public health."[31]

Nevertheless, as the WHO Commission report found, "Most health research (and funding) remains overwhelmingly biomedically focused, whereas the largest health improvements arguably come from improvements in the social determinants of health."[32] Six years later, the Lancet-Oslo Commission on Global Health Governance underscored the importance of addressing specifically the political determinants of health.[33]

Laws, Policies, and Budgets as Social Determinants of Health

A distinguishing feature of a human rights framework, or an HRBA to health, is its emphasis on the rule of law, and in turn, the importance of establishing an enabling legal and policy framework. The operations of power at work in determining patterns of health and illness are reflected in laws that shape the exposures and vulnerabilities to disease faced by different populations. For example, when services or activities are criminalized, the law is shaping— and in many cases hindering—people's opportunities for health and access to care. Imagine the barriers to accessing care that a sex worker or an intravenous drug user faces in countries where those activities are subject to criminal prosecution, and therefore also to extortion and harassment by the police.

The criminalization of abortion—a service only required by women—is another example of how laws, often influenced by religious views, act as social determinants of health and can create discriminatory barriers to access to care. An estimated 13–18 percent of maternal deaths worldwide are attributable to unsafe abortion.[34] These deaths are typically horrendous; women puncture their uteruses from inserting sharp objects into themselves and then face sepsis and hemorrhage from the "home remedies" they inflict on themselves. I recall one case of a woman in Peru who bled to death after an induced abortion and her children then had to sleep in the same bed where they found her body. Had abortion been legally available in her country, she would not have died this way. Yet Catholic and other religious narratives around abortion as "sin" (and murder) in Peru and elsewhere, result not just in moral justifications for laws that lead to elevated suffering and death among girls and women but also remove the issue from the possibility of reasoned public debate, often closing off opportunities for seeking change through political and social forums.

Understanding how laws and policies can act as social determinants underscores, as discussed in Chapter 1, how porous the divide is between the public and private spheres, as well as between private morality and public policy. Take sex, the most intimate private activity possible. If homosexual activity is criminalized, lesbian, gay, bisexual, and transgender (LGBT) people can be subject to police harassment and abuse, as well as confinement or worse. Similarly, if condoms and lubricants are not available through health systems because of discriminatory policies, men who have sex with men (MSM) cannot enjoy sexual relations on an equal footing with heterosexuals. And if heterosexual women do not have access to endowments and information, including comprehensive sexuality education that includes information about pleasure; if marital rape is not criminalized or IPV is not punished; if they have no control over when or with whom they have sex or in what position; or if they cannot use contraception or seek a safe abortion if the contraception fails, it is likewise impossible to expect that these women can fully enjoy sexual pleasure.

Changing laws need not be costly; it may require only negligible additional resources. However, inequitable power relations that determine patterns of disease also are evident in budgetary formulations and allocations. Calling health or health care a right and understanding that budgets function as social determinants of health cannot and should not *always* imply obtaining more resources from public coffers for certain medical treatments. Refusal to acknowledge resource constraints in health can lead to absurdly unjust outcomes even in the wealthiest countries. Imagine, for example, a society spending bottomless resources on an extremely expensive treatment for terminally ill cancer patients when children are going without basic care. Moreover, spending endless amounts on medical care is not the most effective way to improve population health. Budgets for education, infrastructure, and housing also function as social determinants of health. As noted earlier, we now have ample evidence that attention to some of these other social determinants will produce greater benefits than spending on medical care.

But as Peter Uvin notes, however, a human rights approach does not "take resource constraints as natural givens but [treats] them as the result of past choices."[35] In Chapter 2, I noted that CP rights and ESC rights both require resources, but the costs of CP rights are often hidden in general taxation. Social entitlements that relate to many of the social determinants of health—such as social protection schemes, pro-poor housing policies, and monies for public education—are often subject to cuts when countries face fiscal limitations. Just as the conceptualization of rights as merely shields from the state's interference needs to be challenged in a human rights framework, so too do constant refrains of "scarcity" with respect to resources. When "scarcity" becomes a mantra that is not subject to requirements of reasoned justification, it imposes unnecessary restrictions on our ability to think beyond current institutional arrangements and practices.

For example, until ten to fifteen years ago, it was considered impossible to provide ARV therapy in low-income countries. Many arguments were made to justify why what was broadly agreed on as "the right thing to do" could not be done—lack of human resources, failures of compliance, unsustainability—but in the end they all related directly or indirectly to assumptions about resources and budgets. Nevertheless, using human rights arguments, activists challenged the dominant thinking that led to accepting such enormous suffering as merely an inevitable tragedy. In groundbreaking litigation from South Africa, India, and other countries, PLWAs and their advocates argued that failure to provide people with access to ARV medications was a violation of their fundamental rights to health and life. Courts in many countries agreed, and ordered governments to develop plans of action and find the resources to provide ARVs.

In 1997 in Costa Rica, the Constitutional Chamber of the Supreme Court, citing documentation in public health sources such as the Centers for Disease Control and Prevention's *Morbidity and Mortality Weekly Report*, was convinced that recently developed ARV combination therapies were effective in turning what had been a death sentence into a chronic disease.[36] The court upheld the plaintiffs' claim for ARV medications, stating: "What good are the rest of the rights and guarantees, the institutions and programs, the advantages and benefits of our system of liberties, if a person cannot count on the right to life and health assured?"[37] Costa Rica's HIV/AIDS mortality rate went on to become one of the lowest in the region as a result of widespread access to ARV medications. Similarly, in South Africa, a case brought by the Treatment Action Campaign to the Constitutional Court led to a 2002 decision calling for the roll out of prevention of mother to child transmission (PMTCT), which is estimated to have saved tens of thousands of lives.[38] When health—including health care—is considered a right, it makes us think differently about the state's responsibility for providing resources.

Sexual and Reproductive Health and Rights: Struggle and Contestation to Challenge Power Relations That Affect Health

No area more dramatically illustrates the importance of human rights frameworks in expanding understandings of health as well as how contested challenging of the power relations that determine health can be than sexual and reproductive health (SRH). I was in India precisely in the wake of the groundbreaking International Conference on Population and Development (ICPD) held in Cairo, Egypt, in 1994. The messages of the ICPD in underscoring the social determinants and power relations shaping SRH—could hardly be more relevant to any country. The entrenched structural discrimination faced by women in India—and indeed particularly in Haryana—is reflected in, among other things, harmful cultural practices and some of the highest levels of violence against women in all of India, where such violence is widespread.[39] However, India is far from unique.

Prior to the ICPD in 1994, elements of reproductive health (including family planning, maternal health, and sexually transmitted diseases) were treated as fragmented aspects of women's health, while population policy revolved largely around utilitarian goals based on demographic imperatives and control of women's fertility. Women, and their needs and rights, were largely invisible, as were sexual minorities. The ICPD declaration and "Programme of Action" united these disparate aspects under a comprehensive definition of "reproductive health," in wording based on the WHO definition, discussed earlier: "Reproductive health is a state of complete physical, mental and social well-being and not merely the absence of disease or infirmity, in all matters relating to the reproductive system and to its functions and processes."[40] Sexual health was defined as part of reproductive health, with the stated goal being "to promote the adequate development of responsible sexuality that permits relations of equity and mutual respect between the genders; and to ensure that women and men have access to information, education and services needed to achieve good sexual health and exercise their reproductive rights and responsibilities."[41] The ICPD also marked a significant paradigm shift to a view of reproductive *rights* in which women (and men) were the decision makers over their bodies and lives, rather than being instrumentalized by governments as means of reproduction to meet some larger societal objective.[42]

A year later, at the Fourth World Conference on Women (Beijing conference), the vision of SRH and reproductive rights laid out in Cairo was reaffirmed and extended into other spheres of women's health and lives.[43] Thus, the definitions of women's health set out by Beijing and the ICPD reflected a multidimensional view of the factors shaping women's health. These two landmark conferences, building on the Vienna Conference mentioned in Chapter 2, boldly constructed a new view of sexual and reproductive and women's health, based largely on activism in the women's movement, as well as in other communities.

Following the ICPD and Beijing, these conceptualizations of SRH were enshrined in additional documents and instruments under international law. In 1999 and 2000, respectively, the CEDAW Committee and the CESCR issued relevant interpretations related to women and health, and the right to health, which reinforced Cairo and Beijing, and there has been additional standard-setting under international law.[44] Despite an often retrogressive climate in global politics and development over the last twenty years, intensive further work has gone into advancing conceptions of SRH rights in ways that, among other things, reflect an understanding of health as a product of the arrangement of power and gendered relations in society.

At the national level, legislation has been enacted and institutions created to address issues such as violence against women, and policies have been adopted to advance access to contraception and pregnancy-related care in countries around the world. There is now widespread condemnation in law, if not actual enforcement, regarding a number of practices that might have been contested previously on the grounds of "cultural values," such as child marriage.

Other areas of reproductive and sexual autonomy, such as abortion, have a more mixed history, with conservative actors having adopted many of the same strategies as progressives and even appropriating rights language as in "the rights of the unborn."[45] Even hard fought judicial victories regarding abortion have often had substantial normative effects across jurisdictions and yet have gone unimplemented because of resistance from certain social actors including members of the clergy and religiously influenced politicians, as well as a lack of institutional capacity for follow-up in the judiciary, and necessary alliances with civil social actors.

Indeed, it would be misleading to portray these developments as linear. As concluded in the Policy Recommendations for the ICPD Beyond 2014, the High-Level Task Force reports, "The urgency and relevance of ensuring full implementation of the Cairo goals still stand. The Programme of Action has inspired policies and programmes in many countries that have improved millions of lives, but critical gaps and emerging issues that perpetuate discrimination, exclusion, and inequality remain unresolved."[46] Perhaps one of the greatest remaining gaps for progressives is to connect the enjoyment of sexual and reproductive rights, and decisional autonomy in the private sphere, with economic and social justice and access to endowments in the public sphere.

But twenty years after the ICPD, perhaps the greatest vitriol and venom from conservative forces is directed at the concept of sexual rights, which go beyond the brief mention of "sexual health" in the ICPD. At national levels, there have been conflicting trends in relation to LGBT rights, which encompass a broad range of rights that are associated both with protections from harm and affirmations of sexual expression, sexual empowerment, and "sexual citizenship" including, among other things, same-sex marriage, adoption and parental rights, employment discrimination, right to lease and own property, freedom of assembly, hate speech, ill treatment of LGBT persons by state agents, asylum seeking, and legal recognition of gender change.

Notable progress has been made with respect to many of these issues, both in terms of normative recognition and practice over the last twenty years. Same-sex marriage and civil unions have been legalized in a number of countries across Western Europe and in South America, and at least some courts across the United States appear to be overturning state bans. In the 2013 decision *United States v. Windsor*, the U.S. Supreme Court struck down a federal statute that failed to accord the same benefits to same-sex partners under such legal state marriages as to partners in heterosexual marriages.[47] Legal recognition of transgender people no longer calls for surgery in Argentina and many other countries. The rights of intersex people have also achieved significant recognition by legislatures and courts from Argentina to India. In its 2014 National Legal Services Authority (NALSA) judgment, the Indian Supreme Court recognized a third sex and noted the fundamental dignity issues involved in being able to determine one's own sexual orientation and gender identity.[48] The law has both prescriptive and expressive functions and, in these cases, the expressive function creates a narrative that enables the most historically marginalized of people to see themselves as fully human, with equal claims to dignity.

However, in Africa in particular, there has been a sharp rise in anti-LGBT legislation, spawned in large part by transnational actors, including evangelical churches from the United States. The two phenomena are related; as laws and popular opinion change in the West, these conservative forces redouble their efforts to hold their ground in Africa and use "anti-imperialist" and "anti-Western" rhetoric in shamelessly hypocritical ways, especially given that anti-sodomy laws were enacted under Western colonialism. The same week in 2014 that Jason Collins came out as the first openly gay player in the NBA, Uganda passed a draconian antihomosexuality bill, enacted "to prohibit any form of sexual relations between persons of the same sex; prohibit the promotion or recognition of such relations and to provide for other related matters."[49] The act called for life imprisonment for engaging in homosexual activity, seven years for "aiding and abetting homosexuality," and five to seven years plus a fine for "promoting homosexuality." I was in Uganda in February 2014 when the law passed, conducting a human rights seminar. One Ugandan friend, Adrian Jjuko, who had previously litigated some of the most important cases regarding LGBT rights in Uganda, told me that he and other colleagues were challenging the law in court—and eventually they won: it was declared unconstitutional.[50] In this case, however, because the court ruled on procedural rather than substantive grounds of equality and nondiscrimination, the judicial victory may not lead to the social legitimacy for new norms around LGBT rights that we would hope to see in Uganda. Indeed, the law may well be reintroduced. Meanwhile, harassment and other forms of attacks on LGBT individuals have increased in Uganda since the original law was passed.

And as in the case of the Dalit women who would not seek water at the village well, MSM and other LGBT persons are unlikely to seek health care when they fear repercussions. As a result of such stigma—which robs people of a sense of a "normal" identity[51]—the HIV/AIDS rates among MSM across East Africa tend to be far higher (and often undocumented by the government) than in the general population. In a human rights framework, HIV/AIDS is a social phenomenon and not merely an "infectious disease" that can be abstracted in causes or meanings from the context in which it is experienced. Stigmatizing views and discriminatory laws and practices must continually be challenged because conventional public health programs focused on behavior change will not address the underlying causes of ill-health and suffering.

Applying a human rights framework to health forces us to challenge the idea that deprivations of SRH rights are "natural" or inevitable. Applying such a framework changes the narrative through which we understand sexual expression or punishments for violations of divine injunctions. It also shows how illusory it is to think that we can promote SRH through merely behavioral risk modification or biomedical treatment. Sexuality is a fundamental expression of personhood, which needs to be protected but also enabled (rather than criminalized). Thus the goal of adopting a human rights approach is not just about implementing a policy or program to prevent or treat certain conditions, but about explicitly identifying the spaces and opportunities to expand the ability of all people—of whatever gender identity or sexual orientation—to make choices about their lives as well as their bodies. Sometimes such expansion will require changes in laws and policies, or education in the broader society that reflect different narratives about sexuality and who is a full participant in society. Sometimes it will involve specific changes in the health system as well, as I discuss further in Chapter 4.

Concluding Reflections

The Kabliji Hospital and Rural Health Centre in Haryana was founded and run by a Sikh family, including an important feminist in India, and because of this in some ways it was in a good position to intervene with respect to the discrimination against converts to Islam from lower castes, as well as with women. Sikhs do not follow the Hindu caste system. Moreover, the health center was highly valued by the local community, as it became apparent that Kabliji was there for the long term and aimed to promote sustained improvements in the community. In particular because so many cataract operations were performed there, bringing eye surgeons from Delhi once a week and training others, it was known when I was there as "the place that made new eyes" and was even spared when waves of anti-Sikh violence swept across this part of India.

Twenty years later, I found myself visiting another hospital in a place that also was known as a place that "made new eyes." The Comprehensive Community-Based Rehabilitation in Tanzania (CCBRT) sits on a large campus in the middle of Dar es Salaam. Through its outreach and facility-based care, CCBRT reaches about a million disabled people every year, not just for cataract surgeries but also for the treatment of all sorts of conditions. In the early morning, the benches in the waiting area are crowded with patients waiting to be seen—an elderly woman with eyes clouded by cataracts, children with cleft lips and palates, a young man with a disfiguring growth over his eye. It is difficult to walk through CCBRT without reflecting on the incommensurability of human suffering. Abstracted from all social context and meaning, standard public health utility measures pretend to compare what it means to lose our eyesight during adulthood or grow up unable to walk because of a clubfoot that should have been easily repairable in infancy. But that is a very small part of the way humans experience ill-health within the narratives of their lives.

Moreover, even though CCBRT might appear to be a place where the importance of medical treatment comes to mind—to repair bodies and to restore people's dignity—walking through one room after another painfully illustrates the dramatic impacts of the effects of social determinants of health, from the room where prosthetic limbs are fitted to victims of traffic accidents in cities without sidewalks and regulations, to the room for women who have undergone fistula repair.

In the rooms for women who have undergone fistula repair, the beds are filled, mostly with young women, but there are a handful of older women too, and it is remarkably quiet compared with so many health facilities I have been in, given how many people are there. No animated chatter, no yelling from staff, no cries of pain; most of the women sit silently on their beds. Some women move about the room painfully slowly, gingerly holding large, blue, plastic bowls that are collecting their urine through a catheter. Obstetric fistula, which is at the most immediate level caused by prolonged obstructed labor, is one of the most serious of maternal morbidities. The unrelenting pressure from the baby's head in the birth canal causes a hole to form between the bladder and the vagina or between the rectum and the vagina. Virtually always, the baby ends up dying. The woman is left with urine or feces, or both, leaking continuously and uncontrollably.

At another level, fistula is caused by the same problems in health care infrastructure that lead to maternal death, including a lack of available, accessible, acceptable and quality emergency obstetric care. But more fundamentally, fistula is yet another SRH condition caused by social norms that do not value women's dignity, that prevent girls from pursuing education, that entrench a sexual division of labor, and that foster early marriage and pregnancy among adolescents whose pelvises are often very narrow. The women in CCBRT were the fortunate ones; they had a chance to regain their dignity. Too many do not. Obstetric fistula is estimated to affect 3,000 girls and women every year in Tanzania; as many as two-thirds of these girls and women will not have access to repair surgery, and because of the smell of continual leakage, they will face losing their husbands and becoming outcasts in their communities.[52]

In short, how we understand the causes of suffering—whether it is fistula in Tanzania or diarrhea in children in India—is inextricably linked to how we address the problem and how we conceive of the responsibility of the state for preventing and mitigating it. Applying a rights framework to health includes establishing governmental responsibilities with respect to laws, budgets, policies, and programs that underpin a *right to health*. However, a human rights framework is also broader than the right to health. Patterns of health and ill-health are also artifacts of a broad array of social determinants, which relate to equal enjoyment of other rights, including education and gender equality. These are not all part of what should be an enforceable right to health, but they are aspects of interrelated human rights. And in a human rights framework, these social determinants are not distal, background factors but are determining causes, which must be addressed alongside the immediate needs of patients for care.

Applying a human rights framework to health adds a central focus on accountability to other social determinants approaches, converting patients and beneficiaries of programs into claims-holders and the government and other actors into duty-bearers. Using human rights can not only help make visible how social and power structures in society shape unequal health status and lead to conditions such as fistula, as I discuss further throughout this book, they also can provide strategies and tools to challenge those injustices within and beyond health systems.

Chapter 4

Health Systems as "Core Social Institutions"

> The health system is not simply a mechanical structure to deliver
> technical interventions the way a post office delivers a letter.
> Rather . . . [it] functions at the interface between people and the
> structures of power that shape their broader society.
> —Lynn Freedman, "Achieving the MDGs:
> Health Systems as Core Social Institutions," 2005

> Of all the forms of inequality, injustice in health care is the most
> shocking and inhumane.
> —Martin Luther King, Jr., speech to the Second National
> Convention of the Medical Committee for Human Rights,
> March 25, 1966

The day I arrived in Quibdó, in May 2010, was a typically steamy-hot day, which left us drenched in sweat within minutes of leaving the airport. Quibdó is the capital of Chocó, an impoverished, jungle department of Colombia. It is a place that illustrates how "magical realism" in some Latin American literature often merely records observed reality, a place where one feels that "plagues of insomnia and forgetfulness"[1] could surely rival more mundane public health threats.[2]

The enormous army barracks on the outskirts of town were teeming with young soldiers whose menacing automatic weapons and camouflage-covered bravado contrasted sharply with the adolescent roughhousing they could be seen indulging in with each other. But the menace was very real; according to human rights organizations, soldiers posted here had been raping local girls with impunity for years. In the shadows of the barracks stood the recently constructed middle-class homes, with their fake Corinthian columns attached to the cement facades, streaming everything from loud *cumbia* rhythms to FloRida as the owners sat on their fake terraces, drinking real whiskey, heatedly debating for whom to vote in the upcoming election, and erupting into dancing whenever those debates threatened to devolve into fisticuffs. Then there were the rotund, Botero-esque figures[3] crowding through the muddy, unpaved streets in impossibly tight garb and high heels, seemingly unfazed by the extreme heat and humidity. Years of an entrenched drug trade and successive decommissionings of paramilitaries had left the promenade along the river and other public spaces in Quibdó filled with sinister-looking armed men, and gave the unshakeable sensation that one was always being watched.

Chocó is one of the subnational "departments" (states) of Colombia that has been most heavily affected over a half century of armed conflict between the government and guerrilla groups. The long conflict has ravaged the country, killing approximately 220,000 people and internally displacing an estimated 5 million or more. In 2013, the Fuerzas Armadas Revolucionarias de Colombia (FARC) and the Colombian government reached a partial peace accord and as of early 2015, the ongoing peace talks, although extremely contested politically, had advanced considerably.

The population of Chocó is highly Afro-descendant, a result of the slaves who escaped from the slave-trading port of Cartagena in the 1800s and fled eastward into the jungle.[4] Compared to much of Colombia, there are also significant populations of indigenous groups, and they have been particularly adversely affected by the combination of the armed conflict and the mining industries, which have destroyed large tracts of jungle and polluted both soil and water.[5] The area had been relatively peaceful prior to the early 1990s, when an increased presence of the FARC and the Ejército de Liberación Nacional (ELN) drew an army response and brought terror and violence against the indigenous civilian population. The influx of paramilitaries threatened their control over resources, as well as their territorial control and their cultural practices.[6]

A few days before I got there, an indigenous woman, Isabel, had died of obstetric complications in the district hospital. Isabel lived in a small village in the jungle hundreds of kilometers from Quibdó. She had developed protracted labor and in order to reach the district hospital had to be transferred first by boat for two days and then carried through the jungle on a stretcher for the better part of a third. The travel was made all the more treacherous by the landmines that are buried in that part of Chocó and the fact that guerilla and paramilitary operations did not respect standards of medical neutrality.[7] By the time she arrived, Isabel's child had died inside of her. A cesarean section was performed, but it was too late and Isabel passed away as well.

When I asked the director of maternal health for Chocó what provisions were made for people living in remote rural communities in the maternal health plan of the district, she told me that the plan "empowered" local communities to take care of their own maternal health needs by training traditional birth attendants (TBAs) to deliver children. There are indeed some worthwhile programs that utilize TBAs, in conjunction with the formal health system. This, however, was not one of them. These TBAs were not given misoprostol, which can be used to control postpartum hemorrhage, or trained in the use of injectable medicines or intravenous fluids, in order to keep a woman alive until she might reach a health facility. Instead, they received nothing more than simple kits with scissors, sutures, gauze, and the like. They were functionally illiterate and had received minimal training. When I asked about communications and transportation networks in the event of an emergency, I was told : "There are no communications; they'd have to use smoke signals to get help in there!"

Such a program is not really *empowerment* of local communities; it is a cynical abdication of the government's responsibilities to provide health care for all of its citizens. Isabel's death and this state of affairs are particularly scandalous because Colombia is not a poor country, as evident by its 2013 GDP per capita of USD 7,826.[8] It is, however, an extremely unequal society. Between 1996 and 2000, the GDP per capita of Chocó was a little more than USD 450, while that of the capital, Bogotá, was almost ten times that much.[9] And that inequality was—and still is—reflected in its health system. The life expectancy in Chocó is ten years less than that in Bogotá,[10] and women in Chocó face a maternal mortality ratio four times as high.[11]

As discussed in Chapter 3, social determinants, including peace and stability, as well as freedom from the structural discrimination Isabel and her indigenous community faced, are crucial for enabling people to enjoy lives of dignity, along with health and well-being. However, it is equally true that neither the *right to health* nor an *HRBA to health* can be realized without a functioning and equitable health system. As we have seen through previous examples, people often experience their poverty and exclusion through the indifference they face in contacts with the health system. As Lynn Freedman's quote at the opening of the chapter asserts, health systems are far from being simple technical apparatus for the delivery of services; they are part of the fabric of society, reflecting and encoding deeply held social values.[12]

In this chapter, I discuss the implications for health systems of adopting an HRBA to health. After introducing the notion of health systems as "core social institutions," I briefly describe the interrelated elements of a right to health—availability, accessibility, acceptability, and quality (AAAQ)—and explain how these would relate to and be applied to a case such as Isabel's in Chocó. I then explore how human rights has operational implications with respect to planning and budgeting, implementation, monitoring and evaluation, and ensuring adequate remedies. With reference to the United Nations "Technical Guidance on the Application of a Human Rights–Based Approach to the Implementation of Policies and Programmes to Reduce Preventable Maternal Morbidity and Mortality"[13] ("UN Technical Guidance"), which was adopted by the UN Human Rights Council in 2012, I explore the implications of how a human rights framework would change decisions at every stage of the policy cycle. Although the "UN Technical Guidance" sets out the implications of human rights in particular in relation to SRH and maternal health, it can be interpreted more broadly with respect to health generally, in that it sets out a "circle of accountability" in the health system, and beyond. I then discuss how human rights frameworks and principles might contribute to discussions around priority setting and achieving universal health coverage (UHC). Finally, returning to the specific context of Colombia, I note the extraordinary precedent set by the Colombian Constitutional Court in calling for a restructuring of the health system along human rights principles.

Health Systems as "Core Social Institutions"

In a human rights framework, health systems include both care and essential public health interventions that provide the preconditions of health, such as water and sanitation, which, as discussed in previous chapters, make a crucial albeit often largely invisible contribution to population health. In practice, the organization of health sectors often focuses on the delivery of care, with basic responsibilities for water and sanitation or food security and agriculture often left to other ministries.

The World Health Organization has outlined six building blocks of health systems: (1) health-service delivery, which comprises models of health-care

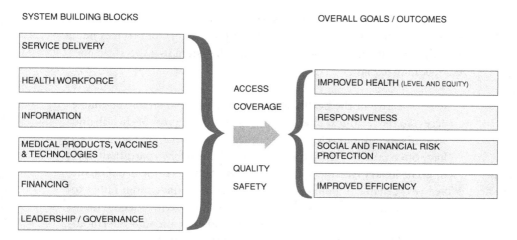

SYSTEM BUILDING BLOCKS

OVERALL GOALS / OUTCOMES

Figure 4.1. The WHO Health-System Framework. *Source:* World Health Organization, "Everybody's Business: Strengthening Health Systems to Improve Health Outcomes, WHO's Framework for Action" (2007).

delivery, infrastructure, and management of delivery; (2) health workforce, which includes national workforce policies and investment plans, advocacy, norms, standards, and data; (3) health information systems, which comprise both facility- and population-based information and surveillance systems, and standards and tools to make the systems effective; (4) access to essential medicines, including vaccines and technologies; (5) health-systems financing, which includes national health financing policies and tools and data on health expenditures; and (6) leadership and governance, which includes questions as to how health is organized politically.[14] In some nations, the ministry of health is combined with "social welfare" or "social protection."

These building blocks are essential in all health systems to the outcomes enumerated by the WHO, in rich and poor countries alike. However, what is notable in the WHO diagram (Figure 4.1) is that people are missing, the users of the health system—the citizens of society. But that is no coincidence. For the most part in global health, health systems and their components are understood in an overly mechanistic way. That is, health systems are defined as being comprised of a series of actors and interventions—as part of each building block, for example—which can be rearranged and applied anywhere.

A rights perspective on health systems is very different; the importance of health systems derives not merely from the delivery of services but also from the way citizens interact with the health system in a specific context.[15] As Freedman explains:

> One objective of the health system is, of course, to ensure equitable access to the technical interventions necessary to promote health and treat disease. But development planners and government authorities have often failed to grasp the extent to which abusive, marginalizing, or exclusionary treatment by the health system has come to define the very experience of being poor. Moreover, they have often failed to grasp that the converse is also true: the health system as a core institution, part of the very fabric of social and civic life, has enormous potential to contribute to democratic development.[16]

In his report on the right of everyone to the enjoyment of the highest attainable standard of physical and mental health, former UN Special Rapporteur Paul Hunt acknowledged the growing recognition of the health system as essential to a democratic and equitable society.[17]

If health systems are understood as core social institutions, it follows that the choices to be made cannot be seen just as technical choices but rather as reflecting and embedding values and norms of the larger society, including in relation to equality, dignity, and human rights. For example, one way in which the health system often reflects social values relates to the provision of different levels of care, depending on whether health coverage is tied to employment or to certain categories of populations versus universal entitlements. The ways in which both patients and providers are treated within the system also mirrors societal norms around discrimination and exclusion, as well as labor rights. The manner in which services are financed—through general taxation or through other means—often reflects the amount of solidarity in a society. The degree of accessibility of pertinent information encodes norms around freedom of information, transparency, and accountability. And finally, the ways in which priorities are set, from the most macro- to the most micro levels of decision making, reflect and sometimes distort social values.[18]

The Millennium Task Force for Child and Maternal Health, co-led by Lynn Freedman, usefully outlined differences between a rights-based ap-

Table 4.1. A Conventional Versus a Human Rights-Based Approach to Health Systems

Item	Conventional Approach	Task Force (Human Rights) Approach
Primary unit of analysis	Specific diseases or health conditions, with focus on individual risk factors	Health system as core social institution
Driving rationale in structuring the health system	Commercialization and creation of markets, seeking financial sustainability and efficiency through the private sector	Inclusion and equity, through cross-subsidization and redistribution across the system
Patients/users	Consumers with preferences	Citizens with entitlements and rights
Role of state	Gap-filler where market failure occurs	Duty-bearer obligated to ensure redistribution and social solidarity rather than segmentation that legitimizes exclusion and inequity
Equity strategy	Pro-poor targeting	Structural change to promote inclusion

proach to health systems and a conventional approach, as illustrated in Table 4.1.[19] The first difference is that in a rights-based approach, the health system is understood to be a "core social institution" whereas in a conventional approach it is generally construed in terms of capacity to respond to specific diseases or conditions. Our understanding of what measures should be taken to achieve equality derives from this basic idea of the health system as part of the foundation of our society, which can exacerbate inequalities and exclusion or facilitate the conditions under which all people can live with equal dignity. In many countries throughout the world today, the health system unfortunately aggravates patterns of discrimination in the overall society—reinforcing inequitable power imbalances in social determinants, rather than mitigating them.

The second difference is that the overarching goal of a health system in a rights-based framework is precisely inclusion and equity as opposed to just efficiency of market creation. Efficiency can enhance equity in some cases, and there is no reason that private actors cannot play a role in the health system. Nevertheless, as discussed in Chapter 2, in a human rights framework, health and health goods, such as essential medicines, are thought of not just as commodities to be allocated by the market but as *rights*. This view has implications for state obligations; the state has an obligation to provide a core minimum, and as discussed in greater detail in Chapter 7, the state also has a role to play in equalizing access to health facilities, goods, and services, including the preconditions of health, to all. Patients are understood not merely as consumers with preferences but as citizens with entitlements, which they must be able to actively claim, at the point of service as well as more broadly. This, in turn, implies mechanisms for accountability, and redress when systems fail to be responsive.

Third, patients are more than consumers of health goods and services in a human rights framework. To say that patients are "citizens" or that exercising claims to health care should be an asset of citizenship in an HRBA immediately raises questions about whether noncitizen residents and undocumented migrants are included. A human rights framework must include those categories of people because they are *human beings*. Nevertheless, in most countries there are currently dramatic differences between the formal entitlements of citizens, qualified legal residents, and undocumented immigrants in terms of health care. These distinctions will vary from one country to another, as will the concept of social as opposed to legal citizenship.[20] Nevertheless, let's consider patients and health-system users as *social* citizens in a broad sense because they reside in, work in, and participate in social, cultural, and political life in a society. In short, they help construct the institutions necessary to make rights real in a welfare state.

Fourth, just as patients are claims holders, the state is a duty-bearer in a rights framework, which goes beyond filling gaps in market or private provision and financing of care to equalizing access and ensuring minimum levels of care and preconditions to health as I discuss throughout this book.

Finally, the UN Millennium Task Force on Child and Maternal Health distinguishes a pro-poor targeting strategy from a structural strategy to increase equity. Pro-poor targeting is sometimes necessary to increase equity and inclusion, as, for example, when water and sewage services preferentially subsidize the poor so that they can become connected to systems. Nevertheless, targeting can also undermine a universal system and even reinforce the social dynamics that underpin health inequities. In this regard, the Millennium Task Force notes: "Narrowly focused but well conceived targeted interventions are sometimes powerful short-term steps that are essential parts of a broader equity-based strategy. But policies that segregate and 'target' the poor can deepen and institutionalize inequality by increasing their marginalization."[21]

In Peru, for example, a certain level of poverty is required to affiliate with the public insurance scheme, which is supposed to provide a certain number of services free of charge. Affiliation requires that participants demonstrate their "condition of poverty" and register in the "System for Targeting of Homes from the Ministry of Development and Social Inclusion." Middle-class people who might like to participate in the scheme cannot do so even if they are willing to pay for affiliation. Middle- and upper-class people need to acquire other insurance through their employment or privately. The public system in Peru and elsewhere, when it is chronically underfunded and divorced from accountability structures, tends to become "poor care for the poor." This in turn reinforces the hierarchies and cleavages in the overall society, rather than mitigating them. By contrast, universal systems can appear less "efficient" if impacts are measured in narrow cost effectiveness terms, but are crucial to human rights because they foster a common sense of ownership and belonging in the system, giving both the wealthy and the poor an equal stake and reflecting a social norm that considers all human beings equal in dignity and rights.

Availability, Accessibility, Acceptability, and Quality of Health Facilities, Goods, and Services

Let's return to the case of Isabel at the beginning of this chapter and analyze more concretely what applying a human rights framework to health systems would require.[22] If empirical evidence indicates that in conjunction with access to contraception, emergency obstetric care (EmOC), skilled birth attendants (SBAs), and referral networks are the keys to preventing and reducing maternal deaths such as Isabel's within a health system, interpretation of the right to health under international law requires that these aspects of care be made available, accessible, acceptable, and of adequate quality for the entire population on the basis of nondiscrimination.[23] Originally adapted from principles in public health, this is referred to as the AAAQ framework under international law, and the CESCR has set it out in relation to various rights, including health.

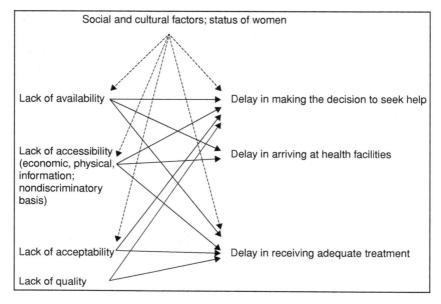

Figure 4.2. The Three-Delays Model and Lack of Available, Accessible, Acceptable, and Quality Obstetric Care: The AAAQ Framework. *Source:* Alicia Ely Yamin, "Maternal Mortality," in *The Right to Health*, ed. Gunilla Backman (Stockholm: Studentlitteratur, 2012).

Even though they are largely unpredictable and unpreventable, most obstetric complications can be treated with a set of interventions (signal functions of EmOC). Thus, just as with ARVs in the HIV/AIDS context, women live or die as a result of getting timely and appropriate EmOC. As Deborah Maine first set out in the early 1990s, maternal deaths overwhelmingly occur as a result of three delays: the delay in the decision to seek care, the delay in arriving at care, and the delay in receiving appropriate care (Figure 4.2).[24] A human rights lens reconceptualizes these delays, which could be treated merely as individual behavioral factors, in terms of a lack of available, accessible (for reasons of economics, physical barriers, poor or no information, and discrimination), acceptable (culturally and ethically), and quality health care. Thus, the focus shifts from individual idiosyncrasy to political failure.

Again, the social determinants discussed in Chapter 3 are key: the low social status of women such as Isabel factors into both of the first two delays in the decision to seek care, primarily because women rarely play a role in either the decision-making process or the (often very low) political priority placed on making the care women need available, accessible, acceptable, and of adequate quality. As the renowned Egyptian obstetrician and campaigner for maternal health, Mahmoud Fathalla, said, "Women are not dying because of diseases we cannot treat. They are dying because societies have yet to decide that their lives are worth saving."[25]

However, providing concrete content to women's rights to health also requires mapping the contextually bound ways in which the AAAQ of health facilities, goods, and services (in this case, EmOC) are at play in creating opportunity structures that lead women such as Isabel to seek care, arrive at care, and receive adequate treatment.[26]

Availability

Under international law, the realization of the right to health has been interpreted to require that a sufficient quantity of health-care facilities, goods, and services—including the underlying preconditions of health, be made available throughout a country's territory.[27]

A lack of availability can influence the decision to seek care when, for example, in a region such as Chocó, health facilities are so scarce that distance is a discouraging factor. At the same time, lack of available medical personnel and shortages of equipment, medical supplies, or drugs create delays in receiving adequate treatment once at a facility.[28]

Accessibility

In interpreting the elements of the rights to health, the CESCR has stated, "Health facilities, goods and services must be accessible to all, especially the most vulnerable or marginalized sections of the population, in law and in fact, without discrimination on any of the prohibited grounds."[29]

Lack of accessibility on any of these dimensions can increase delays. That is, lack of physical accessibility because of distance or difficult terrain can factor into delays in the decision to seek care. At the same time, as in Isabel's case, distance combined with poor roads and poor infrastructure—and the danger implied by the landmines and conflict—can also delay arrival at care. Both explicit and implicit costs of health care, including transportation costs, fees for health services, and medication costs, can produce a lack of economic accessibility and influence delays in deciding to seek care. Failure to recognize signs of obstetric emergencies requiring medical attention can reflect lack of access to information and also lead to critical delays in getting care, as can bureaucratic hurdles.

Acceptability

According to the CESCR, "All health facilities, goods and services must be respectful of medical ethics and culturally appropriate, i.e. respectful of the culture of individuals, minorities, peoples and communities, sensitive to gender and life-cycle requirements, as well as being designed to respect confidentiality and improve the health status of those concerned."[30] According to the CEDAW Committee, the committee that monitors the CEDAW, "Acceptable services are those that are delivered in a way that ensures that a woman gives her fully informed consent, respects her dignity, guarantees her confidentiality, and is sensitive to her needs and perspectives."[31] "Cultural appropriateness," however, cannot be an excuse for inferior services, as it was in Chocó.

Quality

The CESCR has noted that under the ICESCR, "Health facilities, goods and services must also be scientifically and medically appropriate and of good quality. This requires, *inter alia*, skilled medical personnel, scientifically approved and unexpired drugs and hospital equipment, safe and potable water, and adequate sanitation."[32] It also, critically, requires respectful care. Lack of respectful care includes everything from physical abuse and "obstetric violence," to discrimination, to nonconsented and nonconfidential care.[33]

Poor quality of care at health facilities, or even poor perceived quality of care, often leads to reluctance to seek care at a health facility. And inadequate training of medical personnel along with poor quality of equipment, medical supplies, or drugs often produce delays in a woman receiving adequate treatment once at a health facility.

In short, delays that lead to maternal deaths are not idiosyncratic individual decisions. Rather, they are predictable responses to constrained opportunity structures—caused in part by social determinants discussed in Chapter 3 and in part by governmental failures to meet the AAAQ standards for health systems set out in international instruments. When we apply this human rights analysis to maternal health- or to any other issue- we can make visible the political failures and thereby shift the burden of responsibility from individual patients to the government to comply with specific duties.

A "Circle of Accountability" Throughout the Policy Cycle

The AAAQ sets out the interrelated elements of health facilities, goods, and services necessary for a health system to ensure the right to health. However, to operationalize a human rights framework with regard to health, it is essential to understand how doing so would change decisions that are made throughout the policy cycle, and in turn opportunity structures and possibilities for change. The most comprehensive analysis of what applying human rights in the context of maternal health would require was set out in the UN "Technical Guidance" report, which was adopted through an intergovernmental process by the UN Human Rights Council in a 2012 resolution.[34] Implementation of this UN "Technical Guidance" at the national level, as well as its use in countries' mandatory reporting on their human rights obligations under Universal Periodic Review before the UN Human Rights Council, can prove an important precedent not only for SRH but also for the application of human rights approaches to other health and development issues.

This UN "Technical Guidance," for which I was the lead consultant in drafting for the UN Office of the High Commissioner for Human Rights (OHCHR), sets out a "circle of accountability" framework. This policy cycle is shown in Figure 4.3.[35] The fundamental idea is that accountability is not an afterthought in a human rights framework, nor is it limited to adding judicial remedies to a broken health system. On the contrary, accountability needs to be integral to every decision made at every step of the process—from the initial analysis of the situation through the provision of redress.

Enabling Laws and Policies; Planning and Budgeting

Planning in an HRBA goes beyond the technocratic approaches sometimes evident in conventional public health planning. If we recognize that the causes of ill-health often lie in social determinants and power relations in society, human rights planning needs to examine the dominant assumptions underlying the institutional arrangements that maintain the status quo and not just focus on proximate causes of death or disability, as discussed in Chapter 3. Further, if the rule of law is central to human rights, and laws

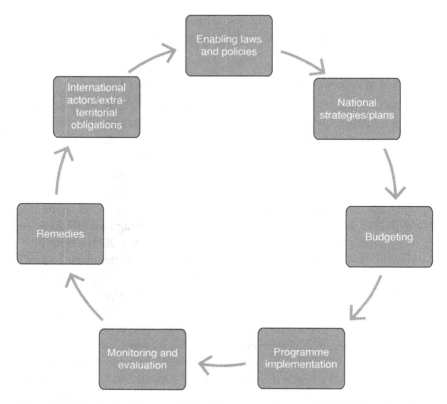

Figure 4.3. The Circle of Accountability Framework. *Source:* Alicia Ely Yamin and Rebecca Cantor, "Between Insurrectional Discourse and Operational Guidance: Challenges and Dilemmas in Implementing Human Rights–Based Approaches to Health," *Journal of Human Rights Practice* 6, no. 3 (2014): 451–485.

function as social determinants of health, planning in an HRBA needs to be based on a robust situational analysis that includes not just epidemiological data but also the legal framework, and institutional capacity of the state. Thus, if there are laws that will impede access to services—such as overly restrictive abortion laws—these need to be addressed from the outset in the planning process, as part of meaningful accountability. Enabling legal and policy frameworks are not sufficient, but they are necessary preconditions to people enjoying their rights to health and other entitlements.

A human rights framework—which, recall, goes beyond just the right to health—also calls for a multisectoral approach to planning, which includes coordination of government ministries, development partners (when applicable), and, crucially, civil society. If there is not coordination among government ministries from the beginning of the planning and budgeting process, it is nearly impossible to get people on the ground to work across ministries after the fact. Further, priority setting in a human rights framework needs to attend to issues of historical discrimination and inequities rather than merely aggregate outcomes. So, for example, indigenous women such as Isabel in Chocó face a conspiracy of inequities and deprivations of rights that call for redress in a rights-based approach. Moreover, there should be a way to hold the government accountable for implementing the national policies and plans that have been agreed, as is the case in some countries.

Plans of action need to be costed, and budgets are where values and visions for society are often most clearly reflected. As discussed further in Chapter 7, attention to formal and substantive equality in a human rights framework may lead to different budgetary allocations than would ordinarily be the case if following a conventional priority-setting process that emphasizes the "biggest bang for the buck." It may not be cost-effective to invest resources in an area such as Chocó, as the cost to save one women's life is much higher than it would be to save more lives in an urban area. But a fundamental notion underlying a rights-based approach is that people have equal dignity and that equality in dignity and rights requires that people have fair chances in accessing health care, as well as other important rights necessary to live a life of dignity.

Thus, just as we would expect the state to ensure that people in remote areas can exercise their rights to vote, so too should we expect the state to take measures to equalize the opportunities people have to access health care, as well as to make available preconditions to health in practice. The Constitutional Court in Colombia has called for the state to assume transportation costs, for example, when there are not appropriate facilities near a person's home. This is a dramatically different approach than assuming that people have "chosen" where to live, so if they happen to be in remote areas, they necessarily must accept the care to which they have access. We would not assume people have less of a right to political participation because they live in rural areas, and if health, including health care, is treated as a right, we cannot treat it that way either.

Further, a human rights framework implies changes to the planning and budgeting *process* as well as to substantive budgetary allocations. That is, throughout budget formulation, distribution, execution, and tracking, there needs to be participation from those who will receive services, depending on what decisions are taken. The transparency that enables meaningful participation is fundamental to the circle of accountability in health systems, which all too often are miasmas of corruption and indifference, as that transparency helps to ensure that monies are actually used as agreed and benefit the intended beneficiaries.

Program Implementation

Despite elaborate planning and policies, without effective program implementation, human rights cannot be realized. An essential part of the circle of accountability is analyzing where barriers to effective program implementation occur, which the UN "Technical Guidance" suggests can only be done through "periodic, bottom up, local diagnostic exercises to ascertain and provide feedback on what is happening to whom and where; why it is happening; who or what institution is responsible for such factors, and for addressing the problem; and how action should be taken."[36] This exercise should provide insight not just into immediate causes and concerns (such as access to EmOC in the case of maternal mortality) but also into broader steps required to address social determinants, such as lack of infrastructure and cultural norms that entrench gender subordination.

The key is not just to identify the problem but also to establish a system in which accountability for follow-up is implemented. It is the system of accountability that has the potential to open spaces for different decisions and in turn to change the relationships between health-system users and providers and between facility-level providers and insurers and policy makers. Otherwise, the diagnostic exercises—which occur in nearly every country through community score-cards and otherwise—remain hollow. This is easy to see in the case of Isabel. It is not hard to identify the lack of transportation and communication as a problem or the structural discrimination faced by impoverished indigenous communities in remote jungle areas. What is far more difficult is being able to use judicial and other points of leverage to ensure that the insurance companies and providers in Colombia, together with the directorate in charge of reproductive health, are held accountable to revise their policies *and practices* to ensure that no more women die the way Isabel did.

Monitoring and Evaluation

Although the "circle of accountability" emphasizes that accountability must be integrated from the very beginning of the policy-making process, monitoring and evaluation are also crucial to ensuring that the health system is responding effectively to people's needs on a nondiscriminatory basis. And what we monitor and measure reflects what we care about. If we do not have the right information on which to make decisions that will improve women's and people's lives, including using *qualitative* indicators to measure changes in laws and policies, as well as public values and perceptions, we may be able to improve health indicators but we will not be able to transform societies.

The selection of *quantitative* indicators is also crucial. I have argued elsewhere that in order to measure compliance with human rights obligations, quantitative indicators should be objective, frequently measurable, subject to disaggregation, and subject to local audit.[37] Frequent measurability can be used to hold specific administrations accountable for "taking all appropriate steps" in accordance with international law; disaggregation—the ability to tease apart different contributing factors—enables government policy makers as well as outside watchdogs to reveal potential discrimination; and being subject to local audit affords some participation and local control in the health system. Imagine how different the situation in Chocó would be if there were the possibility of local audit and if process indicators relating to access to EmOC and other fundamental aspects of sexual and reproductive health care were broken down by race and ethnicity. That would enable detection of patterns of deprivation and discrimination faced by indigenous groups in Colombia and by other marginalized populations elsewhere.

In addition, there is a need for multiple levels of review and oversight. That is, there should be accountability at the professional level (for example, nurses, doctors, professional associations), the institutional level (facility-based supervision and oversight, protocols, appropriately used maternal death reviews), the health-system level, the government level, and even the international level. Each level provides opportunity structures in which relationships can be changed, as discussed further in Chapter 5.

Remedies

Effective remedies are fundamental to meaningful human rights frameworks (I discuss this concept further in Chapter 5). Effective legal remedies help to ensure the implementation of laws and policies, to reform laws and policies that do not protect health rights, and to provide redress and guarantees of nonrepetition for violations to health-related rights in practice.[38] Judicial remedies are also crucial to shifting the balance of power in the broader society in order to put some limitations on the unfettered discretion of executive branches with regard to determining health policies and budgets.

But the theoretical existence of such remedies is inadequate. Raising awareness of different actors—including lawyers, judges, and the public—with respect to examples of and potential for the enforceability of health-related rights from the outset and allocating funds for access to justice and training of legal and judicial officers is fundamental to ensuring that remedies are used effectively and to enhance equity rather than distort priorities by exploiting opportunities within existing systems of privilege. Later in this chapter, I discuss the strengths and weaknesses of judicial remedies in the Colombian context specifically.

International Actors

In Chapter 8, I discuss at length the contours of donor obligations in human rights frameworks, which are critical to include in a "circle of accountability" given the enormous role that so-called development partners often play in determining the parameters for the enjoyment of people's rights to health in aid-dependent countries. These include promoting policies and programs that advance rights, not interfering with health-related rights, and conducting program evaluations that are transparent and open to multiple local stakeholder groups. Development frameworks, such as the SDGs, are crucial to mapping out the extra-territorial and other obligations of donor countries, as are varied sources of international law.

Universal Health Coverage and Priority Setting: Hard Cases, and Principles and Process in Human Rights Approaches

Universal health coverage will be embedded in the SDGs, which will succeed the MDGs and will establish goals and targets in relation to development issues. Under a broader SDG goal related to "ensur[ing] healthy lives and promoting well-being for all at all ages,"[39] UHC and associated indicators for its measurement will become an organizing frame for improving health and

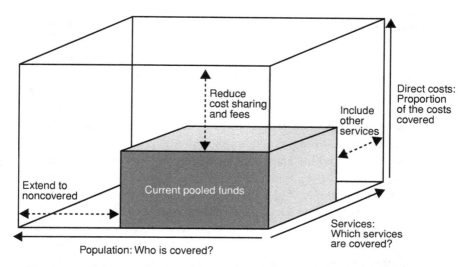

Figure 4.4. Three Dimensions to Consider When Moving Toward Universal Coverage.
Source: World Health Organization, "Universal Coverage: Three Dimensions,"
www.who.int/health_financing/strategy/dimensions/en/.

health systems over the next fifteen years. The WHO defines universal coverage as "all people have access to services and do not suffer financial hardship paying for them."[40] Achieving UHC has been described by the WHO as moving along three axes with which a health system should be concerned (Figure 4.4): including more people in coverage; expanding the services and treatments that are covered; and ensuring against financial loss, as catastrophic health costs can drive people into poverty, including destitution.[41]

A human rights framework does not provide a recipe for how to move toward achieving UHC, but it can contribute to the decisions involved in moving along these axes and along the path to universal coverage—or universal *effective and quality care*, which is what really matters from a human rights perspective.[42] For example, an emphasis on *quality* of care in a human rights framework, which includes respectful care, is part of AAAQ, but it can too often be forgotten in discussions of UHC. Moreover, as we see in Chapter 7, the concern with both formal and substantive equality and nondiscrimination in a human rights framework may not always be the same as "equity," and it carries implications for decisions moving along the different axes.

Applying a human rights framework also influences the nature of the process necessary to come to decisions about setting priorities in health systems, including how to achieve UHC, as it insists on meaningful participation of those affected.

As part of priority setting on the path to UHC and generally, all countries need to allocate resources to different activities, programs, and services. And priority setting invariably implies rationing, whether explicitly or implicitly.[43] Sometimes progressive proponents of ESC rights are averse to discussions of *rationing* on principle, and it is important to address those objections clearly. "Scarcity skeptics," for instance, argue that without the waste, corruption, and inefficiency plaguing the health system, discussions of rationing and priorities would be unnecessary. They point, for example, to the extravagant profits of pharmaceutical and private insurance companies. Indeed, many health sectors are riddled with both transaction costs and rampant corruption. And, as noted, we need not—and should not—take claims of scarcity of resources as a given; applying human rights to health demands that we be able to require justification from the government for budgetary availability and allocations.[44]

Nevertheless, even in the wealthiest of countries resources are finite and, as we have seen, not all monies should be spent on health care; at some point, resources for health services must be rationed.[45] As Justice Albie Sachs of the South African Constitutional Court articulated, "In all open and democratic societies based upon dignity, freedom and equality . . . the rationing of access to life-prolonging resources is regarded as integral to, rather than incompatible with, a human rights based approach to health care."[46] It is when rationing is not done explicitly and deliberately that it is likely to lead to greater injustice. For example, market-based priority setting means that by treating health care as a commodity, certain people are excluded because of financial constraints, thus *implicitly* rationing the care. Yet when we assume that health is a *right*, it should be need, and not ability to pay, that determines a patient's access to care. A health system that relies on out-of-pocket payments or market allocations for care invariably leads to the exclusion of poor patients and their families, which violates the notion of equal concern and respect in a human rights framework.[47]

Priority setting is done through a variety of mechanisms, at a variety of levels. As discussed earlier, national plans of action set broad strategies for priority setting in health care and also reveal the values that inform the health system—such as redressing historical inequalities versus maximizing aggregate health. These broad, national plans of action are then refined through further priority-setting mechanisms that determine which medicines and services will be included in UHC, national insurance plans, or other schemes.[48]

These assessments focus on determining the effectiveness of new technologies or interventions, as well as including cost-effectiveness analysis (CEA) and costs-benefit analysis (CBA). For instance, Britain's health service commonly analyzes health decisions based on the cost per quality-adjusted life years (QALYs), which is an economic measure of how many "quality" life years would be added for a given intervention. Using this measurement, a year in perfect health equals 1.0 QALY; a year in ill-health is proportionally less, depending on people's perceptions; and death is 0.0. As discussed in other chapters, there are a number of questions about measuring subjective health quality in these abstracted terms. Nevertheless, it is important to understand that these calculations are used to determine priority setting *for a service or an intervention*, not for prioritizing one individual patient over another.[49]

Some scholars have argued that using CEA and CBA in assessments of health priorities is anathema to human rights; I disagree, and it is important also to be clear about why. It is true that CEA and CBA alone do not always prioritize care for the worst-off patients, such as those with the most severe illnesses or those who are dying and need palliative care, nor would cost-effectivenss by itself give any priority to interventions to treat disadvantaged populations. Moreover, CEA focuses on single inputs and single outputs and therefore may discount interventions that have broader impacts on multiple outcomes, including through health-systems strengthening. For these reasons, *exclusively* relying on CEA and CBAin priority-setting would in my view conflict with an HRBA.

However, I believe that disregarding cost-effectiveness—which can also be thought of as "comparative effectiveness"—is equally unethical if we are concerned about progressive realization of the right to health, including inclusive and equitable health systems.[50] The constant introduction of new high-technology care and medications inevitably raises trade-offs for spending and raises equity concerns.[51] Think, for example, about what happens in the United States, where inordinately expensive end-of-life care uses a huge percentage of health spending, while younger members of racial and ethnic minority groups suffer from disproportionate unmet health care needs.[52] In the United States, Medicare payments in the last year of life average between USD 24,000 and USD 28,000; and hospital expenses in the last two years of life range from USD 53,432 to USD 105,000 per patient at top hospitals.[53] Because the United States has a health system based on private insurance tied to employment, there is little incentive to invest in preventive care earlier in the life cycle to keep people healthier, reduce chronic morbidities, and compress the time of disability and illness before death. Yet because we are unwilling to have an honest conversation about explicit rationing of care in the United States, neither the reasons for nor the implications of this spending are fully considered by the public.

These are not easy questions. But as the U.S. population ages and long-term health-care costs increase exponentially, they are questions we will need to grapple with. The number of dementia cases is predicted to double in the next few years, costing $379 billion in 2040.[54]

My father's mother died in a nursing home in the Midwood section of Brooklyn, New York. "Palm Gardens" did not bring tropical gardens to mind. The lobby of the nondescript brick building smelled of disinfectant and was entirely empty except around the holidays when the obligatory menorah and Christmas tree would be put up, along with some droopy banners that read "Happy Hanukkah" and "Merry Christmas." It didn't really matter what they said because the message in that institution was clear: "Carpe Diem"—"Seize the day"—for you too will grow old and wither away.

Getting off the elevator was always an assault; the smells of diapers changed too infrequently, the patients lining the hallways in wheelchairs, the droning gibberish punctuated by loud cries. The patients on my grandmother's floor were all women. Indeed, almost all the patients were women, which is not surprising as 67 percent of people over eighty-five in the United States are women, despite the fact that that public discussions of long-term care for the elderly are so rarely gendered.[55]

My grandmother was lucid until she died at age ninety-eight; she refused to sit in the hall. She stayed in her room with the curtain between her and her roommate pulled shut, tending two small plants on a windowsill, and waiting for her visitors. But most of the patients at this institution had moderate to advanced dementia and were either repeatedly acting out or semi-vegetative.

Investments in such care are most often not cost-effective and, as noted, are often inequitable given that other investments in care as well as the social determinants of health could produce far greater results for the disadvantaged or younger and productive members of society. Yet the elderly cannot be discarded and we need to find ways to address their needs and rights so that so many of them do not end up warehoused at the end of their lives.

Applying a human rights framework to health does not provide a formulaic resolution to these complex moral, social, financial, and legal questions. But it does call for such decisions to be based on certain fundamental principles regarding dignity and equality and for priority-setting decisions not to be taken in ways that mask these invariably contested issues. Rather, in designing health systems and in rationing inevitably finite health resources, applying a human rights framework calls for wider societal conversations about what we owe to one another as fellow members of society and across generations, as well as about the values that we want our health and social protection systems to reflect. As former South African Constitutional Court Justice Albie Sachs wrote, citing U.S. Supreme Court Justice John Paul Stevens, "[The right to life] cannot be extended to encompass the right to inevitably evade death. . . . 'Dying is part of life, its completion rather than its opposite.' We can however influence the manner in which we come to terms with our own mortality" both as individuals and as societies.[56] As discussed below, the legitimacy of how we design our health systems and allocate resources within and beyond health—which will inevitably entail life-and-death decisions—require transparent justification and public deliberation in a human rights-based approach to health.

Accountability for Reasonableness: Fair Process in Priority Setting

As the burden of disease from all noncommunicable diseases (NCDs), not just long-term care for the aged, grows throughout the world, creating serious challenges for middle- and low-income countries, in addition to upper-income ones, such as the United States, the equity issues involved at macro-, meso- and micro-levels in decision making on the path toward UHC, and priority setting generally, will likely grow even more acute. According to the WHO, NCDs contribute to 63 percent of the 57 million global deaths annually. Cancer accounts for 13 percent of all deaths, and death rates from cancer are projected to increase.[57] Constant innovation and expensive on-patent medications for NCDs, including cancer, often imply catastrophic expenditures for treatment, which leave families impoverished and can threaten to bankrupt even extensive health budgets.

As noted earlier, a human rights framework does not magically resolve these questions. However, in addition to affording certain principles for making decisions, a human rights framework also demands a process that explicitly recognizes that setting priorities involves contested ethical issues and cannot be decided by technocrats behind closed doors. Together with Jim Sabin, Norman Daniels developed a framework for health priority-setting processes, "Accountability for Reasonableness," which I believe is consistent with human rights principles of pluralism and equal concern and respect for diverse people's dignity. The framework is premised on the idea that priority-setting decisions should be transparent, justifiable, and relevant in the eyes of "fair-minded" people—that is, people who are open to reasoned arguments and are not deciding based on ideology or prejudice.[58] "Accountability for Reasonableness" has been applied in several countries, including the United Kingdom (where it was used to give people the opportunity to participate in decisions on a Citizens' Council)[59] and Mexico (where it factored into decisions about the catastrophic insurance program).[60]

The "Accountability for Reasonableness" framework includes four conditions that must be met to ensure a legitimate process: (1) publicity condition, (2) relevance condition, (3) revision and appeals condition, and (4) enforcement and regulatory condition. The publicity condition states that decisions about rationing and priority setting of health care must be publicly accessible. Decisions must be justified and explained to the public, not merely listed, in order to satisfy this condition.[61] The relevance condition concerns the rationale for limit-setting decisions: rationale must give a reasonable explanation of how the decisions will help meet the health needs of a defined population under resource constraints.[62] Thus, reasons based on discriminatory factors—excluding LGBT populations for example—would fail this condition. The revision and appeals condition considers mechanisms for oversight and review of decisions, and it requires that opportunities for revision and improvement of policies must be in place.[63] If new information comes to light, for example, the decision should be subject to review and appeal. Finally, the enforcement and regulatory condition states that there must be conditions to ensure that the first three conditions are met.[64] In other words, once priorities are set, people should be able to claim their entitlements.

These conditions are closely aligned with human rights principles and with the orders that the Colombian Constitutional Court made with respect to restructuring the health system in that country. Nevertheless, as we shall see in Colombia and elsewhere, the context in which such deliberation about health priorities occurs is crucial for whether it leads to transforming health systems and overcoming inequities in practice.

Colombia: Judicially Led Health-System Reform Based on Human Rights Principles

As noted, the right to health is increasingly being treated by national courts as legally enforceable, and accessible judicial remedies are crucial to applying human rights frameworks to health and to development more broadly. The past twenty years have seen tremendous growth in the number of health-rights cases focusing on issues such as access to health services and essential medications throughout the world. Nowhere has this trend been more pronounced than in Latin America, where judicialization of health rights has led to hundreds of thousands of cases, and has become a contested political issue. Colombia, in particular, stands out as a strong example of judicial enforcement of health rights. Not only were more than a million individual claims for health entitlements brought to date between 1999 and 2012,[65] the Constitutional Court in Colombia has also issued the most sweeping structural judgment related to health systems and the right to health anywhere in the world.

Prior to 2008 when the Constitutional Court stepped in with this structural judgment, the sheer volume of litigation indicated that the courts were being used as an "escape valve" in a health system that was incapable of regulating itself. Between 1999 and 2008, there had been almost 700,000 *tutelas*, or protection writs.[66] The overuse of judicial intervention on matters of health rights created its own set of equity and efficiency concerns. Access to justice is far from equal in Colombia and, despite efforts by the Constitutional Court to unify jurisprudence and to emphasize policy criteria, the courts of first impression were not well-equipped to determine whether medications and other treatments outside the defined obligatory benefit plan should be provided as a matter of *right*. So in 2008, the Constitutional Court took action to address some of the root causes of the litigation.[67]

In the T-760 judgment of July 2008, the court examined chronic failures in the regulation of the health system, reiterated that the right to health was a fundamental right, and called for significant restructuring of the health system based on rights principles.[68] Part of the judgment resolved twenty-two individual *tutelas*, which illustrated problems that the court largely had repeatedly addressed in prior jurisprudence. Part of the judgment also called for structural remedies, including achieving universal coverage; updating and unifying the obligatory benefit plans, which distinguished between a "contributory" regime based on payroll taxes and a "subsidized regime" for those informally employed or earning less than twice the minimum wage; and rationalizing reimbursement from the government to private insurers judicially-ordered care outside of the obligatory benefits plans.[69]

Among other things, the court ordered progressive unification of benefits plans for adults, in accordance with available resources, and immediate unification in the case of children, for whom parental employment status seemed an arbitrary and discriminatory determinant of access to care. Moreover, as the original design of the benefit schemes, and their piecemeal updating through the years, had not been performed with participation from stakeholders or on the basis of explicit and transparent rationales, the court required this. The ruling is notable because although it explicitly adopted the right-to-health framework laid out by the CESCR, including AAAQ, it did not attempt to define the content of the right to health. Rather, it set out what are often called "dialogical remedies."

In the court's order, both unification and updating of the benefits plans were to be performed through a participatory, transparent, and evidence-based process. Indeed, the structured participatory process called for by the court was consistent with the "Accountability for Reasonableness" framework, but it called for broader participation by a wider set of affected groups. The T-760 judgment illustrates the argument that Keith Syrett makes, that courts have an important role to play in fostering "public learning" by imposing transparent and reasoned justifications on criteria used for priority setting.[70] Creating a culture of justification, at all levels, is essential for limiting arbitrary abuse of power and creating space for people to deliberate about their values regarding health and their health system.

However, the highly stratified economic context of Colombia has proven enormously challenging for the "dialogical justice" because some actors in the health-care system are so much more powerful than others, the implications of which I discuss further in Chapter 6.[71] The stark reality of Colombia is that although in Chocó, Isabel and women like her lack the most basic access to care, others have access to the most expensive medications and treatments possible, and the T-760 judgment has not as of yet altered this fundamental underlying reality.

Nevertheless, change can be incremental and the T-760 judgment seems to have destabilized at least some entrenched interests in Colombia's health system and set into motion a series of cascading reactions on the part of the government, as well as other actors, which in itself is an important impact of adopting a rights framework. For example, analysis of media reporting on health from that period of time in Colombia to the present has noted a change in public discourse from one of health care as a commodity to health care as a *right*.[72]

Under the administration of President Juan Manuel Santos there has been more openness to the decision, supervision of the health system increased, the benefits were unified and overhauled, and a grand-breaking Statutory Law on Health that enshrined health as a fundamental right was enacted, as well as pharmaceutical regulation being expanded.[73] The extent of the final reform of the system, which is based on a managed-care model that creates certain incentives for insurers, however, remains to be seen.

Concluding Reflections

Colombia is a country of remarkable paradoxes and extreme contrasts. Ravaged by decades of violence, the country also a long tradition of the rule of law. Extraordinary wealth coexists with abject destitution. And, in the health system, private insurers and providers have repeatedly been exposed for massive pillaging and corruption, even as poor people are denied basic care. It is in that context that the court tried to step in and that the health system was being reformed. Not long after the T-760 decision, I was in Bogota at a panel discussion. At this event, an eloquent older woman representing patients with rare diseases requiring expensive treatment not covered by the obligatory health plan spoke up. She spoke carefully and slowly but passionately, and said she would be willing to forego treatment, leading to inevitable death, if she believed that the money saved in not treating her were going to needy children or some other worthy cause, other than lining the pockets of the insurance companies. But she did not trust the insurance companies, or governmental supervision, to ensure the fairness of the process.

From this and many other similar experiences, I have come to believe that fair-minded deliberation about health is possible but not in the absence of a legitimate process and justified trust in the health system, which needs to be built and sustained over time, as the Colombia case demonstrates. Just as citizen trust and perceptions of equity are essential to a justice system or an electoral system in a democratic society, so too is it critical to a health system.

At the Maternal and Child Institute (Instituto Materno-Infantil) I saw other challenges to adopting a rights-based approach to health in Colombia. The Maternal and Child Institute was where "kangaroo care"—the idea of wrapping premature infants to a mother's chest to increase survival—was first tested and shown to be effective.[74] Yet now the institute was a hulking shell of its former self. Formerly a public hospital that served any woman or baby who needed to be referred for care, it was now being taken over by a private, for-profit company.

The former labs were in the basement, still filled with glass jars of every possible human deformity imaginable. There were some reminiscent of "Aureliano Buendia" the seventh-generation child in Gabriel García Márquez's *Hundred Years of Solitude*, born with a pig-like tail, in addition to children with multiple heads, reptilian bodies mixed with human parts, and various permutations of semi- and wholly anencephalic fetuses.

But perhaps equally surreal were the health-care workers—some with quite severe health issues themselves—who had been encamped for months in this windowless basement, taking turns sometimes sleeping on cots. Since 2006, there had been successive "liquidations" of employees in order to "rationalize costs," and increasing use of flexible contracts in Colombia, as is the case wherever governments are relying on market-based systems, and increasingly private providers, for health care delivery. On the one hand, it was clear that their fight was doomed; the forces aligned against them in the Colombian health system were far stronger than they were.

And yet, this small band of men and women was inspiring. These were health workers standing up not just for their own labor rights and dignity but also for a vision of a health system where truly public hospitals—those hospitals in which care for the poor was the same as for the rich—and research and innovation were valued, even when not profitable, had an important role. They were standing up for the idea of a health system that mitigated some of the inequities in the larger Colombian society, and contributed to promoting greater social inclusion and dignity even for women in abject poverty. They were standing up for the idea that the state had fundamental obligations with respect to ensuring universal access to essential maternal and child health care, beyond filling in gaps left by private providers.

By the next time I visited Bogota, the health-care workers with whom I had spent much of the day years before were gone; I heard that the woman who had stood up to argue for transparency in priority setting and spending had died.

It remains to be seen in Colombia in the wake of T-760, and the subsequent adoption of the Statutory Law, whether the health system can build up legitimacy through the ways in which priorities are set, and what norms and values regarding social solidarity and dignity of providers as well as patients will be encoded in practice. And it remains to be seen whether, as a fundamental social institution, the health system can play a constructive role in social reconciliation in a postconflict Colombia. The fight for the soul of the Colombian health system shows vividly what is at stake in terms of a rights-based approach versus one that reduces health care to a commodity and users to consumers. However, Colombia is not unique. Many of these same issues will be played out across many countries—upper-, middle-, and low-income—as health care costs continue to rise and reforms are instituted to achieve universal health coverage.

PART II

Applying Human Rights
Frameworks to Health

Chapter 5

Beyond Charity: The Central Importance of Accountability

Charity is no substitute for justice withheld.
  —St. Augustine, as quoted in Sydney J. Harris, *Majority of One*

I am not interested in picking up crumbs of compassion thrown from the table of someone who considers himself my master. I want the full menu of rights.
  —Desmond Tutu on the *Today* show, January 9, 1985

I was privileged to be able to help shape Amnesty International's "Demand Dignity Campaign," especially in relation to its work on maternal mortality. Launched in 2009, the Demand Dignity Campaign signaled a watershed in international human rights. Previously, Amnesty had eschewed ESC rights, focusing instead on a narrow slice of CP rights, involving, for example, political prisoners and freedom from torture.[1] As the oldest and by far the largest international human rights organization, Amnesty International's reticence with respect to ESC rights had ripple effects throughout the field. So when, under the leadership of then-Secretary General Irene Khan, the organization changed course and boldly embraced addressing poverty as a human rights imperative requiring accountability and not charity, it signaled a huge shift in the international human rights movement. With Amnesty including issues such as maternal mortality and slum dwellers—right to health and housing questions, respectively—as central to its mandate, the entire human rights movement was presented with the opportunity to re-think itself.[2]

In 2009, while in Sierra Leone on a fact-finding delegation with Amnesty for the maternal mortality campaign, I met the family of Yerie Marah, who had died in childbirth the year before. In Sierra Leone, if a girl is especially diminutive, she may be called "Kinkini" in Krio, which connotes that she is petite. Yerie was like that. She was twenty-two when she died by the river near her home in Koinadugu district, in northern Sierra Leone. But judging from photos, she looked as though she had barely entered adolescence; a reality not uncommon for a country with widespread malnutrition.

Yerie's story was all too typical for Sierra Leone. She and her husband, Mahmoud, had been together for six years, since both of them were teenagers. Neither Yerie nor her husband had ever attended school. They were both Mandingo and came from the same community. Mahmoud and Yerie lived in a very small, one-room structure in the center of the village of Sokralla, amid relatives on both sides of the family.

Yerie died of a postpartum hemorrhage, which was almost surely either caused or significantly exacerbated by malaria. Although the placenta was delivered intact, she began to bleed after the delivery. But according to Rebecca, the maternal child health (MCH) aide who attended her delivery, it seemed to be mostly lochia—the normal discharge from the uterus that occurs after childbirth—and by mid-afternoon, after a shot of ergometrine,[3] Yerie had permission to go home with her baby. Mahmoud and Yerie walked home and everything seemed all right. Yerie took a nap and when she woke up she and Mahmoud were talking and joking about what to name the child. They decided to name the little girl Mariama Sawanah.

But everything was not all right. Later that evening, Yerie went to the latrine and her mother, Sirrah, saw that she was bleeding heavily. Sirrah knew something was seriously wrong. The bleeding continued all night, and in the morning Yerie left for the river to try to wash some of the blood away. Finding her there, her uncle summoned Yerie's mother and sister for help. They came running, but it was too late.

Yerie's antenatal record showed that she had been diagnosed during her second trimester with malaria, which can greatly exacerbate bleeding postpartum. Although the Global Fund to Fight AIDS, Tuberculosis, and Malaria was providing insecticide-treated bed nets (ITNs) to Sierra Leone to be distributed free of charge to all pregnant women and children, Yerie had never received one.

It turned out that Yerie did not receive an ITN because Rebecca had (she admitted to us) sold the primary health unit's (PHU's) bed nets on the private market. According to Rebecca, Yerie had been referred to a district hospital for malaria drugs but had not gone because Mahmoud would not pay for the transportation; Mahmoud told us, however, that Yerie had never been referred. In any case, as there were no malaria drugs at the PHU, she had just been given paracetamol for the pain.

How does applying a human rights framework affect how we react to Yerie's death from a perspective concerned with human rights? As I emphasized in Part I, the principle of *accountability* is "the raison d'être of the rights-based approach" and what human rights most distinctively add to other approaches to health equity based on social determinants.[4] But what does *accountability* require in Yerie's case? Should Rebecca be suspended, fired, even prosecuted for her likely role in Yerie's death?

Before you make your judgment, let's think about the health system where Yerie died. Sierra Leone is now of course known to have a health system decimated by the Ebola crisis, but it was dysfunctional long before Ebola hit. At the time of Yerie's death, Rebecca had been working for four years without a salary, a reality all too common across the country. According to the district medical officer in Koinadugu, almost half of the MCH aides and community health officers at the PHUs were not on salary as of the end of 2008. Rebecca worked six days a week and she was forced to live away from her own family and three children, whom she saw approximately once a month. Without a salary, Rebecca's survival depended on her ability to sell the drugs she dispensed at the PHU for a small profit and to tack on charges for attending patients. Her sale of the PHU's ITNs on the private market was a means of survival, however ethically dubious it may have been.

This chapter continues the discussion of accountability begun in the last chapter in respect of health systems. In the first part of this chapter, I look at the *what*, *who*, and *how* of accountability in a human rights framework. I discuss *what* we should mean—and not mean—by accountability, *who* is accountable at different levels, and *how* different mechanisms can be engaged to promote accountability in human rights frameworks. As accountability refers to holding duty-bearers to account for meeting certain obligations under international and domestic law in a human rights framework, the second part of the chapter explores how we should understand the *obligations* for which we seek accountability. I argue that there are three aspects of obligations toward progressive realization of health and related rights: (1) *what* the state is doing (whether it is taking the appropriate measures in terms of legislation as well as programs, as evidenced in part by outcomes); (2) *how much effort* the state is expending in terms of policy implementation and resources; and (3) *how* the state is going about the process (for example, whether it is showing concern for equality, nondiscrimination, and participation).

The What, Who, and How of Accountability in a Human Rights Framework

What Do We Mean by Accountability? Beyond "Naming and Shaming"

A human rights framework identifies who has rights (rights-holders) and what rights they have under international human rights law (freedoms and entitlements), as well as who is responsible (duty-bearers) for making sure rights-holders are enjoying their rights (obligations). As the OHCHR and Center for Economic and Social Rights (CESR) report titled, "Who Will Be Accountable?" notes, "Accountability has a corrective function, making it possible to address individual or collective grievances, and sanction wrongdoing by the individuals and institutions responsible. However, it also has a preventive function, helping to determine which aspects of policy or service delivery are working, so they can be built on, and which aspects need to be adjusted."[5] Thus, accountability principles and mechanisms can be used to improve policy making by identifying systemic failures that need to be addressed in order to make service delivery is more effective and responsive.

Another way to think of the "circle of accountability" set out in Chapter 4 is that an HRBA, or human rights framework more broadly, changes the relationships between legislators/parliamentarians who enact laws and policy makers who set national plans, between policy makers and health programmers who implement those plans, between programmers and health-care providers, between providers and patients, and between citizens and their elected representatives (Figure 5.1). At every stage of this circle, establishing new relationships based on claims held by rights-holders in relation to duty-bearers, as opposed to discretion by those in power which produces different opportunity structures based on balances of resources and barriers, for exercising choices. It is these changes in opportunity structures that afford

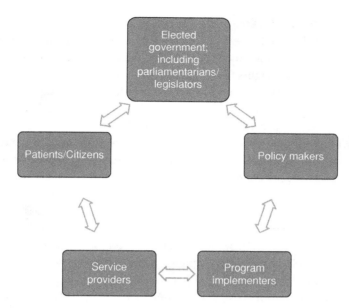

Figure 5.1. Changing Relationships and Power Dynamics Through a Circle of Accountability. *Source:* Alicia Ely Yamin and Rebecca Cantor, "Between Insurrectional Discourse and Operational Guidance: Challenges and Dilemmas in Implementing Human Rights–Based Approaches to Health," *Journal of Human Rights Practice* 6, no.3 (2014): 451–485.

potential spaces for people to relate to each other differently, and in turn for broader social transformation.

Understanding accountability as potentially transformative requires looking beyond "naming and shaming" the frontline health-care workers to the system itself. As we reflect on Yerie's death—and the deaths of countless others like her—Rebecca's behavior perhaps cannot be justified, but it can be explained. When health professionals are either unsalaried or underpaid, these under-the-table payments and side sales become one of the survival mechanisms by which health workers who were not adequately compensated earn a living. In 2009 in Sierra Leone, at least, it had become a system that bred corruption at every point; it also set the stage for patients' suffering and death, as in Yerie's case.

Indeed, to give you some sense of how dire things were, the WHO recommends a minimum of 23 health-care workers for every 10,000 people; in Sierra Leone, however, there were just 0.2 physicians and 1.7 nurse-midwives for every 10,000 people at the outset of the Ebola crisis.[6] Thus, if Rebecca were fired, it might have led to even greater suffering among the patients in the large catchment area for which she provided the only basic health care.

Applying human rights frameworks cannot mean simply punishing the frontline health workers who need to be our allies in the struggle to transform health systems. In deeply broken health systems, the actions or decisions of an individual provider can be vitally important, but those providers may have very limited power to save a life in a given situation. In the case of Yerie's death, for example, in addition to the systemic problem of fair remuneration and working conditions for an adequate number of trained health workers, the PHU had no malaria drugs and Yerie had no way to get to a larger hospital; her transportation and other cost barriers to access were also rooted in governmental failures to provide available, accessible, acceptable and quality care. As Leslie London argues, "Front line health workers are frequently unable to provide adequate access to care because of systemic factors outside their control and because of management systems that disempower them from acting independently and effectively."[7] Focusing on individual health practitioners' conduct, divorced from context in such a situation, "frequently makes little headway and gives a human rights approach a bad name."[8]

This is not to say we should condone negligent or abusive treatment or malfeasance of individual actions; there is a valid sanctioning aspect to accountability. I have investigated maternal death cases where, for example, a doctor on duty was making love to his girlfriend instead of responding to urgent calls to attend a woman who was dying from eclamptic seizures down the hall; in another case, a doctor whose indifference meant that a patient who by protocol should have been kept at the hospital and treated was sent home to die; and, in another, a nurse who promised to attend a delivery went home instead, leaving the family to search desperately for her as the young woman bled to death. In all of these cases, the health system covered up the abuses. Files went missing and key records were disappeared; doctors and nurses were transferred; colleagues were silenced. The families suffered a double injustice, failed by health systems and by justice systems that would not even provide them with the truth about why they had lost the person they loved. Thus, not only is punishment sometimes appropriate, it is essential that all providers are aware that professional standards will be enforced and that information necessary for patients to vindicate their rights will not be withheld.

However, as Lynn Freedman notes, it is important that individual sanctions have "not been used to scapegoat a doctor, pacify the public, and cover up wider, deeper problems."[9] Freedman suggests an alternative understanding of "constructive accountability" within health systems in which a "new dynamic of entitlement and obligation" is established.[10] Patients all too often see themselves as beggars and accessing services is, in turn, treated as a matter of largesse by providers. Establishing a circle of constructive accountability is aimed at shifting that relationship and other relationships throughout the health system and society (see Figure 5.1).

Who Is Accountable?

In order to transform power dynamics, we must identify accountability gaps at every level of the health system, and even beyond. For example, at the facility level, there is a need not only for effective oversight of staff in terms of quality of care as well as management of supplies, medicines, and funds but also for leadership with respect to values that determine accessibility on a basis of nondiscrimination. Whether a client is disabled, LGBT, of an ethnic minority, or anything else, no one should face discrimination or disrespect and abuse, as happens far too often. Nor should anyone face denial of care on religious or ideological grounds. "Conscientious objection" is a right held by individual providers but not by institutions, which have a responsibility to ensure that all legal services, including abortion, are available to the patient population in a catchment area.[11]

Health professionals also have individual accountability, for example, through licensing procedures as well as through medical and dental boards. These boards and associations are extremely important because without such professional accountability it would be impossible to uphold reasonable standards of ethical and scientific conduct by health workers. When associations become politicized or if they are used to cover up responsibility by their colleagues rather than to promote best practices and foster a culture of responsibility, relationships of trust between the public and the health system are undermined. Alternatively, those associations can serve as essential forms of peer pressure in maintaining quality standards.

There is also accountability at the health-system level, at every stage of the "circle of accountability." That is, from the initial situation analysis through the development of national policies and plans of action; the budgeting process; program implementation; and ensuring effective monitoring and evaluation processes that support a culture of transparency—responsiveness and a culture of justification need to be built in. As the UN "Technical Guidance" emphasizes with respect to SRH, the system itself is accountable for ensuring sequencing and coordination within and between systems, including appropriate alignment of laws, policies, budgets, programs, and training.[12] As a human rights framework is necessarily multisectoral, other sectors are also accountable for follow-up on plans of action corresponding to their related remits, such as the ministry of education or the community development ministry.

Private actors play increasingly important roles in the provision of services in many health sectors, and human rights law is clear about their accountability as well as the accountability of the state to regulate these actors. As noted in the CEDAW Committee report on the case of Alyne da Silva Pimentel Teixeira, an Afro-African Brazilian woman who died in 2002 of preventable causes while in labor, "Private institutions . . . are subject to the principles of the health system and the national audit system in respect of evaluation of service quality." The CEDAW Committee found that the government of Brazil failed to exercise "due diligence" and oversight with respect to "the mechanisms used to contract private health services and, by extension, the inspection and control thereof."[13]

Finally, as discussed at much greater length in Chapter 8, we must locate the capacities of states to fulfill their ESC rights and obligations, including their health rights obligations, within the context of a global political economy in which multinational corporations, international financial institutions, and donor states are often the ones calling the shots. We need look no further than Sierra Leone to note how, on top of a brutal colonialist legacy, the rapacious global demand for precious minerals fueled the civil war that disrupted family units and livelihoods and migration patterns, and left a country with emasculated and unaccountable political institutions that are incapable of responding adequately to people's immediate survival needs and unable to establish forward-looking policies and programs to fulfill ESC rights, as has become all too tragically apparent in the Ebola crisis. Just as it can be misguided to focus on the failures of individual health-care workers, it is counterproductive to focus exclusively on the accountability of governments in the global South for unfair global rules that lie beyond their control.

How Do We Hold Actors Accountable? Forms and Mechanisms of Accountability, and the Central Role of Remedies

Human rights accountability can be judicial, political, social, or even administrative, and mechanisms include "institutions as varied as parliaments, civil society, the judiciary, and Ombuds and independent national human rights institutions (NHRIs).[14] These forms of accountability do not operate in isolation from one another. For example, in the context of governance—which is directly related to basic service provision—accountability requires the ability to hold public officials responsible for their performance as well as for the results of their decisions. However, political accountability through periodic elections is greatly enhanced by ongoing social accountability efforts by collective actors, such as NGOs, community-based organizations, and the media.[15] A prime example is India's Right-to-Food Campaign, which is organized through a decentralized network of civil society and grassroots organizations, in which rural women have played a central role. The campaign has organized a wide range of activities, including public hearings and rallies, media advocacy, and lobbying of members of Parliament. Their efforts have been critical in persuading several state governments to provide hot lunches in primary schools, as well as instrumental in pushing national legislation, such as the National Rural Employment Guarantee Act.[16]

In many countries, networks and broad popular movements for social accountability relating to health issues emerged as a reaction to autocratic governments. These governments had pushed through neoliberal sector reforms and privatizations of basic services, such as water, with almost no consultation, and often largely by executive and ministerial decrees.[17] Efforts at social accountability highlight the importance of decision-making processes, as well as outcomes, and of increasing the voices of marginalized or excluded communities with respect not only to the diagnosis of institutional failures that most directly affect them, but also to the negotiation of social policies and health budgets. However, successful models of social accountability also point to the importance of creating coalitions and networks across class and between grassroots and professional organizations.[18]

It is also misleading to draw a strict distinction between litigation and political strategies in struggles for health rights. Evidence shows that litigation for health rights, and ESC rights more broadly, need not straitjacket social demands into narrow formalistic claims, but can be and often is used creatively as a political tool when embedded in broader strategies.[19] Lisa Forman argues that, although settled, the 2001 Pharmaceutical Manufacturers Association (PMA) case in South Africa, relating to legislation that gave the government powers to import or manufacture cheaper, generic versions of brand-name drugs, "facilitated a tipping point [in social consciousness] for the emergence of a human right to AIDS medicines and acted as a catalyst for broader legal *and political* changes around AIDS medicines" (emphasis added).[20]

Similarly, the Indian Right to Food Campaign began in April 2001 when a case was brought to the Indian Supreme Court, demanding that the government use its large food stocks to prevent mass hunger and starvation.[21] The Supreme Court has since held regular public hearings and has issued important interlocutory orders in the case, which is ongoing. However, activists soon realized that the litigation itself was insufficient, so they organized the much larger public campaign for the right to food; this has placed the right to food at the center of discourse regarding India's development policy.[22] The involvement of civil society and grassroots organizations has also played a central role in pushing for the right to freedom of information to help curb corruption, the right to employment, women's empowerment, social security pensions, and integrated child development services.

Thus, as Siri Gloppen asserts, in evaluating the impact and value of courts' roles in bringing more justice to health, "It is important to keep in mind that this is part of a larger picture," including broader accountability processes in which multiple actors and stakeholders' behaviors are at play.[23] Nonetheless, throughout this book, I spend quite a bit of time on different judgments because it does not make sense to talk about a *right to health* or applying human rights to health without talking about remedies, and judicial remedies in particular. First, it is a double violation of a person's right if she cannot seek redress for a wrong committed regarding her health. But more broadly, rights are fundamentally legal vehicles and require certain assumptions about the use of law for social transformation, for shifting narratives of social meaning, and for shifting relationships between citizens and governments to dynamics of entitlement and obligation. Indeed, for good and for ill, our notion of *rights* is to a large extent the product of courts' actions and the rise of constitutionalism as the preeminent form of social transformation in the second half of the twentieth century.[24]

And, as noted in Chapter 2, in the last twenty years or so we have witnessed a dramatic shift in the possibilities of enforcing rights relating to health through courts. Beginning with cases revolving around access to ARV medications in the 1990s, which were based on arguments relating to the right to life as well as health, courts in a number of countries throughout the world have increasingly enforced access to health goods and services.[25] Colombia is but one example. Across very different contexts and legal systems, courts have required the political branches of government to better regulate health systems; to reform discriminatory laws, policies, and practices affecting health; to provide access to health-related information, as well as both care and preconditions to health; and require public justification for the "reasonableness" of their policies and practices in relation to health.

But we still need to understand better the conditions under which courts can bring more justice to health.[26] For example, when does the pattern of judicialization of health rights lead to emphasizing individualized access to curative treatment over public health preventive measures? When is litigation captured by the urban middle class or, worse yet, by pharmaceutical companies pushing their own drugs? Can judges be educated and enabled to consider broader equity and system concerns when making judgments?[27] What kinds of judicial orders and supervision lead to improved regulation of the health system in practice? And, given the importance of social determinants of health and the role of health systems as core instutions, what is the impact of judicial enforcement on broader equity concerns?

We also need to acknowledge that although the use of courts and litigation can be misused and undermine equity, often few alternatives are available to challenging the discretion of government institutions when it comes to health-related policies and programs, and to creating relationships of entitlement and claims, rather than discretionary largesse. When there is chronic democratic failure, and politics become largely transactional rather than based on the representation of diverse interests, this is particularly true. When courts subject laws, policies, and regulations to scrutiny as to whether they are *reasonable*, there is evidence that they can contribute to systemic accountability and a culture of justification where patients can claim their health rights.

Reasonableness can be a very low standard, requiring merely that laws and policies be rationally related to a stated objective. And courts can be very deferential regarding the budgetary decisions of the political organs of government.[28] But a judicial review of the government's actions can inquire more deeply into the justification for a given law, procedure, or budgetary allocation, especially where there may be suspicion of discrimination or failure to consider the impact on the most disadvantaged. As Bruce Porter writes, "The ability and willingness of the Court to engage in a meaningful review of government decisions . . . is largely dependent on an understanding of how they engage not only explicit [rights] but also central constitutional values and principles of dignity and equality."[29]

Moreover, as discussed in Chapter 4 with respect to the Colombian Constitutional Court's reform of the health system, new understandings of how courts can contribute to transformative accountability are emerging from current practices. For example, in an Argentine case involving the highly polluted Riachuelo River Basin, the Argentine Supreme Court called on multiple levels of governmental actors to devise and implement a clean-up plan and involved various civil society groups as well as the Human Rights Ombuds Office in the monitoring of compliance.[30] Almost ten years have passed since the 2006 ruling, and the results have been mixed, with almost no chemical changes in the river quality.[31] Nevertheless, as discussed in relation to the T-760 case in Colombia, the judicial intervention arguably has disrupted political dynamics and opened opportunities for new actions by some actors.

Through these more "dialogical" remedies, as opposed to "black letter" rulings, courts may be better able to preserve their own constitutional legitimacy in addressing complex policy questions, as well as foster processes that catalyze democratic participation, and dialogue with the executive and legislative branches of government regarding spending priorities and critical health-policy questions.[32] Through these sorts of decisions, as discussed in Chapter 4 in relation to Colombia, courts can sometimes promote broader deliberative discussion regarding health-related rights by overcoming "burdens of inertia" or "destabilizing" institutions that have been insulated from normal political accountability.[33]

Such destabilization is extremely important to consider when we are thinking about the impacts of applying human rights frameworks to health, as unsettling entrenched power dynamics is crucial to changing the patterns of health and ill-health within a society, and of transforming health systems. Thus, in assessing the contribution of courts in applying a human rights framework to health, we need to go beyond narrow studies of compliance and direct effects on litigants to consider indirect impacts on processes, institutions, and society. For example, if marginalized populations' perspectives are meaningfully included in the priority-setting process or in debates about the right to food, it matters. We also need to consider that César Rodriguez-Garavito refers to as "symbolic" impacts: "changes in ideas, per-

	Direct	Indirect
Material	Designing public policy, as ordered by the ruling	Forming coalitions of activists to influence the issue under consideration
Symbolic	Defining and perceiving the problem as a rights violation	Transforming public opinion about the problem's urgency and gravity

Figure 5.2. Types and Examples of Effects of Judicial Decisions. *Source:* César Rodriguez-Garavito, "Beyond the Courtroom: The Impact of Judicial Activism on Socioeconomic Rights in Latin America," *Texas Law Review* 89, no. 7 (2011): 12.

ceptions, and collective social constructs relating to the litigation's subject matter"[34] (Figure 5.2). Thus, for example, if people appropriate a sense of entitlement with respect to health goods, and services as a result of a given judgment, such as T-760, and begin to behave differently as a result, that can play a role in social transformation. Ultimately, we want to see changes in people's actual enjoyment of health rights, but these sorts of institutional and political changes, which enable people to exercise different choices in their lives, are also fundamental to the social transformation we are seeking through applying human rights frameworks to health.

National human rights institutions can also potentially play important roles in providing remedies and fostering systemic accountability for violations of health-related rights. For example, in Peru, the Defensoría del Pueblo (Human Rights Ombuds Office) has actively pursued monitoring and oversight of health rights for the last ten years, which has led to, among other things, revised regulations and policies relating to issues ranging from informed consent to the free distribution of birth certificates to all children.[35] Other NHRIs, such as those in India, Kenya, and Argentina, have also assumed work bearing on health and related rights, including monitoring implementation of structural judgments by courts.[36]

However, an NHRI's enforcement power rests on its legal mandate and, for the most part, NHRIs currently lack these powers. Therefore, the impacts of policy recommendations as well as case adjudications can be haphazard and depend on the independence and political authority of the NHRI in question, as well as on social mobilization around an issue. A minority of NHRIs actively engage in ESC rights work, and fewer still do so in relation to health rights. Those that are tasked with health rights work often face insurmountable barriers to performing effective oversight. In late 2013, in connection with a project examining how HRBAs are implemented on the ground, I interviewed a number of NHRI representatives from Eastern and Southern Africa. As one NHRI representative remarked, "It's hard to monitor government institutions when [the officials] don't know about the [NHRI's] mandate, don't know their obligations, and don't know people's rights." It is fair to say that NHRIs in most countries are not currently playing as strong a role as they could in filling accountability gaps in health systems, and in relation to health conditions.

Unpacking Obligations

In a human rights framework, accountability requires compliance with meeting certain obligations and standards under international, as well as national, law. Therefore, promoting accountability with respect to laws, policies, and programs that bear on health rights requires defining those normative obligations.[37] One way of understanding obligations is to enumerate the rights that are entailed in resolving a given health issue, such as maternal health. Think back to Yerie's life, or to any of the examples provided throughout this book; all of those women were deprived of multiple rights, both CP and ESC, which led to a series of events culminating in their unnecessary deaths. Indeed, effectively addressing *any* health issue requires protection of a wide array of both CP and ESC rights.

As discussed in Chapter 2, the enjoyment of these CP and ESC rights is inextricably intertwined. Especially since the Vienna Conference, international law has affirmed that these rights are truly "interdependent and indivisible."[38] For example, in international law, the right to life should not be interpreted restrictively as the right to be free of extrajudicial execution, for example, or considered in isolation from the positive measures required to fulfill the right to health.[39] And various national courts around the globe have expansively interpreted the right to life to include the conditions necessary to live a life of dignity, including access to health care.[40] In India, in a landmark Supreme Court case in 1981, the right to life was interpreted "to include the right to live with human dignity and all that goes along with it, namely, the bare necessities of life such as adequate nutrition, clothing and shelter."[41] All ESC rights, including the right to health, entail both freedoms and entitlements. Health requires freedom from coercion and discrimination; it also requires entitlements regarding care and preconditions of health. The tripartite framework set out in the CESCR's General Comment 14, "The Right to the Highest Attainable Standard of Physical and Mental Health," provides a useful conceptual framework for understanding states' obligations. Debunking the outdated notion that CP rights are "negative rights," which demand only state restraint, and that ESC rights are "positive" rights, which require positive programmatic measures, General Comment 14 followed others, which had established that all human rights give rise to three dimensions of state obligations: to respect, to protect, and to fulfill.[42]

The obligation to *respect* the right to health requires that states refrain from actions that interfere with individuals realizing their rights to health, such as discrimination against certain classes of people including women, as I have discussed in relation to services that only they require, such as abortion. The obligation to *protect* the right to health demands that states prevent interference by third parties with the enjoyment of the right to health. Such interference might relate to private actors' pollution or to domestic violence, as discussed in Chapter 1; the obligation to protect requires that the state ensure clarity with respect to the legal obligations, as well as regulation, in relation to private actors. Finally, the obligation to *fulfill* the right to health requires states to take "appropriate" steps, legislative and otherwise, toward the progressive realization of the "right of everyone to the enjoyment of the highest attainable standard of physical and mental health," as the right is phrased in the ICESCR.[43] Under the ICESCR, this includes issues relating to preconditions of health, but it also calls for states to create the "conditions which would assure to all medical service and medical attention in the event of sickness."[44]

Of the three dimensions of states' obligations described here, I am concentrating most explicitly in this chapter on accountability for the "obligation to fulfill." Not all obligations to fulfill health-related rights are subject to "progressive realization in accordance with available resources" under international law or under some domestic constitutional law. As noted in Chapter 2, states have obligations to provide minimum threshold levels of rights, as well as to take certain basic measures—such as developing national plans of action—which are arguably not subject to resource constraints or to progressive realization under international law, and at the very minimum, impose a burden of proof on governments to justify why they have not met such core obligations.[45]

But I am focusing here on the state's obligations to take steps toward the progressive realization of the right because it links most clearly to the practical application of human rights in the context of development and social policy and in the circle of accountability discussed previously. Establishing accountability for obligations to fulfill progressive programmatic obligations also poses the most difficult challenges to traditional human rights approaches, which tend to announce absolute principles. These principles are critical, as coercive measures that violate rights and dignity—from forced evictions that allow dams to be built, to involuntary sterilizations to control population growth—have too often been justified in the name of economic development.

Nevertheless, as I have emphasized throughout this book, if human rights frameworks are to be relevant to development and public health practice, they also need to have something to contribute with respect to the very real questions of trade-offs, and they need to make clear the implications of the abstract normative concepts for practice. Here I argue that progressive obligations for which states, as well as other duty-bearers in some circumstances, should be held to account in human rights framework include *what* they do, *how much effort* they expend, and *how* they achieve their goals.[46]

Accountability for *What?* Linking Normative Obligations to "Take Appropriate Steps and Measures" to the Best Evidence from Public Health.

As noted in the previous section, under international law, states are responsible for taking steps, individually and through international assistance and cooperation, especially economic and technical, to the maximum of its available resources, "with a view to achieving progressively the full realization of [ESC rights] by all appropriate means, including particularly the adoption of legislative measures."[47] We have already discussed the critical importance to the "circle of accountability" of creating an enabling legal and policy framework, which entails enacting legislation to promote rights, as well as rescinding legislation that impairs rights. Laws and policies are necessary but not sufficient, for people to enjoy their health-related rights in practice. Programmatic interventions are also required, and this is where defining what steps and measures are "appropriate" becomes more complex.

In CP rights, we generally have clear ideas of how to evaluate, for example, whether due process standards were sufficiently complied with to ensure the fairness of a trial. Indeed, the quality of a criminal justice system, as a core social institution, is judged by whether it is arranged in such a way as to

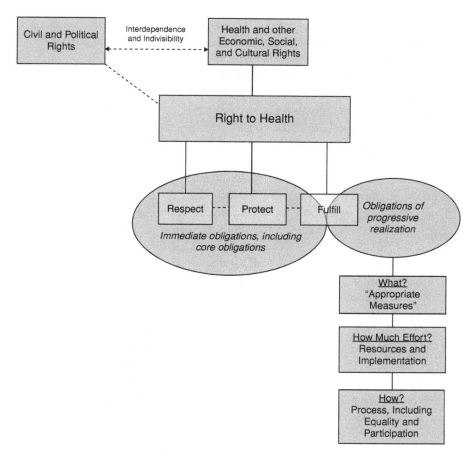

Figure 5.3. Obligations Relating to Health Rights

provide for the right to a fair trial. Yet standard setting has proven exceptionally difficult with respect to programmatic obligations to fulfill ESC
rights, including health. Sometimes this is because there is no consensus as
to the starting premises about what justice requires with respect to a health
system—how do human rights prioritize different categories of disadvantage
in defining what an enforceable right to health demands?

At other times, however, the necessary standard setting has been slowed
by the need to look beyond the traditional legal domain of human rights advocacy. This is particularly true in the technical realm of health. For example, in relation to maternal health, CEDAW requires states' parties to report

on the measures they have adopted "to ensure women *appropriate* services in connection with pregnancy, confinement and the post-natal period."[48] However, the appropriateness of services to address maternal health—or any condition—does not spring forth inevitably from immutable principles of human rights law. The CESCR has specifically called for governments to devise national strategies and plans of action "on the basis of epidemiological evidence."[49] Thus, standard setting for accountability in an HRBA to health requires reaching out to the medical, public health, and broader scientific communities for their knowledge.

It is not the function of courts to establish all the steps that are appropriate. Rather, courts have turned to scientific evidence to determine whether the content of government policies and actions is *reasonable* in the light of desired outcomes.[50] For instance, the South African Constitutional Court, in the case of *South African Minister of Health v. Treatment Action Campaign*, considered studies by both the WHO and South Africa's Medicines Control Council regarding the safety and efficacy of nevirapine to prevent mother-to-child transmission. On the basis of the scientific evidence, the court found that the state's claims about the need to limit the use of nevirapine to eighteen pilot sites in order to control for and study side effects was not reasonable. The court, in turn, ordered the state to devise a national plan for the rollout of prevention of mother-to-child transmission (PMTCT) treatment.[51]

Moreover, the advent of effective ARV therapy, including PMTCT, in the HIV context also illustrates that what measures are *appropriate*—and what is considered *reasonable*—must necessarily evolve with scientific knowledge. For example, the existence of resistant strains of malaria or multidrug-resistant tuberculosis challenges many governmental responses where those diseases are prevalent. What was once appropriate in terms of health policy, as well as normative requirements—for example, providing only chloroquine for malaria treatment or introducing one new tuberculosis drug at a time—can no longer be considered so because it will not enable effective enjoyment of rights in practice.[52] What *should be* done as a matter of obligation needs to be based on what we know works.

Finally, defining what is appropriate in terms of prioritizing interventions requires an examination not just of clinical effectiveness but also of cost-effectiveness, or comparative effectiveness, of different medications, interventions, and treatments. As discussed in Chapter 4, without an institutionalized way to judge whether certain medications are as or more effective for the same or less money, it is impossible to establish a rational system to determine what should be covered in a national insurance plan or to undertake a path toward UHC. And in a world and societies in which we need to honestly grapple with questions of resource availability, the comparative effectiveness of different services and treatments, and in turn how a specific use of resources will benefit the population, is relevant to whether a government is taking appropriate measures to realize the right to health for everyone in its territory. Despite all of the problems with data availability and interpretation, as the WHO Consultative Group on Equity and UHC notes in their "Final Report," "Even an imperfect application of the cost-effectiveness criterion—combined with other relevant criteria—is likely to be better than ignoring cost-effectiveness entirely, as suggested by the huge variation in cost-effectiveness across services" that are included in health systems today.[53]

Accountability for *Effort*: Implementation and Resources

If obligations for progressive realization of health rights are to be meaningful, in addition to defining what steps a state should be taking to achieve the desired outcomes, we must also determine whether the state is expending sufficient effort. As suggested in the "circle of accountability," this requires looking at whether laws are effectively regulated and policies are effectively implemented. Laws and policies do not apply themselves. A statute such as the Affordable Care Act in the United States, for example, implies the need for thousands of implementing regulations and the creation of entire institutions, programs, and monitoring frameworks. Even narrower legislation relating to, for example, exceptions to criminalization of abortion, requires regulation and clinical protocols to enable women to effectively enjoy their rights. These can take years to put into place. However, states are not free to indefinitely defer taking such steps to implement laws and policies—such as assigning a budget to strategies and plans of action relating to the various aspects of health. Moreover, as the South African Constitutional Court held in the PMTCT case, and other courts have held elsewhere, the reasonableness of a state's actions goes to the implementation of policies as well as to their existence.[54]

Rights require resource expenditures, and budgets often reveal whether states are expending adequate effort toward the progressive realization of health rights, including UHC. Under the ICESCR, as well as other treaties containing ESC rights, a state needs to take steps "to the maximum of [its] available resources, with a view to achieving progressively the full realization of the rights recognized in the present Covenant by all appropriate means."[55] As discussed in previous chapters, this does not mean taking as a given whatever a particular government decides to spend on health.

Sometimes lack of spending on appropriate items is a result of outright systemic corruption, not just the petty individual corruption demonstrated on the front lines by people such as Rebecca in Sierra Leone. Throughout the world, health-sector corruption can be so egregious as to seemingly reflect an inability on the part of those responsible to see their fellow citizens—whose lives are at stake—as fully human. In the wake of the Ebola crisis, for example, a report by the country's national auditor stated that government minsters in Sierra Leone has lost track of USD 3.3 million to fight the disease, while another USD 2.5 million in disbursements had incomplete documentation.[56]

Although corruption has long been considered an accountability and a human rights problem, larger economic questions relating directly to budget-allocation decisions have traditionally fallen outside the purview of human rights advocacy.[57] But including such issues is critical to transforming systems to overcome entrenched discrimination or marginalization of certain groups. This omission is beginning to change, as human rights activists are increasingly recognizing the need to learn how to monitor budgets and advocate not just for catching leakage but also for promoting substantive equality.[58] Innovative examples of budget analysis, from Latin America to Africa, have been used to highlight state inaction and failure to fulfill human rights obligations relating to health.[59]

Lack of appropriate effort toward realizing health and other ESC rights because of low social spending, including health spending, can often be traced at least in part to insufficient tax revenues. Under international law, the obligation of the state to maximize available resources has been interpreted to include the maximization of internal revenue. Moreover, fiscal policy affects compliance with both CP and ESC rights. For example, Guatemala—a country with notoriously bad fiscal policy—has health indicators that are among the worst in the region.[60] But Philip Alston, then-special rapporteur on extrajudicial, summary, or arbitrary executions, also pointed out to the Human Rights Council in 2007, "The reason the executive branch of the Guatemalan state has so little money to spend on the criminal justice system is that the Congress resist the imposition of all but the most perfunctory taxes. To put this in perspective, as a percentage of GDP, Guatemala's total tax revenue in 2005 was 9.6 percent of GDP."[61] The International Monetary Fund argues that adequate fiscal space requires tax revenues that total at least

15 percent of GDP.[62] In my view, and as I discuss further in Chapter 7, it is not a stretch to argue that applying a human rights framework to health that demonstrates concern for enabling everyone, including the worst off, to live lives of dignity, requires transforming regressive and discriminatory fiscal and monetary policies.

The opposite of adequate progress is "retrogression," or backsliding.[63] Retrogression can refer to a specific policy change that is not supported by scientific evidence, such as a reduction in access to contraception, because of ideological inclinations. At other times, however, retrogression can relate explicitly to financing and resources. Under international law, before making any cuts to public expenditure or introducing other fiscal austerity measures that could lead to retrogression in ESC rights enjoyment, including health, governments are supposed to seek out and exhaust all possible alternatives, which includes both tax and budget alternatives.[64] National courts have subjected retrogressive budgetary measures to high-level, or "strict," scrutiny, especially regarding potentially disproportionate effects on poor or marginalized groups.[65] Thus, for example, when the Colombian government sought to reduce spending with respect to the subsidized health insurance scheme as part of a "rationalization of public spending," the Constitutional Court held that the drastic reduction of spending for the needs of the poorest segments of Colombian society was inconsistent with the government's legal obligations under a *social state of law*.[66]

Accountability for *How*: Processes That Promote Participation and Nondiscrimination/Equality

As I have stressed throughout this book, applying a human rights framework to health invests significance in the process through which health goals—and outcomes—are reached. Two principles that are widely agreed to characterize procedural aspects of an HRBA to health are nondiscrimination/equality and participation/agency. Both of these merit separate discussions and will be addressed in Chapters 6 and 7, respectively, so I will merely introduce them here.

Under various international human rights instruments and documents, the central importance of participation has been emphasized in relation to the right to health in and of itself, as well as to sexual and reproductive health, children's health, indigenous health, and health for people with disabilities.[67] However, participation goes beyond questions of promoting health in a human rights framework; participation is sometimes called "the right of rights" because it allows us to claim our other rights. Indeed, as stressed in Chapter 1, participation is critical to our most fundamental understanding of being human and having dignity.[68]

A fundamental part of human rights is the conversion of passive beneficiaries into active agents, people who participate meaningfully in the decisions that will affect their well-being. As the UN "Technical Guidance" notes with respect to SRH, participation and "engagement by civil society is necessary [to] hold Governments to account."[69] This includes engagement throughout the policy-making cycle, from identifying needs in budgeting discussions to contributing to social accountability methods like community scorecards.[70]

Further, as noted in Chapter 4 in relation to health systems, we cannot assume that matters of health are merely technical, to be decided by experts and technocrats. Rather, setting priorities in health and negotiating the social parameters of a right to health involve fundamentally contested ethical claims. Thus, in a human rights framework the government needs to be able to publicly and transparently *justify* its decisions as reasonable—given competing social values as well as the best scientific evidence.

In Chapter 4, I also discussed the importance of a legitimate process in terms of priority setting in health and argued that Daniels's "Accountability for Reasonableness" could be consistent with human rights principles such as those underpinning some of the Colombian Constitutional Court's orders in T-760. In this chapter, I have also I emphasized that courts in various settings have shown they can play an important role in enhancing public deliberation and, in turn, promoting greater systemic accountability.[71] In Chapter 6, however, I add some caveats, noting that the extent to which participatory processes—whether "Accountability for Reasonableness" or judicially triggered dialogue regarding health-related rights issues—can subvert asymmetries of power depends on how the contours and boundaries of public participation and agendas are set.

Nondiscrimination and equality are also cross-cutting principles in human rights law, and a government is accountable for addressing what are often intersecting forms of discrimination—including gender, race, ethnicity, class, and the like—on individual, institutional, and structural levels. For example, at the individual level, it is common in many countries for discriminatory attitudes and coercive practices on the part of health providers to be reflected in the poor treatment of minorities. The Roma, or Romani people, are an ethnic group centered in Europe that has faced discrimination stretching back several centuries. As a report on Slovakia by the Center for Reproductive Rights (CRR) and its local partner found, there were, "clear and consistent patterns of health-care providers who disregarded the need for obtaining informed consent to sterilization and who failed to provide accurate and comprehensive reproductive health information to Romani patients."[72]

Indeed, in 2011, the European Court of Human Rights issued a judgment in *V.C. v. Slovakia* in favor of a Romani woman who was sterilized without her consent, on the grounds of the state's failure to institute measures to ensure her freedom from intersectional discrimination, as well as from inhuman and degrading treatment and the right to respect for private and family life. Discrimination and inequality can be the result of laws, policies, or practices that deliberately differentiate, such as against the Romani. But discrimination can also be based on a failure to take into account the differential effects in practice on diversely situated groups or disadvantaged populations. For example, if no provisions are made in laws or policies for health personnel to speak the local indigenous population's language or for cultural adaptation for birthing traditions, these constitute barriers to accessible and quality care for those populations.[73]

Structural discrimination can also be the result of budgeting processes. In an investigation I led while director of research and investigations at Physicians for Human Rights, we were able to show how structural inequalities in resource allocation resulted in de facto discrimination against indigenous women in Peru.[74] Greater health-related resources are available on a per capita basis to Peruvians in areas with low indigenous populations, compared to areas such as Huancavelica, Ayacucho, and Puno, with high indigenous populations.[75] We were able to show how this translated into fewer health facilities, doctors, and specialists per capita, and that as a result of this structural discrimination in spending, interventions such as the support of skilled birth attendants, were substantially lower in disproportionately indigenous areas.[76]

Concluding Reflections

After the research and advocacy that Amnesty International undertook in Sierra Leone, described at the beginning of this chapter, the British Department for International Development (DFID) and other donors worked with the government in an effort to make free care for pregnant women and children a reality, including underwriting salary support for a number of health care cadres in the country and topping off those salaries in order to reduce incentives to charge for medicines and sell bed nets.[77] This was real, although incremental change, although even before Ebola devastated the country it was unclear whether national resources would be deployed when donor funds inevitably shifted to other priorities.[78] In the wake of the Ebola crisis, it may seem impossible to contemplate how to begin to apply a human rights framework to health in such a setting. Yet there are lessons we can learn from Sierra Leone precisely because of the lack of accountability mechanisms, and indeed we must.

First, we need to begin to think differently about health as a matter of rights. For example, it is true that accountability for mass atrocities and grave violations of CP rights in Sierra Leone was also anemic. In 2012, Charles Taylor, the former president of Liberia, was convicted by the Special Court for Sierra Leone of war crimes and crimes against humanity for his role in fostering the atrocities in Sierra Leone.[79] When I was there with Amnesty, the effects of the civil war were still evident at every turn. The rebels had been especially brutal, hacking off hands and cutting off women's breasts. The roadblocks where they had previously strung human intestines to block traffic were still marked. The only surgeon performing cesarean sections at the time in Koinadugu was an orthopedic surgeon by training, who told me he had become burned out by operating on so many mutilation victims. In many parts of the country it would have been hard to find a family that had not been affected.

Although Taylor's conviction was met with great fanfare around the world, only thirteen people were ever indicted. Of these, nine were convicted and four either died or were thought to have died before a judgment could be made.[80] A deliberate strategy was put into place to go after the "big fish" in order to send a message, leaving the majority of the local commanders with impunity and Sierra Leone required political and social justice as well as criminal justice for reconciliation.

Although these initiatives on CP rights were radically insufficient, the idea that the suffering experienced by victims resulted from war "crimes" was indeed an essential change to make in the narrative of the country as well as their own lives. By contrast, the deaths of women such as Yerie—and health issues experienced by people like her—were relegated to being "humanitarian" rather than justice questions in crisis and postconflict settings, as well as development more broadly. Let me be clear: humanitarian relief was essential in Sierra Leone during the war and during the Ebola crisis, and it is essential in this world wracked by senseless cruelty and conflicts. Nevertheless, humanitarianism is inherently conservative; it is about putting bandages on the world's wounds.

Applying a human rights framework to health, by contrast, should be about remaking the world, reshaping the power relations that underpin conflict and humanitarian emergencies, as well as calamities such as Ebola. The Ebola outbreak vividly demonstrates, as discussed in Chapter 4, that health systems are not just a means for the technical delivery of goods and services; they can either encode norms of solidarity and equality or they can exacerbate social exclusion. In Sierra Leone, as well as in Guinea and Liberia, the health systems were all dysfunctional before Ebola hit, and it was entirely foreseeable that there would be enormous mistrust of the government and the health systems when a crisis broke out. Further, it is not a coincidence that Liberia and Sierra Leone are two countries that have been ravaged by brutal civil wars, which destroyed institutions and social cohesion. Nor is it a coincidence that more than half the population in each heavily affected country lives in abject poverty, with little or no possibility for self-governance or dignity, as discussed in Chapter 2.[81]

Applying a human rights framework to Ebola would not be about building temporary structures staffed largely by foreigners, which will disappear like sandcastles when the crisis is contained, just as they did after the wars in the region, or see the primary lesson as being to develop contingency plans to allow the WHO and others to contain such catastrophes in future.[82] A human rights framework would not accept the status quo ante as "normal"; it would instead involve the international community as well as the national governments in making long-term commitments to strengthening health systems, and other core social institutions needed in a democracy, but also in changing the rules of the game that disadvantage countries such as Sierra Leone, as I discuss further in Chapter 8. Such measures would be aimed at promoting the "circle of accountability"; that is, promoting people's own voice and agency in decisions affecting their lives and well-being, changing relationships within the health sector and beyond to one of entitlement and obligation, and taking the time to build and strengthen mechanisms that are not beholden to the political organs of government—including courts—so that the reasonableness of policies and actions can be assessed.

Second—and this is a central message of this book—even amidst the devasatation of Ebola and even in a country as poor as Sierra Leone, when we think differently it is possible to begin to act differently and to apply aspects of human rights frameworks. In 2012, a former student at Harvard's T. H. Chan School of Public Health, Dr. Mosoka Fallah, came to me with the idea that he wanted to establish a health facility focusing on the needs of women, including maternal health, in neighboring Liberia, whose suffering and deaths he clearly saw as the result of human rights deprivations and structural violence against women—laws, policies, customs which were made worse by the indifferent unaccountable health system in his country.

Against all odds, Fallah persevered, establishing Refuge Place in early June 2014 which remained open throughout the Ebola crisis to attend to the health needs that women and children continued to have, even during the outbreak. The staff of Refuge Place delivered babies, treated sexually transmitted, urinary tract, and other infections, as well as malaria and diarrhea. They also undertook thousands of Ebola-related interventions, such as distributing chlorine and hand-washing buckets.

In 2014, Fallah along with other health professionals were named *Time* magazine's Person of the Year.[83] He implicitly took accountability very seriously. He not only monitored and provided monthly reports accounting transparently for all activities throughout the crisis in Liberia, he further engaged with the government, donors, and international institutions to propose concrete ways in which they could not only "get to zero" in Ebola but also create sustainable systems and institutions, showing that each part of the "circle of accountability" affords an entry point.

During the height of the Ebola crisis, I also participated in a webinar for donors, organized by the International Human Rights Funders Group. These were donors committed to supporting local initiatives, promoting women's voices and empowerment, and strengthening the accountability of governmental institutions, in both the short and long term. And there was no shortage of examples of courageous work, such as Fallah's, being done on the ground. Thus, if we fail to learn the lessons of Ebola and repeat the mistakes of the past, it will be a failure of imagination to see past the way things have been, and to imagine a world where the people, like Yerie, in Sierra Leone and West Africa more broadly, are entitled to justice, not just charity.

Chapter 6

Power and Participation

Participation and active involvement in the determination of one's own destiny is the essence of human dignity.
—Mary Robinson, former UN High Commissioner for Human Rights

Participation is a means of challenging forms of domination that restrict people's agency and self-determination.
—Magdalena Sepúlveda, former UN Special Rapporteur on Extreme Poverty and Human Rights

In 2007, as director of research and investigations at Physicians for Human Rights, I led a field investigation into maternal mortality in Peru.[1] I had lived in Peru for years before and knew the country well. As part of the follow-up to that investigation, I worked with CARE Peru to develop a program to strengthen the capacity of local health promoters in the subnational "department" (state) of Puno, to accompany pregnant women to their antenatal checks and delivery care, and to ensure that their rights were respected. Among other things, the health promoters recorded such things as whether the women received respectful treatment from the health personnel, whether there were significant delays before they received care, whether they were spoken to in their own language and their customs were respected, and whether they were asked to pay for supplies or services that should have been provided free of charge. All of the women in the program were volunteers who had chosen to participate on their own initiative, members of the indigenous communities spread over the *Altiplano*.[2] Most of them had participated in another community-based reproductive health initiative in the past. The volunteer program gave them a formal opportunity to develop further knowledge and capacity with respect to human rights.[3]

We connected these local women volunteers with the Defensoría del Pueblo (the National Human Rights Ombuds Office), which is decentralized and has offices in each department of Peru. In this way, the women could channel any complaints to the Defensoría, who could then advocate on behalf of women in Puno. But they did not need to simply depend on the Defensoría to speak for them; rather, these local health promoters were also invited to personally share their findings and recommendations with local government and in doing so, they had a personal voice and played a direct role in shaping and altering district-level policy and programming. They had real power to effect change.

On one occasion, over breakfast with a group of these health promoters, Lupita—a destitute widow who spoke only broken Spanish—described to me her experiences of monitoring her local health center.[4] An obviously hostile *mestizo*[5] doctor, annoyed that this woman was interfering in his treatment of the patient, yelled at her, "Go home; this is my house. I don't go to your house and tell you what to do; don't try to come to mine and tell me what to do." Lupita smiled a great toothless grin as she recounted how she had responded: "This is not your house; this is a public health center and you are a public servant. As long as this patient wants me here, I have a right to be here—as a citizen." The doctor—undoubtedly taken aback—allowed her to stay. And, along with her colleagues, Lupita later presented her findings to the district-level health authority.

To understand how significant it was for an illiterate, indigenous woman to stand up to a male, *mestizo* doctor, you need to know something about the deeply hierarchical Peruvian context, in which indigenous women sit at the bottom. For example, Peru's Truth and Reconciliation Commission, which examined the brutal armed conflict with Shining Path (Sendero Luminoso) between 1980 and 2000, underscored that a true national reconciliation would need to be based on "full citizenship for all Peruvians," oriented toward overcoming the historical fragmentation and discrimination in Peruvian society.[6] As health outcomes and the relationships between providers and patients at health facilities reflect that historical fragmentation and discrimination, it was extraordinary when Lupita and the other impoverished and largely illiterate indigenous women could begin to change that dynamic to one of "entitlement and obligation."

In addition, this participation in the health system and the new way of relating to providers led to empowerment in the Peruvian health promoters' personal lives as well. These women had to negotiate with their husbands to care for their children while they were away from home accompanying the pregnant women. Many of their relationships with their husbands began to shift, albeit with the expected opposition and difficulties along the way. Most fundamentally though, their relationships with themselves also evolved, as for the first time in many of their lives, they perceived themselves to be subjects who had rights to expect and claim as members of Peruvian society.

Indeed, sometimes the most transformative impacts of applying rights frameworks lie in permitting people to conceive of themselves as full human beings. And when they do so, everything else has the potential to change. Once people appropriate a sense of themselves as having dignity and believe themselves worthy of being treated that way, it shifts not only the way they relate to service providers but also the way service providers relate to them. As suggested by the circle of accountability among different relationships, as outlined in Chapter 5, that appropriation of rights can also transform expectations of justice in relation to the wider conditions of our lives.

The Peru program was aimed specifically at fostering "social accountability," which is an aspect of meaningful participation in a human rights framework. Social accountability refers to the idea that governments should be able to justify their decisions and policies to the people who are ostensibly being served by them. It is fundamental to changing not only relations between patients and providers but also relations between citizens and their elected governments, from one of largesse for passive beneficiaries to one of active claimants and duty-bearers, as discussed in Chapter 5.

Indeed, the CARE Peru program has been cited by the World Bank as well as the UN Independent Expert Review Group as a model of social accountability and is being replicated elsewhere in Peru.[7] Sometimes "social accountability" programs only relate to the monitoring and review aspects of accountability, such as tracking public expenditures in health to identify malfeasance or corruption in health sectors. In this case, however, we also created spaces for participation in shaping policies and decisions, thus promoting changes in opportunity structures across a greater part of the policy circle of accountability.

Participation, more broadly, is inextricably related to our understanding of rights and of what being human means. As the quote from Mary Robinson at the beginning of this chapter stresses, participation is both expressive of and instrumental to human agency and self-government. In a human rights framework, as discussed elsewhere in this book, human beings are not targets of projects designed to benefit our health or to rescue us in disasters such as Ebola. Rather, we have some objective interest in dignity, in developing our own "life plans," and rights are tools that enable us to do so.

Thus, our approach to participation in a bold and empowering human rights framework may be quite different from the ways in which "participation" is promoted in mainstream public health and development practice. Participation is stressed in the discourses of a wide array of actors, from grassroots social movements to the World Bank. Yet the rhetoric masks deep divisions about the concept and practice of participation. In practice, participation can mean the simple provision of basic information or tokenistic consultation—or even the opportunistic use of community resources, such as using local people to build latrines, without paying them for their labor. That is not the kind of participation that can challenge power relationships.

I argue in this chapter that a meaningful approach to participation in an HRBA to health not only requires going beyond these instrumental uses of people and communities to achieve health outcomes but also demands more than access to information and spaces for pluralistic voice, as important as these are. If we want participation to present an effective challenge to the different ways in which power relations are organized that leave people without choices over their lives and their health, we need to understand the multiple levels, forms, and spaces in which power operates and how it can constrain opportunities and agency. As set out in John Gaventa's power cube (Figure 6.1), these include the ways in which spaces for participation are controlled or defined by governments and other actors and the ways in which conflicts over choices are hidden or suppressed through contextually determined power relations. In order to understand where there is leverage for change, a human rights framework must be applied that requires analyzing power across multiple sectors, not just health, as well as at local or community, national, and global levels. Finally, an empowering approach to participation also requires that we understand what I referred to in Chapter 1 as internalized domination—which causes people to assimilate a view of themselves as inferior to others. It is this invisible power that can be the most insidious way to prevent people from taking social action to challenge

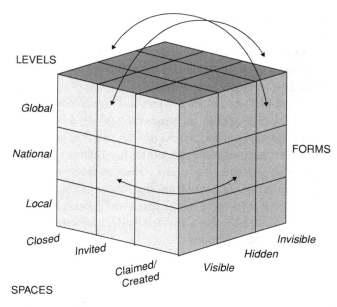

LEVELS

Global

National

Local

FORMS

Closed *Invited* *Claimed/ Created* *Visible* *Hidden* *Invisible*

SPACES

Figure 6.1. The Power Cube: The Levels, Spaces, and Forms of Power. *Source:* John Gaventa, "Finding the Spaces for Change: A Power Analysis," *IDS Bulletin* 37, no. 6 (2006): 23–33.

injustice, in health and beyond. In short, in shifting our understanding of power, we can better understand what forms of meaningful participation we need to facilitate through applying rights.

Conventional Liberal Conceptions of Participation and Power

Our notion of participation, and agency, reflects our notion of human beings and the contexts in which they act as agents. As discussed in earlier chapters, in a narrow, conventional liberalism, people are taken to be "autonomous and rational actors faced with a feasible set of choices, more or less aware of the external constraints they face, sometimes cooperating and even collaborating with those who dominate them, and resisting, even rebelling when the opportunity arises."[8] Thus the obligations of the traditional liberal state were confined to a narrow slice of CP rights, intended to protect people from a limited set of abuses of power involving "external coercion and constraints" that restrict otherwise free people's options to live as they choose.[9]

Political participation is one of those rights. Participation to promote "pluralistic" voice is fundamental to liberal democracies—the notion that people with many competing perspectives can express their views and be heard. Establishing a dynamic of entitlement and obligation between citizens and their elected representatives is critical to the circle of changing relationships for accountability set out in Chapter 5. Pluralistic voice is similarly fundamental to the rule of law. The process by which a law is drafted has an impact on its moral claim on citizens of a country.[10] If laws are passed by decree, or without a meaningful opportunity for different viewpoints to be heard in the legislative debate, those laws cannot be taken as a legitimate reflection of the transfer of authority from the people to their representatives in a democratic society. Likewise, as we discussed previously in the context of priority setting for health, those affected by decisions should have an opportunity to express their opinions.

As an empirical matter, we have long understood that authoritarian regimes that disregard people's voices with impunity can have especially disastrous consequences for health. In studies comparing famine in China and India, Jean Drèze and Amartya Sen illustrate how the democratic governance in India, and the freedom of information, association, and movement that stem from it, enabled India to avoid the catastrophic famines that gripped China.[11] As they note, it is difficult to imagine how it is possible that "the Chinese famine raged on for three years without it being even admitted in public that such a thing was occurring."[12] Measured in terms of "extra deaths," "the Chinese famine was about five to ten times as large as the largest famine in India in this century."[13] In short, freedoms of expression, association, information, movement, and other civil rights are crucial to health and development, although the mainstream development community rarely makes these connections.

And placing limits on the capacity of elites and autocratic governments to impose their will on individuals and groups; protecting rights to information, expression, and the like from governmental interference; and democratizing health-policy making through opportunities for pluralistic voice are critical in *any* human rights framework more generally. Nonetheless, I argue in this chapter that just as we discussed with respect to the intimately related conceptions of rights and state obligations, we need to move beyond the conventional liberal frameworks of what power means, the spaces in which it resides, and how power is exercised. Confining our understanding of power to a narrow liberal view that focuses exclusively on forums for pluralistic choice undermines the possibility of applying a human rights framework in a transformative manner.

The conventional liberal view of power is that "A has power over B to the extent that A can get B to do something that B would otherwise not do."[14] This is the power of the torturer who extracts confessions, as described in Chapter 1. And we are all familiar with this kind of power in our daily lives. Imagine, for example, at a family meal, a parent physically prevents one child, say a daughter, from eating the meager food in the household so that another child, say a son, can have it. We would all agree that the parent has exercised power over the girl.

Such decisions are taken all the time in both private and public spheres, including the provider-patient setting.[15] Think, for example, of an HIV-positive woman such as Paula in Kenya, discussed in Chapter 2, who depends on the health facility for ARV medications for herself as well as infant formula for her child. If the health provider threatens to withhold ARV medications or formula unless the woman undergoes bilateral tubal ligation, and then the woman agrees to do so despite not wanting to, that is a form of coercion that deprives the woman of meaningful choice over her body and life. Historically, in accordance with the first two dimensions of Jonathan Mann and colleagues's paradigm of the linkages between health and human rights, whether addressing the health effects of torture and other civil rights abuses or the need to preserve autonomy and informed consent in health policies, the health and human rights movement was largely focused on protecting weaker actors from exactly this form of domination.[16]

In *Participation and the Right to the Highest Attainable Standard of Health*, Helen Potts stresses the need for all affected parties to have an equal opportunity to be part of the participatory process and for the process to be transparent with information that is rationally related to the issue at hand.[17] These conditions resonate closely with what I discussed in Chapter 4 in terms of legitimate national planning and priority-setting processes for health, as well as the conditions of "Accountability for Reasonableness," and these process issues are key to applying human rights to health.

Examining the Application of the Liberal Model of Participation in Health: Decentralization

Support for decentralizing governmental responsibilities for health, which has occurred across the world, has been based on this logic of opening spaces for democratic participation. If health sectors (and governments generally) are brought closer to the people they serve, the idea was that they would afford more opportunities for pluralistic voice, and therefore be more responsive.[18]

Decentralization has occurred in myriad ways, with varying degrees of budgetary and programming control shifting from central governments to state or provincial governments, while policies generally remain in the remit of central governments. Decentralization continues to be ongoing in many countries, including many in sub-Saharan Africa.

Evidence regarding the effects of decentralization on the health rights of the poor is mixed,[19] and it demonstrates that health sectors and their building blocks cannot simply be "unbundled" as technical apparata but need to be considered in the light of the role they play within specific social and historical contexts. In many instances, decentralization has not led to authentic democratic space or participation but rather to enhanced local control by elites and the reproduction of national inequities at the regional level.[20] In Kenya, for example, early experience with devolution has been poor, with a dramatic mismatch between the demands placed on local health systems by national policies and guidelines and the budgets obtained by the county governments, together with obfuscation of accountability from different levels of government. The result of misalignment between national policies and local programs can be even greater inequity. For example, in the case of free maternal and child health care, patients may be forced to pay retail prices, often with markups, for basic maternity kits and other supplies and medicines if there is not effective monitoring and oversight of decentralized implementation.

In an account of what has happened in Guatemala, Walter Flores and colleagues laud the significance of the Urban and Rural Development Councils Law, which created mechanisms for "participation in the allocation of public budgets from community to central government levels."[21] Yet they conclude that, although spaces are necessary, they are insufficient to adequately address the ESC rights, including the health rights, of the poor in Guatemala. Likewise, in Mexico, a 2006 study that monitored the effects of health decentralization in four states cited similar problems. From the user's perspective, there was a "lack of opportunities for participation in decision making to establish health care priorities of communities jointly with health services."[22]

In sum, it turns out that "opening spaces" for pluralistic voice, whether in the context of decentralization or otherwise, does not always shift people's real opportunity structures or guarantee that people are meaningfully empowered. In the next sections, by exploring the ways in which power relations structure (in)action, I hope that we can better understand the less visible ways of securing compliance from disadvantaged groups and individuals, which have enormous impacts on both dignity and well-being.[23]

Hidden Power: The Need to Challenge Agendas and Boundaries of Participation

Underlying many of the progressive critiques of so-called participatory approaches to health and development are criticisms of the liberal understanding of what power means and how it is exercised to control and exclude disadvantaged groups.[24] For example, a leading critic of participatory development, Bill Cooke, has argued that, "because participatory processes prioritize what happens *within* the participatory group, [they] foster the assumption that they represent a natural, uncontestable way of things. . . . Simultaneously, important and malign structural forces outside the cognizance and/or influence of participants are ignored and sustained."[25] That is, allowing people to participate within certain forums can actually obscure the less visible or indeed, hidden, ways in which they are disempowered outside those forums.

Let's return to our example of a family dinner table. Once again, imagine there is not enough food for everyone in the household. Let's say that the spoken or unspoken rule is that the boy eats before the girl. The girl dislikes this rule and wishes she could be fed first sometimes. But she does not perceive the rule about who gets to eat first as open to challenge. There is no overt conflict either with her parents or with her brother, simply because the issue of who gets to eat first, and how much, is not open for discussion. It is organized out of debate; left "off the table," as it were. In the first example, illustrating the first dimension or form of power, food was physically withheld from the girl by her mother, who exerted power over her daughter by preventing her from doing something she otherwise would have done. In this example, control—over the terms of debate, the "rules of the game"—illustrates a second dimension or form of power that is essential to understand if we care about changing people's opportunities to exercise effective agency.

That is, the often hidden power to decide *what* gets decided can be a greater constraint on choices and people's capacity for self-government than the ability to overcome open resistance. Consider that it shows much greater control over the girl if she never challenges the family food policy, even though she would like to, than if the mother has to remove the food the girl has already shoveled onto her plate at every meal. The same is true for health policy.

For example, imagine a somewhat different scenario than Paula's in Kenya, where she was coerced into accepting a bilateral tubal ligation because she was HIV-positive. Imagine a health policy in which impoverished rural women were only offered permanent (such as bilateral tubal ligation) and long-acting methods of contraception (such as implants and injectables). This is indeed the reality for women in many communities across the global South, not just because of stock-outs and supply-chain problems but also because of deliberate policies that promote these methods, as the most cost-effective manner in which to provide "couple years protection." Naturally, many women and girls would—if given a real choice, with meaningful information as well as availability of methods—prefer to use some other form of contraception. Yet because of the objective established and the assumptions about impoverished women's ability to comply with other methods, women's options about their own fertility regulation have already been preset before they even get to the forum to express their views. It is not coercion from the health provider at the facility that is the real health rights issue here; the real issue is the definition of what the women get to decide about their own bodies and lives.

The Agenda-Setting Power of Private Actors

If it is important to consider not just who gets their way within decision-making settings but also how the agenda and the boundaries of agency are set, we need to look at who and what factors prevent many issues that have an enormous impact on health from ever arising in decision-making arenas in the first place. In the health sector and in relation to some social determinants, those whose interests are best organized are often private actors, even though private actors' power is generally not conceived of as relevant in the traditional liberal framework of democracy. These private actors exercise enormous control over what issues ever come up for contention within political forums.

All political organization involves "a mobilization of bias . . . in favor of the exploitation of certain kinds of conflict and the suppression of others . . . some issues are organized into politics and others are organized out."[26] For example, the saga of health care reform in the United States that led to the passing of the Affordable Care Act speaks to how provider and insurer organizations managed to mobilize certain biases to define the terms of what could be debated. The universe of possibilities for reforming the system was largely established outside the public, traditionally "political" sphere.[27] Despite polls that indicated strong public support for a universal single-payer plan, only one subcommittee hearing was held on the single-payer option, and that plan never came up for a vote.[28] The active lobbying of pharmaceutical and insurance companies and managed-care and provider organizations, together with a mainstream media, mobilized a bias against a universal single-payer plan so effectively as to suppress even the possibility of an overt conflict or public debate on the issue.[29]

The pharmaceutical and insurance industries exercise a similarly great influence in the Colombian health system, in contrast to patients who have little or no economic means and are unorganized, which drastically affects possibilities for further structural reform and regulation in the wake of T-760. Indeed, the highly unequal Colombian social context illustrates how meaningful deliberative discussion—and, in turn, the democratic legitimacy of the results that emerge—depends to a great extent on the context in which it occurs and what is up for contention. Nancy Fraser argues that in "stratified societies"—societies in which the basic institutional framework systematically generates unequal social groups—"full parity of participation in public debate and deliberation is not within the reach of possibility."[30] Thus, we need to think carefully, in Colombia and beyond, about what the preconditions are for the kinds of dialogical judicial remedies discussed in Chapters 4 and 5 to contribute to meaningful democratic transformation of health systems.

In general, so-called public–private partnerships (PPPs) and the private sector more broadly are increasingly touted as a solution to underfinancing in health sectors and development programs. Private actors are not anathema to HRBAs, or human rights in general. However, in a human rights framework, the state has an obligation to ensure that their conduct meets certain standards, relating to quality and equality. Moreover, overreliance on the private sector may change the nature of outcomes sought. For example, there is a risk that the "efficient delivery" of health care, such as contraceptive methods to women, can drive a technocratic, target-led "fix" approach—which in turn may limit the method mix available, as discussed earlier—over a more complex understanding of women's SRH rights that seeks to empower women to have choices in multiple domains.[31]

As discussed in previous chapters, failure to adequately regulate private actors in health systems tends to convert health care into a commodity to be allocated by market mechanisms—that is, price—rather than in terms of rights and entitlements of citizenship. Profit-making agendas can also discount the rights-based concerns with reaching marginalized populations; neglecting unprofitable public health interventions, such as sanitation; and converting health care workers into instrumental cogs, as we saw in the example of the Maternal and Child Institute in Bogotá.[32]

It is not just within the health sector that private actors define agendas relating to health; the commercial activities of private actors across an array of industries also dramatically affect health. Sometimes, of course, these are positive, but sometimes they are negative, ranging from issues of intellectual property in agricultural seeds, which affect access to food security—to plain old pollution. And in many cases, such private actors end up defining the boundaries of political action through inaction—not even active lobbying, as in the case of insurance or pharmaceutical companies within the health sector. In his now classic study, *The Unpolitics of Air Pollution: A Study of Non-Decision Making in the Cities*, Matthew Crenson documented how "US Steel influenced the content of the pollution ordinance without taking any action on it, and thus defied the thinking that political power belongs to political actors."[33] In a 2006 study of participation and health rights in a community in rural Peru, Mario Rios and Henry Armas came to similar conclusions with respect to the large mining company that has historically dominated economic activity there, again challenging liberal assumptions and showing how power is exercised by nontraditionally "political" actors.[34]

The Importance of Context in Determining Possibilities for Meaningful Participation and Social Change

In Chapter 5, I stressed that applying a human rights framework to health calls for changing specific relationships in ways that can lead to broader social transformation—relationships between politicians and policy makers, between policy makers and service providers, between service providers and patients, and between health-system users and their elected governments. But changing those relationships and in turn people's opportunity structures for acting differently requires understanding their specific contexts and how power dynamics function within those contexts. Take the example at the beginning of this chapter, of the indigenous health promoter defying the doctor. There were very specific, contextualized ways in which power asymmetries based on gender, ethnicity (*mestizo* and *criollo*[35] people are heavily privileged in Peru), class, and role (the doctor's position of authority) affected the role relations between doctor and the indigenous woman, and in turn the possibilities for indigenous women such as Lupita to enjoy their health rights. As Lynn Freedman warns, "Imagining a structure for participation is fairly easy; developing meaningful engagement with a community and a process that is truly participatory can be enormously difficult."[36] Formulaic designs or indicators of participation in health are likely to ignore the complex realities of such power relationships that shape and constrain people's lives.[37]

In contrast, when we situate participation in a specific social and historical context, we can begin to see how power, and in particular this agenda-setting power, gets built up over time. For example, Flores and colleagues have described how Guatemala's decades-long, brutal internal conflict generated a "climate of generalized terror that gripped the population," leading to such fear and intense insecurity that people stopped seeking spaces for social participation, even though they could not explain exactly why they did so. Flores and his colleagues conclude that there is a need for specific ways of regenerating the social fabric as "essential and basic elements that cannot be separated from the processes of social participation" in health, and beyond.[38] Rebuilding the social fabric need not mean naive faith in the beneficence of the state.

On the contrary, we need to have more trust in an emancipatory, confrontational politics that encourages and sustains open conflict over health *as a deeply and an inexorably political issue*, without resorting to violent suppression.[39] We in human rights may tend to feel more comfortable in "neutral" roles, talking about demystifying human rights for health policy makers and other government officials and providing them with objective "tools." But the depoliticization of participation—as a neutral process occurring in a neutral space—is deeply problematic. A transformative approach to applying a human rights framework, as I have been arguing in these pages, is invariably political and should indeed be profoundly threatening to those politicians who seek to hold onto the privileges and power that they have as a result of the status quo. Participation in such a framework is inherently messy and unpredictable because it is aimed at bringing suppressed transformative possibilities, suppressed conflicts—such as that between the doctor and Lupita—into the open.

Where Do Decisions Get Made? "Invited" Versus "Claimed" or "Demanded" Spaces

If we understand the goals of applying a transformative human rights framework to be inherently political in this way—which is not the same as being cynically politicized or aligned with fixed political parties—it is important to distinguish between participation in decisions affecting health rights that occurs in "invited" and participation that occurs in "claimed" spaces.[40] An invited space is one that is created and substantively controlled by health planners and policy makers, where participation is induced—supported by governments or aid agencies, or both. The government or some other "authority" effectively controls the spaces and defines at least the preliminary agenda. By contrast, claimed or demanded spaces are those demanded, created, claimed, or chosen by communities or social movements themselves.[41] We need not think of a rigid dichotomy between the two. Under some circumstances, such invited spaces and induced participation can open greater opportunities for authentic agency to be exercised, as in Brazil's constitutionally created health councils, which have allowed for some genuine transfer of control over priority setting and budgeting to affected populations.[42] However, they can also close possibilities, reinforce existing privileges, and preclude alternative perspectives.[43] As Uma Kothari has argued, some initiatives "designed to bring the excluded in often result in forms of social control that are more difficult to challenge, as they reduce the spaces of conflict and are relatively benign and liberal."[44] For example, spaces that might be used for creating meaningful change can be converted by the government or other controlling power into being merely administrative, precluding precisely the political dimension that would allow agenda-setting power to be challenged.

Thus, although within a liberal framework on rights, legislating the creation of "participatory spaces" for health policy making is unequivocally a positive indicator, we should be cautious about applying such so-called "rights-based indicators" abstracted from political context. We cannot assume that the creation of officially sanctioned processes for participation guarantees meaningful opportunities for empowerment.[45] At times, a government's claim to establish a priority-setting process in health can be a means to legitimate political and social control over groups that would otherwise have articulated bolder demands.[46] Thus, for example, for "Accountability for Reasonableness" to be used in politically emancipatory, rather than managerial, ways, we need to be conscious of the manner in which the agendas for deliberation are set and controlled by different actors.

We also need to critically reflect on the spaces for and quality of participation supported by donor funding. The sorts of "log frames" and time-bound projects that many donor-funded "participatory" initiatives entail tend to favor working with reliable elites in invited spaces rather than grassroots groups and social movements. An independent study by Ghazala Mansuri and Vijayendra Rao of the participatory initiatives in which the World Bank had been involved over the past decade, for example, concluded that there is little evidence that induced participation leads to greater civic engagement or collective action, although it may under certain circumstances have a positive impact on service delivery.[47]

At What Level Do Decisions Get Made That Affect Health Rights? Looking Beyond "the Community"— and Beyond Health Care

In a human rights framework, participation should not just be at the project or program level but "in all health-related decision making at the community, national and international levels."[48] Often it is precisely the restriction of where and when people can meaningfully participate in decisions that allows those with power to decide which issues shall be open for discussion— when and indeed if those in power allow those most affected by the decision to "have their say." Thus, if approaches limit participation in health to the local community level or to delivery of health programs, as often happens in conventional public health, certain key decisions never come "up for contention."[49] True participation in decisions such as resource allocation, health-care workforce, structuring of health systems, and paths chosen toward universal health coverage is what drives the possibilities for people to realize their rights to health.

For instance, had the program in Peru, which I described at the beginning of this chapter, not connected the community health promoters to the Defensoría, their "participation" would have been toothless. It was because they had an interlocutor at the policy and programming level, with national-level authority—and both they and the personnel at the local health centers understood that—that local people were able to have meaningful voice. Moreover, at the same time, we were able to connect the accompaniment of pregnant women to broader advocacy by a Citizen Forum on Health (*ForoSalud*) in Peru. Among other things, *ForoSalud* was instrumental in advocating for a revised law on Committees for the Local Administration of Health Care (CLAS, by its Spanish acronym), which in turn gave communities some degree of power to audit and oversee their local health facilities and quality of care in many parts of the country.[50]

These initiatives were in no way a magic bullet to transform what remains a very hierarchical and exclusionary health system and society. Nevertheless, connecting the local and the national, and the grassroots or community level with the "tree-tops" level of advocacy, was critical to achieving some meaningful participation and social accountability in Peru. When initiatives ignore this need to connect local engagement to higher levels of power, "participation" in development and health practice often means incorporating marginalized people into preconstructed agendas that they are unable to question in fundamental ways.[51]

Sometimes the very notion of "community participation" can obscure power imbalances within communities, such as between men and women.[52] Participatory approaches that emphasize "consensus" at the community level tend to ignore the ways in which group dynamics, just as participatory spaces, are invariably embedded in power structures. As a result, subordinate perspectives are often not articulated.[53] For example, discrimination against MSM or the health needs of transgender people are rarely raised in "local community" discussions of sexual and reproductive health. Similarly, in discussions of disabilities at the community level, the needs of persons with physical disabilities or psychosocial problems are often raised, while the needs of those with psychiatric disabilities often are neglected.

Examining nonissues and silent spaces—where conflict has been suppressed in ways that prevent social action from making change—can be more telling in terms of assessing whether real opportunities exist for participation to be empowering. And when group identities and dynamics exclude or actively harm certain people's health interests, the human rights concerned with dignity and empowerment places parameters or criteria on what may be classified as "participation."

Also, there is not just one "community" to which any of us belong, and projects aimed at "community participation" can be overly rigid in defining identity by local geographical boundaries. In a human rights framework, as I emphasized in Chapter 1, it is understood that all human beings are part of multiple communities—based on different parts of our identity, which include our religion, class, national origin, employment and unionization status, ethnicity, race, gender identity, and sometimes health status, among other factors. And we know communities can exist within communities and across borders. For example, in what were often explicitly rights-based advocacy initiatives, PLWA advocacy at multiple levels—local, national, and international—was essential in changing global and governmental policies with respect to HIV research and treatment.[54]

Invisible Power: Challenging "Internalized Domination"

Throughout this book, I have given examples of how suffering that is caused by injustice is allowed to persist unchallenged, precisely because it is construed as inevitable or "God's will." Think back to Happiness's desperate situation in Malawi or Pilar's in Baborigame. Indeed, Pilar reacted differently to the military's violations of CP rights than she did to the government's neglect of her health and other social rights, precisely because she understood them differently. I have argued that adopting a human rights framework demands that we think differently about the causes of our own suffering and that of others. Further, doing so is a form of appropriation of agency, and empowerment.

The British sociologist Steven Lukes suggests that the greatest form of domination is "the power to prevent people, to whatever degree, from having grievances by shaping their perceptions in such a way that they accept their role in the existing order of things, either because they can see no alternative to it or because they see it as natural and unchangeable, or because they value it as divinely ordained and beneficial."[55] In the example of the family dinner table, imagine that the girl not only never challenges the food distribution in her household, but she herself does not feel it is unjust; she has internalized the idea that her brother should eat before she does or have access to more food. In these cases, the exercise of power is neither an overt conflict of wills nor a suppressed or hidden conflict. It is not that the girl's demands do not get contested openly; they are not even felt. That is, she believes, perhaps fervently, that she does not deserve as much food as her brother because she is a girl. Moreover, in accepting the way things are, as divinely or culturally ordained, she is likely internalizing a sense of her own inferiority—in this case, because of her gender, and the socially prescribed role and demonstrations of affective attachment she reenacts every day that come along with it.[56]

As I discussed in reference to gender-based and domestic violence in Chapter 1, this cultural and ideological domination—which produces not just inaction but willing compliance in the face of stark injustice—is the most insidious and prevalent way in which people are prevented from controlling their own destinies and furthering their health and dignity. As Frantz Fanon recognized, the greatest power of colonialism was not global exploitation but rather its capacity to colonize the interior worlds of its subjects.[57]

Internalized Domination and Living a Life of Dignity

Asserting the existence of such internalized cultural and ideological domination is profoundly controversial because it inevitably appears to be passing paternalistic judgment about those who suffer from the inequities that they themselves participate in maintaining. But we don't need to resort to the Marxist language of "false consciousness," with its exclusionary focus on class, to assert that everyone is not the best judge of his or her own interests, as the utilitarian Jeremy Bentham may have claimed.

No form of domination is ever complete and indeed part of applying rights frameworks to health resides in enabling people to construct themselves as more than "victims." Yet, an empowering human rights framework in relation to health needs to acknowledge the pervasive yet invisible ways in which, in Martha Nussbaum's words, "habit, fear, low expectations, and unjust background conditions deform people's choices and even their wishes for their own lives."[58]

A "participatory" process that focuses only on tallying people's preferences may be meaningless if we do not recognize the impact and barriers created by internalized domination. This is acutely apparent when we think of gender subordination.[59] As Nussbaum has written about women, "[When] someone who has no property rights under law, who has no formal education, who has no legal right of divorce, who will very likely be beaten if she seeks employment outside of the house . . . says that she endorses traditions of modesty, purity and self-abnegation, it is not clear that we should consider this the last word on the matter."[60] Similarly, as noted in Chapter 1, studies in societies as diverse as Peru and Swaziland have found that women often believe that their husbands or partners are entitled to be violent with them if the women fail to please them in one way or another, including such trivial things as having a meal be late.[61] Imagine what life is like for a woman who not only lives in constant fear that she will be beaten for talking to another man in her village or chatting with girlfriends or failing to fetch water on time or burning the food she is preparing or any number of other items but also believes she *deserves* to be treated in this way. This invisible power, which operates through structuring internal thought, undermines the very possibility of dignity, and needs to be taken seriously in a human rights framework that seeks to change people's opportunity structures and transform patterns of health and ill-health. And it calls for distinct approaches to participation.

Critical Thinking to Overcome Invisible Power and Internalized Domination

If we need to change the way people are thinking about themselves in relation to others and to society, participation needs to begin by fostering critical consciousness. As I emphasize throughout this book, applying rights frameworks to health in truly empowering ways calls for making visible and challenging precisely what is taken for granted as unchangeable.[62] This applies to the hegemony of neoliberal economic models through which we organize our institutional arrangements at national and international levels. It applies equally to our individualistic understandings of health in biomedical and conventional public health models, as described in Chapter 3.

Focusing on internalized domination again calls our attention to the porousness of the public and private spheres in the socialization that precedes and perpetuates the systemic inequalities in societies and in patterns of health, and the need for a concept of participation that addresses them.[63] Think of the girl at the dinner table at home who absorbs social understandings of gender roles through her interactions with her family, even before she is affected by societal differences in access to entitlements and endowments. Or think of how we talk about and treat children so that those who have minority sexual orientations or gender identities come to internalize self-hating views of themselves. Laws and judicial decisions are essential to creating and revising social meanings, but these invariably interact with the ways we learn to identify ourselves in relation to others, beginning in infancy.

A number of leading thinkers in "empowerment approaches" to participation in health have come to advance the work of Brazilian Paolo Freire, who spent much of his life developing forms of popular education to promote critical thinking to confront structures of oppression.[64] "Reflect," a model of participation used by ActionAid, is explicitly based on Freirian principles,[65] as are some of the International Budget Partnership's projects on participation in health and education.[66]

Freire's pedagogy rejected what he termed a "banking notion of education," in which reality is treated as static and unchangeable, and knowledge is deposited into students by the teacher. Rather, he calls for a constant humanizing praxis—*conscientizao*—of progressively engaging students in dialogical practice to transform the injustice, exploitation, and oppression that dehumanize not only them but also their oppressors.[67]

Dialogue, in a Freirian model, is not merely a tactic of participatory approaches—a way to engage community members in a particular task, for example.[68] Rather it allows for people to deliberate collectively and come to decisions that reflect recognition of others as equals. Further, the process of dialogue should recognize how their environments shape their attitudes toward themselves, which in turn may affect risky or health-seeking behavior, for example. A rights framework can then provide tools to change those attitudes—not as conventional individual behavior modification but as part of a larger challenge to the structures that condition the way we think about ourselves, or treat ourselves, with less than dignity. And educating young children, before their minds are hardened with hatred and learned indifference, is the best way to promote a future that does not merely repeat the past.

Concluding Reflections

At an international meeting relating to participation in HRBAs in the context of maternal health, one participant noted that some donors and governments are wary that rights-based approaches are really about "radicalizing the poor and re-making the world." I would argue that this is indeed what HRBAs and human rights frameworks more broadly *are*—or should be. Yet recognizing the complexity of the ways in which different forms of power keep us from seeking the change that justice would demand, the true demands of meaningful participation, can be daunting and leave us feeling that no effort is enough. Nevertheless, just as I suggested at the end of Chapter 5, we should not allow the complexity of the challenge to discourage taking action within a rights framework. And Peru is a good example of what can be done.

Imagine if instead of needing to tell the indigenous women going to health facilities in Puno to "stand up for your rights" against a doctor or other provider, these women were raised in homes, taught in schools, and lived a society where they were already treated in law and practice as full human beings with rights. That culture of rights and equality is the ultimate goal of applying a human rights framework to health. It was because we recognized this was not the case in Peru that we designed a model of accompaniment so that these women would not be alone. Of course, addressing the root causes of those deep social inequalities calls for much broader strategies, including fostering critical rights consciousness from childhood. Yet meaningful incremental change can be achieved over time, and setbacks and violations can also destabilize entrenched interests and spur positive change.

Where you start the story has theoretical commitments, and it is important to note that Lupita's standing up to the doctor did not begin in that interaction. I was living in Peru at the end of the 1990s when my friend the late Giulia Tamayo, a human rights lawyer, led a human rights investigation revealing that the autocratic regime of President Alberto Fujimori was responsible for systematically sterilizing more than a quarter of a million, overwhelmingly indigenous, women. The brutal conditions under which the sterilizations took place were matched by brazen measures used to secure massive numbers of women in the program, including the "sterilization fairs" and the imposition of quotas on health providers across the country.[69] These offenses were detailed in reports by the Peru office of Latin American Committee for the Defense of the Rights of Women (CLADEM Perú) and the Defensoría. In conjunction with the reports, Giulia and colleagues brought a case, *Mamérita Mestanza v. Peru*, to the Inter-American Commission on Human Rights, which in turn led to successful law-reform campaigns.[70] *Mamérita Mestanza v. Peru* ended in a friendly settlement, with the government of Peru promising both reparations and policy changes.[71] To date, few reparations have been paid and the intellectual architects of this scheme have so far eluded criminal culpability.

The sterilization revelations did, however, create an enormous scandal in Peru and abroad, which led to the destabilization of deeply entrenched interests and the surfacing of conflicts that had been suppressed in Peruvian society. For example, USAID, which had underwritten the government's family-planning program, hired the Population Council to write a report that feebly concluded that there had been lapses in quality of care.[72] Human rights advocates would have none of this, however, asserting that the sterilizations were representative of pervasive structural violence and discrimination against women—in particular indigenous women—in public health services across Peru which, in turn, reflected the deep divisions in the broader society.

The exposure of forced sterilizations also led to tremendous social mobilization of *campesina* women. In one particularly affected area, an Association of the Victims of Forced Sterilizations (Asociación de Mujeres víctimas de esterilizaciones forzadas de Anta) was formed and the Broad Movement of Women (Movimiento Amplio de Mujeres, or MAM) took on a far more visible role in Peruvian society. Moreover, reproductive rights and health became part of the public agenda for democratization, which eventually led to Fujimori's resignation.

It is hard to calculate the overall impacts of this case, given the combination of noncompliance and the dramatic indirect material and symbolic impacts that were triggered. Yet it is a powerful illustration of a number of the themes in this chapter and this book: how ESC and CP violations are inextricably intertwined; how patterns of health are related to social determinants; how health systems reflect the values and norms in the overall society; how human rights approaches differ from conventional ones, which might categorize these abuses as lapses in quality of care; how the accountability in a rights framework goes beyond individual providers to systemic issues that are both legal and political; and how participation must be combined with information, as well as effective redress, if it is to produce transformation rather than alienation.

It took an outside investigation to trigger the destabilization of structures long insulated against political accountability—to reveal to indigenous women the degree of injustice to which they were being condemned by social norms, the animal-like treatment they received at the hands of those entrusted with their care, and the distorted mirror being held up to them in the larger Peruvian society. However, just as a judicial decision may trigger a reconfiguration of expectations and actions in India or Colombia, in this case the reports, litigation, and law reform contributed to thousands of indigenous women from throughout Peru, appropriating a sense of their own subjectivity, of being part of that society, and of having claims to rights. In some cases, indigenous women even ran for and won parliamentary seats and were able to participate in the public decisions that affected the lives and well-being of the people living in their communities.

It was in the wake of the forced sterilization revelations that women's health and rights groups began more systematic programs to raise awareness among *campesina* women about their reproductive rights. The health promoters we worked with in Puno, as noted at the beginning of the chapter, had been collaborating on such a program, "ReproSalud" previously, and then had self-selected to obtain even greater knowledge with respect to human rights through the CARE program. The Defensoría, in turn, had the institutional mandate, expertise, and capacity to address SRH rights.

Thus, as I have stressed throughout this chapter, meaningful participation that fosters social accountability and critical consciousness does not occur in a vacuum. It occurs in a specific social and historical context. Revelations of abuses can create moments of societal epiphany, but those moments need to be built on to change opportunity structures and, in turn, the way people act. Transformative social change requires changing relationships across the circle of accountability and creating spaces for participation in institutions and networks at local, national, and even global levels. And it takes time to develop critical consciousness—critical consciousness about the way our societies are organized, how our health systems are functioning, and ultimately what we as diverse people in diverse communities need in order to live lives of equal dignity.

Chapter 7

Shades of Dignity: Equality and Nondiscrimination

The law, in its majestic equality, forbids the rich as well as the poor
to sleep under bridges, to beg in the streets, and to steal bread.
—Anatole France, *Le Lys Rouge*, 1849

The position of women will not be improved as long as the
underlying causes of discrimination against women, and of their
inequality, are not effectively addressed. The lives of women and
men must be considered in a contextual way, and measures adopted
towards a real transformation of opportunities, institutions and
systems so that they are no longer grounded in historically
determined male paradigms of power and life patterns.
—UN Committee on the Elimination of Discrimination
Against Women, 2004

I met Nomkhosi's mother, Zondi, in 2013, in an impoverished, semirural area
of KwaZulu-Natal province in South Africa. KwaZulu-Natal is the birthplace
of the Inkatha Freedom Party (IFP) and Zondi lived not far from some of
the battles and massacres that had taken place in the early 1990s between the
IFP and African National Congress (ANC) members. Political violence in the
region, referred to as the "unofficial war" between the IFP and ANC, killed
an estimated 20,000 people between the mid-1980s and the late 1990s. The
violence had a drastic impact on the everyday lives of the people living in
KwaZulu-Natal and is a reality often overlooked in the sometimes overly

plasticized versions of South Africa's peaceful transition from apartheid to democracy.[1]

Zondi was sixty-two when I interviewed her; she supplemented her pension by selling sweets and chips at a local school. When I came to interview her at her house, we met her along the way. She moved slowly and deliberately on the hilly, unpaved road, her heavy body showing some of the toll that her difficult life had taken. Her daughter, Nomkhosi, had died a senseless death caused by childbirth complications. Seven years after Nomkhosi's death, Zondi's husband had been gruesomely murdered—his body mutilated and parts removed in what the family believed to be a ritual *muti* killing, not uncommon in certain parts of rural South Africa.[2] Zondi was left to raise her granddaughter alone, in addition to caring for other children. There was no accountability for her husband's murder or even the slightest official acknowledgment of the senselessness of her daughter's death. In a life lived largely under apartheid, however, Zondi seemed well-accustomed to impunity.

Nomkhosi had appeared to be healthy at birth; she started to crawl at a normal age and was beginning to walk at close to a year. But the muscles in one of her legs did not function properly, making that leg drag behind her when she walked and preventing her from running normally. When she was a toddler, her parents sent her to a government hospital for six months, and she returned with special shoes and crutches that allowed her to get around. But there was no improvement in the underlying condition, and her parents were never given a formal diagnosis. Despite her disability, Nomkhosi was by all accounts very active. She cooked and did the washing and, according to Zondi, was the most helpful of her children in doing household chores.

Nomkhosi's disability resulted in her getting little education. Because Zondi and her husband were worried about Nomkhosi navigating along the hilly dirt roads and through the traffic to get to the school, she started her studies only as a teenager and she got only three and a half years of schooling. School cannot have been easy for Nomkhosi, physically or emotionally. Starting so late had placed her at an enormous disadvantage. And, by all accounts, the other kids at school teased and bullied her relentlessly because of her disability and comparatively older age. Her mother said she was able to protect herself when the other kids physically tormented her, but no doubt the daily dose of cruelty took an emotional toll.

Yet when Nomkhosi became pregnant, the decision to drop out was not her own. In South Africa, it was not official policy that pregnant girls could not attend school, as it is in many neighboring African countries.[3] However, Nomkhosi's parents, like many others, stopped her from going to school, fearing stigma and further marginalization. Zondi didn't know, or didn't want to say, whether Nomkhosi was forced to have sex with the boy—who lived in the same impoverished semirural area—or whether it had been consensual, the result of efforts to attract a boy's desire and affection in spite of her physical difference.

The fine line between being treated as asexual versus being victimized by sexual abuse is a reality that girls (and boys) with physical and mental disabilities navigate throughout their lives. A 2012 global study published in the *Lancet* found that children with disabilities are almost three times more likely to experience sexual violence than their nondisabled peers.[4] Yet disabled adolescents should be able to explore and enjoy their sexuality just as any others do. In this case, whatever the reason for her pregnancy may have been—whether consensual or forced—by the age of eighteen, Nomkhosi was pregnant and had dropped out of school.

The ill-informed preconceptions of health providers in South Africa further disadvantaged Nomkhosi. Although gains have been made in recent years to improve the number of women using prenatal services in public facilities in South Africa, the quality of such services continues to be low.[5] Further, a high incidence of disrespect and abuse in health facilities in South Africa has been documented.[6] Given that Nomkhosi had the additional and stigmatizing disadvantages of being both young and disabled, it is unsurprising that she did not attend prenatal checkups during her pregnancy.

Recall the discussion in Chapter 4 regarding how an HRBA transforms consideration of the lack of AAAQ of care from being a matter of individual idiosyncrasy to a responsibility of the government. The findings of a 2012 pilot study conducted in Tanzania revealed a fascinating dichotomy in this regard. Although community perceptions attributed lack of use of reproductive health services by disabled women to lack of physical accessibility, the disabled women themselves regarded stigma and discrimination as the greatest barriers.[7] In this case, the combination of marginalization related to disability and a lack of youth-friendly, quality SRH care, may have proven fatal. Had Nomkhosi attended prenatal checks, the doctors at the hospital where she delivered would have been more familiar with her case and risk factors, and it is possible that the critical mistakes that cost her her life might have been prevented.

The surgical option of cesarean delivery is not necessarily indicated for a disabled woman, unless there is further evidence of physical inability to use the necessary muscles. Yet the doctors at the public hospital where she delivered simply assumed Nomkhosi would not be able to push the baby out vaginally and scheduled her for a cesarean delivery. Nomkhosi gave birth to a healthy girl but died of complications four days later. Nomkhosi may have had pregnancy-induced high blood pressure or some other condition detectable during antenatal care, which predisposed her to thromboembolic events,[8] such as strokes. She was left to lie in bed without any effort to ambulate her for four days after her cesarean surgery, mobilization that would be required for any person who was unable to get up and walk on his or her own, in order to prevent the risk of circulation-related complications. In the end, it appears that Nomkhosi may have suffered an ischemic stroke, which was exacerbated by or produced fluid on the brain. She became incoherent, calling out repeatedly to her mother in muddled, panicked tones that would become permanently etched in Zondi's memory.

Nomkhosi's death was the result of a series of deprivations of choice in her life, coupled with an indifferent and unresponsive health system. Nomkhosi's short life had been marked by intersecting discrimination on the basis of race, gender, and disability, compounded by poverty, which left her parents with few options for providing education and health care. Her story is not atypical—for South Africa or elsewhere. As has been discussed throughout the examples in this book, it is invariably women, racial and ethnic minorities, disabled persons, and other marginalized populations who are not only disproportionately represented among the most economically disadvantaged but also consequently denied agency and effective enjoyment of rights.[9] And in the context of South Africa, inequalities based on gender and class and other axes of identity are exponentially aggravated by the still everprevalent racial discrimination.

Postapartheid South Africa is a country of extreme contrasts, and seemingly incompatible truths. One of the most progressive constitutions in the world coexists with entrenched racial, social, and economic inequalities. Even having the highest Gini index in the world (63.1 in 2009)[10]—a measure of economic inequality—cannot convey the starkly visible extremes of ostentatious consumption and abject poverty. Under apartheid's brutal regime, forced evictions, relocations, and segregation kept the rich and poor, as well as different racial groups, tidily separate. Slums and informal settlements still separate the rich and poor, but today you can also find posh neighborhoods, just minutes away from the unbearably bleak squalor of slums.

Twenty years after apartheid was formally ended, South Africa remains a profoundly unequal and divided country. Apartheid was an intricate, multifaceted economic, political, legal, and social system built over decades, through which racial superiority and inferiority were systematically instilled alongside political and economic oppression. And, unfortunately, in today's South Africa, as the Constitutional Court found in a case involving housing rights, "the Constitution's promise of dignity and equality for all remains a distant dream."[11]

The foundational principle of human rights is that all human beings are equal in rights, dignity, and worth.[12] As noted in previous chapters, the right to health requires some equalization in both care and the preconditions of health, for which the state is responsible. Moreover, health reflects the enjoyment of many other human rights, including social determinants of health. Therefore, as we have discussed, in a human rights framework, the state has an obligation for leveling the playing field, as well as addressing underlying inequalities and discrimination.

In public health, there is increasing evidence that social inequality, not just the absolute deprivation we focused on in Chapter 2, is bad for our health.[13] That is, the steeper the gradient of the social ladder, the worse the outcomes are in terms of life expectancy, infant mortality, crime rates, and a host of other indicators.[14] Thus, the WHO Commission on Social Determinants of Health has suggested that addressing health inequalities requires a two-pronged approach, which includes (1) reducing exposures and vulnerabilities linked to position on the social ladder and (2) reducing the social gradient itself.[15]

Historically, human rights law has been most concerned with identifying those who are consistently kept low on the proverbial "social ladder" and with reducing the exposures and vulnerabilities—because of subordination based on gender, race, or disability, for example—that keep them there. In so doing, as I have discussed, a human rights approach highlights that poverty is not only about lack of income, as it was traditionally conceived in development practice but also about relations that discriminate against and disempower certain people. "The poor" have individual faces, and it is no coincidence that 70 percent of those faces belong to women—women like Nomkhosi and Zondi.[16] Further, a rights perspective enables us to see that the ways in which certain people are kept low on the ladder represent not inherent vulnerability but active processes of exclusion and marginalization through laws, institutional arrangements, and cultural norms, as well as the responses of social systems. Thus a human rights framework calls for attention to disparities—including disaggregated data—as opposed to merely aggregate advances in health and development.[17]

In the first part of this chapter, I set out how concepts of formal and substantive equality and nondiscrimination are presently understood under international human rights law and how they relate to some of the questions we currently face in public health and health systems. Just as we saw with respect to other key concepts of a human rights framework—accountability and participation—the application of these concepts is far from formulaic. Interpretations of equality and nondiscrimination necessarily reflect deeply held understandings about justice and how we are the same as and different from one another. And they have implications for priority setting and state obligations to "level the playing field" in a rights approach to health.

The demands of human rights with respect to reducing the social gradient itself—that is, creating greater social and income equality in society—are less well developed. Conventionally, the human rights community has been reticent with regard to economic prescriptions. Nevertheless, I argue in the second part of this chapter that a human rights framework must concern itself with these broader questions of social and economic policy if we hope to transform some of the power relations that systematically deprive certain people and groups of their health and other rights.

Finally, in the third part of this chapter, I explore more deeply some of the principles mentioned in earlier chapters, in terms of the demands for equality in health-planning and priority-setting processes. In health, how badly off a person is in terms of health status matters as well. For example, as we saw in Nomkhosi's case, a disabled person may not be able to translate income into effective enjoyment of rights in the same way as a nondisabled person.[18] Moreover, competing interests, as well as values, need to be balanced in setting health priorities. Therefore, we need to consider fair processes for weighing these other dimensions of inequalities as part of setting priorities in health justly.

Unpacking the Demands of Nondiscrimination and Equality Under International Law

The concept of equality and its relation to nondiscrimination is complex as well as comparative. Law and ethical theory, as well as other fields, contest what is important about equality. Determining what differences should be taken into account between individuals and populations and in what ways—in short, what is fair—is not only controversial but speaks to deep-seated assumptions about us as human beings, as well as about the responsibilities of the state. For example, should deaf patients have the right to sign-language translators in any health establishment they choose to attend, or is that an extra concession for which the state is not responsible? Is there a difference in providing such a service to deaf patients versus the responsibility to ensure access by all patients to language interpretation at the point of care, including for those languages very rarely found in the catchment area? Should a patient with a rare, life-threatening condition receive treatment when the state may still not be providing everyone with basic water and sanitation and primary health care? Is it permissible for HIV/AIDS patients to be treated in newly built, air-conditioned buildings, with better staffing, medical supplies, and laboratories, while other patients amass in the crumbling decrepitude of government health facilities across much of Sub-Saharan Africa? Is it acceptable to have different quality of care for paying versus free patients at a facility, if at least in theory the paying patients are subsidizing the indigents? These issues are playing out in countries across the world to define the contours of a right to health in specific countries, and rights-based approaches to health more broadly. My aim in this chapter is to explore how these legal concepts—nondiscrimination, formal equality, and substantive equality—relate to different real-world issues that we face in health systems and public health today.

Elements of Nondiscrimination

Under international law, all human rights—including the right to health—are to be guaranteed "without discrimination of any kind as to race, colour, sex, language, religion, political or other opinion, national or social origin, property, birth or other status."[19] "Other status" has been interpreted to include characteristics such as caste, disability, and sexual identity, which I discussed as critical axes of identity in previous chapters. For example, South Africa's constitution makes explicit that "prohibited grounds" also include disability, along with pregnancy, marital status, ethnic or social origin, sexual orientation, age, conscience, belief, culture, language, and birth.[20]

The CESCR has defined discrimination as "any distinction, exclusion, restriction or preference or other differential treatment that is directly or indirectly based on the prohibited grounds of discrimination and which has the intention or effect of nullifying or impairing the recognition, enjoyment or exercise, on an equal footing, of [ICESCR] rights."[21] The scope for understanding that it is the effect of discrimination, without a requirement for intent, that is crucial to whether people can enjoy their rights, is broader under international law than under some domestic law, including the laws of the United States. For example, a health policy that requires out-of-pocket payment may be neutral on its face but have the effect of discriminating against women because of a "disproportionate impact" on them—as women tend to have less access to formal employment and earn lower wages than men.

Prohibited Grounds

Under international law, health status and disability can both be "prohibited grounds" of discrimination. The idea that differentiation must be "based on" a "prohibited ground" in order to count as discrimination has been criticized. As Gillian MacNaughton argues, determining whether differential treatment occurs because of a specific trait can be complicated and may impose undue burdens of proof. For example, in a case of forced sterilization in Namibia, the court found that plaintiffs had not demonstrated that the women were sterilized because they were HIV positive.[22] Similarly, in trying to establish national-level culpability in Peru, civil society advocates have had difficulty persuading prosecutors that the women were sterilized because they were indigenous.

However, as Catharine MacKinnon has written, "Group membership does not simply distinguish humans; it is part of being human."[23] In practice, focusing on individual as opposed to group rights is often not the best way to achieve meaningful empowerment of people from disadvantaged groups. The factors that allow people to convert resources into the effective enjoyment of the right to health generally often need to be addressed structurally. For example, development programs based on equalizing individuals, such as through cash transfers to promote individual behavior change, can at times preserve and even legitimize structural inequalities. A study of the impact of conditional cash transfers (CCTs) in Latin America found that in disbursing monetary awards to poor individuals, governments were given an alibi to actually scale back on the provision of goods. The study author concludes that in Latin America, the idea that CCTs, "might facilitate a broader process of redistribution, reducing inequality and all but eliminating poverty, does not hold in principle, and still less in practice."[24]

The UN committees that monitor compliance with international human rights treaties have generally adopted a flexible approach to nondiscrimination, examining treatment of individuals, groups of individuals and collectivities. A committee might examine, for instance, whether people within a group receive similar treatment, and then compare it to treatment of other groups in society.[25]

In a number of countries, including South Africa, there is a constitutional presumption that discrimination on one of the listed grounds is unfair unless a defendant establishes the contrary. Moreover, courts in South Africa and other contexts, as well as treaty-monitoring committees at the international level, have applied different levels of scrutiny to assess the reasonableness of differentiation when they believe fundamental issues of human dignity are at stake.[26]

But how far might the concept of nondiscrimination be applied to wealth-based differentiations relating to health-care access or background social conditions? For example, can we consider user fees or premiums that are uniform across incomes to constitute discrimination against poor people (as well as the potential disproportionate impact on other defined groups)? The CESCR has clarified that payment for health-care services has to be based on the principle of equity, ensuring that poorer households are not disproportionately burdened with health expenses as compared to richer households.[27] Uniform fees that pose unduly high burdens on the poor violate equity principles. Arguably, they also discriminate against poor people under some circumstances because of their effect in producing obstacles to accessing even essential care.

Formal Equality: Connections Between Equality and Universality

A claim for formal equality is a claim for equal treatment under the law in relation to another individual or group and not a claim in relation to a particular outcome. Individuals or groups that are alike should be treated alike, according to their actual characteristics that are relevant, rather than assumptions or prejudices. For example, in *United States v. Windsor*, the U.S. Supreme Court found the federal Defense of Marriage Act unconstitutional, as it discriminated against same-sex couples in relation to federal benefits they could obtain.[28]

Formal equality has been pivotal in human rights struggles—from anti-slavery to civil rights, from women's suffrage to LGBT movements. As discussed in Chapter 1, achieving formal equality for different groups has in many ways reconfigured our socially constituted understanding of who is fully human and who therefore possesses all of the dignity accorded to those already recognized as full human beings. The law's recognition of equal rights has a crucial effect on the diffusion of social norms, as well as on people's self-perceptions, as those who have been historically denied them readily assert. For example, when laws change to become more progressive—as happened with the 2014 Indian Supreme Court's NALSA decision regarding the acknowledgment of a third gender—they inscribe a new understanding not just of others as fully human but also of what being human means and, in turn, require us to think about who we ourselves are.[29]

Formal equality implies that the right to health is only meaningful if its content can be universalized within a specific polity, as in Kant's prescription for dignity in the "categorical imperative"—that the rules we make to govern our behavior be universally applicable.[30] That is, all patients with a given condition should be treated the same. This has enormous implications in terms of staging governmental efforts to achieve UHC, as well as for judicial enforcement of health rights, imposing a presumption that everyone should be entitled to a certain level of care before some people get access to expanded sets of interventions, as a government moves toward providing UHC.[31]

In addition, when a court enforces a right to a given treatment or service, it should be something that can reasonably be provided to everyone who is similarly situated. This does not necessarily imply that we need to accept resource constraints as a given, or what the state is currently providing within its current health budget. However, it is also not "just" for medical care decisions to be allocated without any attempt to think of similarly situated patients within the society and the inherent opportunity costs of enforcing one individual's health rights. In his studies of judicialization of health rights in Brazil, Octavio Ferraz has argued that judicialization has led to a "first-come first-served" approach—that is, those who know their rights and take steps to claim them through the courts—which favors people who are relatively better off financially—criteria that should be morally irrelevant in determining access to health benefits and which have the effect of compounding, rather than ameliorating, layers of exclusion.[32]

Prior to the T-760 structural judgment on the health system, then-Associate Justice Rodrigo Uprimny, commented in a 2004 concurrence (T-654/04) that the Colombian Constitutional Court should consider the question of treatment universalizability—whether all people can access a treatment in similar circumstances—in order for the decision to be consistent with principles of equality and the realization of social rights. Otherwise, Uprimny argued, a judicial decision was sanctioning a "privilege" rather than a "right," as few could access the treatment because of its cost.[33]

Substantive Equality: What Counts When We Are Measuring Fairness?

Formal equality, although critical, is radically inadequate to achieve equal enjoyment of ESC rights, including health, and indeed can give the illusion that fairness exists "without addressing underlying inequalities in power, access, and socioeconomic and political circumstances."[34] Prohibitions on substantive discrimination therefore call for adopting "measures to prevent, diminish and eliminate the conditions or attitudes which cause substantive or de facto discrimination."[35] The question in achieving substantive equality is not "How do we treat all people in the same way?"; rather, it is "What is required for people in fundamentally different circumstances to actually have equal enjoyment of their rights?"

Linking the distinct notions of equality to the obligations of the social state of law, as opposed to the traditional liberal state, the Colombian Constitutional Court articulates the distinction:

> Formal equality requires equal treatment under the laws and regulations and starts from the premise that everyone is free and equal. . . . It requires impartiality from the state and proscribes any unjustified differentiation. . . . Substantive equality, on the other hand, starts from the recognition of inequalities in society that are not merely a result of natural causes, but also of social, cultural, and political arrangements, which constitute obstacles to the substantive enjoyment of constitutional rights. . . . The principle of substantive equality demands that the state adopt measures to counter such inequalities and offer everyone opportunities to exercise their liberties, develop their talents and overcome economic hardship.[36]

Table 7.1 Some Considerations in Formal Versus Substantive Equality

Formal equality	Substantive equality
• Are all people accorded full dignity and the same health and other rights under the law, regardless of their race, gender, ethnicity, sexual orientation, and other factors?	• Does the legal and policy framework recognize that because of background conditions, historic power relations, and personal characteristics, differently situated people have differential needs in order to effectively enjoy their health and other rights on an equal footing with others in practice?
• Does the legal and policy framework treat everyone with a given condition or health need in the same way by universalizing the health-related entitlements to preconditions and care in the health system?	• Does the legal, policy, and institutional framework provide for affirmative measures to ensure disadvantaged groups' effective enjoyment of health and other rights on an equal footing with others in practice?

Under international law, the importance of substantive equality has also been recognized. For instance, in the Alyne da Silva case, described previously in this book, the CEDAW Committee found the government of Brazil responsible for a lack of appropriate maternal health services, which had a "differential impact on Alyne's right to life" and a failure to meet Alyne's "specific, distinctive health needs" during her pregnancy. The committee also found Brazil responsible for a failure to address "her status as a woman of African descent and her socio-economic background," thus articulating the importance of examining intersecting patterns of discrimination based on race and gender, for example, in assessing substantive equality.[37] The CEDAW Committee has also articulated a model of "transformative equality," which calls for addressing the causes and consequences of substantive inequalities, and for redistributing power that favors men and disadvantages women.[38]

Achieving substantive equality often requires adopting temporary or permanent "positive measures"—for example, with respect to racial and ethnic minorities, women, people from scheduled and lower castes, and people with disabilities—to combat the constraining effects of socially constructed disadvantage and hierarchies.[39] The failure to take such measures—inaction—has been interpreted under various constitutions to constitute substantive discrimination. Similarly, under the Convention on the Rights of Persons with Disabilities (CRPD), discrimination includes the "denial of reasonable accommodation," which is defined as "necessary and appropriate modification and adjustments not imposing a disproportionate or undue burden, where needed in a particular case, to ensure to persons with disabilities the enjoyment or exercise on an equal basis with others of all human rights and fundamental freedoms."[40]

In Nomkhosi's case, such accommodations would not have been hard. A human rights framework goes beyond issues of quality of care during her delivery and even her prenatal care, including seeing Nomkhosi's needs from her perspective, as a whole person, who required education, including sexuality education, and other rights to be able to exercise full self-governance.

However, more generally, what constitutes "reasonable accommodations" and "disproportionate or undue burden" is contested. For example, in *Eldridge* (decided under Canadian law before the CRPD entered into force), the Canadian Supreme Court determined that the government's failure to provide for sign-language interpreters when hearing-impaired people receive health care infringes on the equality guarantee in the Canadian Charter of Rights and Freedoms.[41] Yet the majority of such cases have not prevailed in Canadian courts; the claim has been interpreted as relating to a benefit that the law has not conferred—as something different and "extra"—rather than as something that enables substantively equal access to a benefit that the law has already recognized.[42] That may change. Virtually all initial cases brought to the Committee on the Elimination of Discrimination Against Persons with Disabilities under the CRPD have involved this issue in relation to employment, with implications for health.

These are not always easy questions. Stating abstract principles about the immediate obligation to redress discrimination and substantive inequality may be helpful for litigation and advocacy in some cases, but it often does not facilitate the kinds of changes in social perceptions and reframing of social contracts that are necessary to realize diverse people's health rights in the long term.

Further, health inequalities are not always inequities. The CESCR sets out that states that have ratified the ICESCR have a core obligation to ensure an "equitable distribution of health facilities, goods and services."[43] To determine which inequalities are inequities in a human rights framework, we need to examine how those inequalities are produced and, in turn, whether governments and other actors can be held accountable for redress. For example, in developed countries, women have higher life expectancies than men. According to data from the WHO in 2012, the life expectancy at birth of a man in Japan is 80 years, while that of a woman in Japan is 87, and in the United States, 76 compared with 81.[44] That does not imply injustice.

Goran Dahlgren and Margaret Whitehead's famous argument that "health inequalities count as inequities when they are avoidable, unnecessary and unfair"[45] does not get us terribly far because there is little agreement as to what is avoidable, unnecessary, and unfair. From a human rights perspective, an "equitable distribution of health facilities, goods, and services" arguably would be the one necessary condition to enable disadvantaged groups to effectively enjoy health rights on an equal basis with others. This approach, which would require dramatically restructuring institutional arrangements in many countries, diverges greatly from what is generally done in public health and development under the rubric of "equity" in health financing or programming.

But the human rights community has not always been forthright about how to approach the tensions between public health maximization and distributive justice. For example, in maternal health, because of the added cost of overcoming inherent limitations in infrastructure, transportation, and staffing, providing remote populations with substantively equal care would require substantially more resources per person compared to providing services for urban women. If budgets remain fixed and additional resources are not available, shifting resource allocations in a budgeting process to address the compounded inequalities that Alyne and others like her face would mean that more women would probably die in the short and medium term, and the aggregate goal of reducing deaths would not be accomplished as quickly. Again, we need not defer to governments reflexively about expenditure decisions. However, some resource constraints are a reality. I believe that in human rights we can go beyond incantations of abstract principles, and we can make valid arguments with respect to the path to UHC and, more broadly, based on both normative considerations of what is required to produce fair chances and engage in frank discussions with other disciplines about tradeoffs.

The Social Gradient: Income and Wealth Inequality in a Human Rights Framework

Historically human rights has focused on nondiscrimination as a CP rights issue, and more recently, with the burgeoning of ESC rights work, has applied the lens of nondiscrimination to examine why certain people are kept at the bottom of social structures. Questions relating to the social gradient itself and to the economic policies and tradeoffs that shape income and wealth inequality—which in turn influence different people's possibilities for enjoyment of health—have remained far less explored.[46] These are typically thought of as "economic questions," beyond the appropriate purview of human rights, although some progressive economists have begun to look at macroeconomic policies and their effects on rights.[47] In this section, I explore what kinds of social and income inequality are of greatest concern from a human rights perspective, as well as how a human rights framework might guide steps to address those inequities.

The Case for Income Equality from Public Health

Patterns of income and wealth equality and inequality are social determinants of health, as noted by the WHO Commission on Social Determinants of Health.[48] And there is ample empirical evidence that equality is generally better for a society's health, as it appears that greater social equality facilitates long-term economic growth as well as other societal benefits. For example, a 2009 meta-analysis of how inequality affects health suggested "the existence of a threshold of income inequality beyond which adverse impacts on health begin to emerge" within countries (Gini 0.3 in this study).[49] The Gini coefficient contrasts actual income and property distribution in a society, with a perfectly equal distribution, and the value varies from zero (complete equality) to one (complete inequality). The authors of this study, as well as others reaching similar conclusions, have argued that the impacts of increased inequality are not just the result of a relatively larger portion of the population living in poverty but also the result of "spillover effects" that affect the health of the better off in society as well as the worse off.

In their review of research, Richard Wilkinson and Kate Pickett also found that "almost all problems which are more common at the bottom of the social ladder are more common in more unequal societies."[50] It is not just ill-health and violence—measurable by indicators such as life expectancy, infant mortality, homicides, and imprisonment rates—but also level of trust, mental illness (including drug and alcohol addiction), children's educational performance, teenage births, and social mobility.[51] Evidence suggests that "even a 'modest' association can amount to a considerable population burden" compared with the countries having Gini coefficients lower than 0.3.[52]

Consider that South Africa had a Gini coefficient of 0.631 in 2009, more than twice as high as 0.3, the level at which adverse effects become evident in society.[53]

However, the Gini coefficient measures relative, not absolute, wealth. So it is possible for the Gini coefficient of a country such as South Africa to rise (because of increasing inequality of income) while the number of people in absolute poverty decreases. Changing income inequality, measured by Gini coefficients, can also be caused by factors such as changes in population (baby booms, demographic transitions and longer life spans, the division of extended family households into nuclear families—as poverty is counted at household level—or emigration and immigration) in addition to income mobility.[54] So policies aimed at changes in the coefficient may not necessarily improve the lot of the poorest and most disadvantaged members of society, or their health, as we would want from a human rights perspective concerned with substantive equality.[55]

Equality and Justice

Understanding the relationship between social equality and dignity is complex, and this book in no way pretends to set out comprehensive economic or ethical arguments for specific models of equality. Nonetheless, I do believe that it is essential for the human rights community to grapple with what is normatively acceptable in terms of a social gradient and with the tradeoffs to be made in moving in that direction. I also believe that the principles and elements of a human rights framework, which have been outlined in this book, do indeed allow some judgments in that regard.

We must understand that both relative inequality and absolute deprivation are important. As I have discussed, deprivation of a minimum core of ESC rights, including health, in turn deprives people of the ability to exercise meaningful self-government in their lives. For example, Bangladesh had approximately the same Gini index (which is the Gini coefficient multiplied by 100) as Switzerland in 2010—Bangladesh, 32.1; Switzerland, 29.6—yet the very poor in Bangladesh face far greater deprivations of their health rights.[56]

Anthony Atkinson, however, has argued that as the general level of income rises in a country, we should be more concerned about inequality precisely because a rich nation can better afford to implement policies that promote equality.[57] For example, in South Africa, Zondi's living situation was nowhere near as desperate as that of Happiness, in Malawi. Zondi lived in a two-room house with a cement floor, a tin roof, a door, and furniture; she had electricity and even a television; and a water tap and latrine were both within 100 meters of the house. But in 2012, South Africa's GDP per capita was more than 27 times that of Malawi.[58] In human rights, the concept of using "maximum available resources" to realize health and other ESC rights points to expanded obligations as countries become wealthier.

The liberal philosopher John Rawls outlined a prioritarian theory of distributive justice, which underpins much thinking about contemporary human rights as well as constitutional interpretation.[59] Rawls proposed that for a society's institutional arrangements to be considered fair, in addition to every person having an equal claim to basic liberties, social and economic inequalities that are permitted by institutional arrangements must satisfy two conditions: (1) they must be attached to positions and offices open to all under conditions of fair equality of opportunity and (2) they must be to the greatest benefit of the least advantaged members of society.[60] Under this view, if through the tax and other regulations minimum health- and social-protection packages can be offered to the poor in South Africa as a result of economic growth, it is acceptable that the same regulatory schemes allow for greater enrichment by the already well-off.

But this does not mean that so long as the poorest in South Africa are a little better off, policies that greatly improve the lots of the best off, thereby vastly increasing income inequality, are fair or consistent with a "just ordering of society."[61] For example, average household income tripled between 2000 and 2007 in South Africa, but it was disproportionally distributed to the very top of the social ladder.[62] Indeed in all of the so-called BRICS countries (Brazil, Russia, India, China, and South Africa), which are hailed for their strong economic growth, the evidence of growing inequalities is dismal from the standpoint of human rights. For example, in Russia, average household wealth has increased over sevenfold since 2000, and yet it has one of the greatest income inequalities in the world, with 110 billionaires owning 35 percent of all capital. In India, despite consistent economic growth of more than 5 percent annually over the same period, ActionAid reported that a shocking 47 percent of children under six face chronic malnutrition.[63]

Rawls put a limit on how much social inequality is acceptable by stating that there needs to be equality of opportunity attached to any positions of difference and it must be tied to equal enjoyment of liberties, which are essential to enable people to choose how to use resources. Many philosophers feel Rawls's theory did not go far enough toward establishing equality. For our purposes, the point is that placing limits on private greed as well as public lassitude is neither an "economic concern" beyond the purview of human rights nor merely a matter of individual moral debate untethered to principles that are central to a human rights framework.

Indeed, economic and social equality are inextricably linked to all of the elements of a human rights framework. In Chapter 6, for example, I noted that the preconditions for effective participation require, in Nancy Fraser's words, "the sort of rough equality that is inconsistent with systemically-generated relations of dominance and subordination."[64] As discussed in Chapter 5, accountability is also undermined by great income and wealth inequality.

And it is not a stretch to argue, based on the concept of everyone having equal dignity, that a human rights framework that takes substantive equality seriously calls for certain fiscal and economic policies, including the structure and level of taxation in a country, that reflect equal concern and respect for all.[65] As I discussed in Chapter 2, once we recognize that regardless of the legal and regulatory framework in place, there are implications for who gains and who loses and that there is simply no pre-societal—or pre-legal—distribution of goods, it frees us to see that we can reshape our institutional arrangements that are better suited to promoting the dignity and rights of all people in society.

Choices can be argued about on political or economic grounds and based on reliable evidence, but it is misleading to think of changing the tax structure as "taking from the wealthy." As Ronald Dworkin argues, "Taxation in many countries now is unjust, but because it takes too little, not too much. It does not deprive people of what is rightfully theirs; on the contrary it fails to provide the means of granting them what is rightfully theirs."[66]

Equality and Dignity

Enormous wealth inequalities, as well as absolute deprivation, undermine our capacity to see and treat our fellow citizens as full human beings. Think of the invisibility of the beggars at street corners or the doormen who hold doors open or the custodians who clean our public buildings. And just as the wealthy suffer health consequences in societies with great wealth inequality, so too do they suffer from dignity deprivations. As Dworkin writes, "the value of a life that is led with other people's money" often cannot make up for a dignity shortfall.[67]

It may be easier to see in societies that are not our own the repulsiveness of untrammeled material accumulation and the injustice that allows some people to use others as instruments for their own ends. South Africa is an easy target—the Ferraris racing past slums to get home to their mansions, the mine owners' wealth built on the backs of exploited workers. Yet in societies across the globe, including increasingly the United States, the rich build ever higher walls—both external and internal—to protect themselves and their wealth, and they end up imprisoning themselves in lives and politics that breed contempt for their own dignity as well as that of others.

As noted in Chapter 4, in Colombia, as in South Africa, extreme wealth inequality coexists with an emancipatory vision for substantive democracy laid out in the constitution of 1991. A judgment in 2013 interpreted legislation in such a way as to hold that no benefit in the pension regime for former legislators, judges, prosecutors, and certain others could exceed the equivalent of twenty-five minimum wages (about USD 7,610 each month in 2013) and held that permitting untrammeled relative inequality ran counter to the "social state of law" enshrined in the constitution:

> It is precisely in the context of macroeconomic and social decisions that different sectors of the population, by virtue of the principle of solidarity, assume reasonable burdens in order to permit excluded sectors to progressively be incorporated into the effective enjoyment of social progress, which will only be possible to achieve through the growing awareness of the necessity of cooperation and acting collectively to improve the lives of all Colombians and gradually overcome existing inequalities.[68]

In short, the sophistry that economic policy is beyond the concern of a human rights framework condemns human rights to a very restricted and palliative role in the face of egregious social inequalities that shape the possibilities for people to live lives of dignity and, in turn, have dramatic health consequences.

When Is One Situation Worse Than Another, and How to Decide?

Domains of Equality

What makes judging equality demands in health so complicated is that to figure out who is "worst off" and what inequalities are injustices requires going beyond socioeconomic questions. For example, although Rawls's theory of justice as fairness was undoubtedly the single most influential theory of distributive justice in the twentieth century, Kenneth Arrow and others pointed out that Rawls assumed for the sake of building his theory that everyone was in good health; consequently, it was impossible to ascertain from his theory whether a poor person in good health should be considered better off than a slightly economically better-off person who is ill.[69]

Amartya Sen has argued that income—and even Rawls's concept of primary goods (education, employment, and the like)—are not the right spaces in which to measure social inequalities. Rather than focusing on the means of living, Sen suggests, we should focus on the actual opportunities for living, doing, and being. He has proposed that we should measure inequalities in terms of capabilities—"the ability to achieve various combinations of functionings that we can compare and judge against each other."[70] Thus, for example, a disabled person such as Nomkhosi with the same income as a nondisabled person does not enjoy the same capabilities because he or she suffers from a "conversion handicap," a differential ability to convert resources into actual opportunities to enjoy good living—and to effectively enjoy rights.[71]

As Sen's argument implies, relative differences in income can translate into absolute differences in capabilities or in effective enjoyment of rights, including the right to health. That is, it is not so much what you have but what you can do with what you have. Capabilities are influenced by individual states of health and disability, but they are also heavily influenced by the nature of societal responses. That is, are schools, health facilities, goods, and services fully accessible in practice to persons with physical as well as mental disabilities? Are employment, housing, and transportation readily available to them? Thus, as human rights law recognizes, it is not just the incidence of a certain condition or disability but also the penalty that the person faces in his or her community and society that causes the suffering, as we saw in Nomkhosi's case.[72]

Judging Health Inequalities within a Human Rights Framework

I believe Sen's capability theory is generally compatible with a rights framework, and they both contrast with the utilitarian forms of priority setting that prevail in public health, as discussed earlier. For example, in judging inequalities in health, cost-utility analysis might compare the cost of treatment A with treatment B, where treatment is needed to generate one additional quality-adjusted life year (QALY). As explained in Chapter 4 in relation to a similar measure, disability-adjusted life years (DALYs), to calculate the QALYs of an intervention, each year in perfect health is assigned the value of 1.0 down to a value of 0.0 for death. Years that would not be lived in full health because of some impaired functioning are assigned a value between 0 and 1. Put very simplistically, the goal in public health is to select cost-effective interventions in order to maximize QALYs and to design public health plans based on the burden of disease in order to minimize DALYs.

The use of QALYs occurs at many levels, from hospitals and health insurance organizations to priority setting in national health systems.[73] Although they are unquestionably useful, QALYs will always favor treatment for relatively minor conditions that in aggregation sum up to lots of QALYs; conversely, they will always disfavor treating people who suffer from costly conditions who cannot achieve full or near-full recovery. Think, for example, of a patient with ALS or Huntington's disease or of a child with a rare degenerative disease. But disfavoring treatments for people with very serious conditions runs counter to other values we hold in society. And, as I point out throughout this book, a rights framework does not allow us to simply discard people whose care is not cost-effective in order to meet some fiscal objective. Moreover, not financing care for seriously ill people can have dramatic socioeconomic consequences as well, as patients with very serious conditions see themselves and their families driven into poverty, trying to pay for care that the state is not subsidizing.

Another reason we cannot rely solely on cost-utility measures in an HRBA to priority setting has also surfaced in previous chapters. The QALYs and DALYs reduce all suffering to a single quantitative scale based on survey data. As Jennifer Prah Ruger, a proponent of capabilities theory in health, notes, "One cannot quantifiably compare one individual's inability to hear or see with another's inability to bear children or to walk. These reductions in individuals' capabilities for functioning are qualitatively different and different people will have widely diverging views on which functional capability reduction is better or worse than the other."[74] And what of other dimensions of illness? How can we compare the suffering of a person with paranoid schizophrenia who struggles against the voices in his head day after day with that of a young amputee, who struggles every day to find new ways of relating to his body? As I noted in Chapter 3, our notions of health and illness, and in turn of suffering, are inherently contextualized. The loss of different capabilities has different meanings in different social contexts, and those differences will invariably inform how diverse people perceive the "badness" of their conditions, which sometimes involve multiple diseases or forms of disability.

Finally, as I discussed in Chapter 6, given certain conditions or internalized experiences of disempowerment, some people may not perceive their disability or impairment to be as great as it objectively is. For example, numerous studies comparing clinically observed with self-reported ill-health among pregnant women have found that women tend to "take for granted" even quite profound levels of fatigue, which are actually evidence of anemia.[75] Therefore, a credible rights (or capabilities) theory requires some objective account of how both biological and social conditions impede certain people from effectively enjoying their rights to health, as well as other rights.[76]

In his writing in the context of the great Bengal famine, Sen discusses how widows reported less ill-health than widowers, concluding, "Quiet acceptance of deprivation and bad fate affects the scale of dissatisfaction generated and the utilitarian calculus gives sanctity to that distortion."[77] That is, people's understanding of their own suffering are mediated by unjust power relations, including internalized domination, which may make them value themselves and how much they are suffering less than they should.[78] Thus, relying solely on subjective assessments of preferences and rating, through cost-utility measures, means that our evaluations of progress and priority setting in health may reinforce underlying inequalities.

The Importance of Fair Processes

If health and health inequalities are necessarily multidimensional concepts in a human rights framework and reasonable people can disagree about how to allocate scarce resources in health, then, as discussed in Chapter 4, we require a process for arriving at priority setting in health that does not depend solely on cost-utility measures or other technocratic measures that pretend to be value-free. Norman Daniels, Sen, and others all suggest the need for a process that allows for "reasoned public-policy decision-making in the face of multiple, and even conflicting, views on health."[79] I have discussed Daniels's framework for "Accountability for Reasonableness" previously, and argued that the criteria for a legitimate process that it sets out—publicity and transparency, relevance of reasons, opportunity for revision and appeals, and regulation and enforceability—are compatible with human rights.[80]

All of these ethical theories about making fair decisions—whether based on Rawls (as "Accountability for Reasonableness" is), Sen, or Jurgen Habermas—invest importance in the process of deliberation. Moreover, these processes are all based on the conception that human beings are capable of fair-minded and reasoned decision making under the appropriate circumstances and are not simply driven by preassigned identities. I have also noted that courts can, under certain circumstances, can play important roles in advancing deliberative democracy by requiring justification from the executive for its health decisions to those who are affected and in creating a space for broader public learning about societal values in relation to health-care rationing.[81]

It is important to stress, however, that assigning values and weights to different kinds of inequalities in health is not a one-off exercise. Processes for deliberation need to be institutionalized along with health-technology assessments and other evidence-based evaluations used in priority-setting resources. Moreover, institutionalization of those processes needs to be carefully designed and executed so that it does not merely provide a patina of participation to an otherwise closed process. In a rights framework, as discussed at length in Chapter 6, processes for determining which inequalities are truly inequities require not just "relevant grounds" for decision making, "partial rankings," or "incompletely theorized agreements." They also crucially demand justification to and meaningful participation by the people who will be affected. And empowering, as opposed to managerial, participation depends to a great extent on the context in which it occurs and what is up for contention. Thus meaningful participation is necessary to foster legitimate and fair outcomes in health decisions in a human rights approach. At the same time, as mentioned earlier, some degree of background equality in society is necessary to enable meaningful participation.

Concluding Reflections

Nelson Mandela's vision for a postapartheid South Africa as a society in which there would be human dignity, freedom, and equality staked a claim that the hatred between racial groups was not inevitable: "No one is born hating another person because of the color of his skin, or his background, or his religion. People must learn to hate, and if they can learn to hate, they can be taught to love."[82] Indeed, to believe that all people are born equal in dignity and rights, and in the possibility of a social and an international order in which everyone can enjoy their rights, requires that we believe that the hatred and dehumanization that underlies so much of the most egregious discrimination in the world is not inevitable. It also demands that we understand what it is to be a human being with dignity in a way that both incorporates and allows us to transcend our group identities, precisely so that we can engage in the kinds of reasoned deliberation that underpin rights-based priority-setting processes discussed in this book, and democracy more generally.

I was in Bosnia in 1996, shortly after the signing of the Dayton Peace Accords, which ended the three-and-a-half-year bloody civil conflict that had wracked Bosnia-Herzegovina, Croatia, and Serbia in the former Federal Republic of Yugoslavia.[83] The graves in Tuzla, where the army of the "Republica Srpska" had bombed civilian sites and killed dozens of young people, were still fresh. The toll was still being calculated from the genocidal massacre at Srebrenica, where a UN "safe haven" had become a death trap for Muslim men slaughtered under order from the maniacal Ratko Mladíc.[84] On a day I was in Mostar, a bomb went off in the Christian side of town. We quickly fled across the ravine that separated the Muslim and Christian sides of the town, using the rope bridge that international troops had built to replace the real bridge that gave the city its name, the "Stari Mostar." The original bridge had been built by the Ottomans in the sixteenth century and had previously been bombed. The apartment of the family I stayed with in Sarajevo bore the scars of sniper fire and shelling, and they reflexively stayed away from the windows.

It would have been easy to believe that the way the elections were set up, which in effect cemented the population dislocation caused by the "ethnic cleansing" of the war and ratified by the Dayton Accords, was the "natural" or "inevitable" solution to the religious and ethnic hatreds that had wrought so much horror. But just as seeing people as free-floating autonomous beings is a myth, so too are these clichés of sociology, which do not give credit to the capacity of humans to reinvent both ourselves and our social institutions.

The truth is, just as with the outbreak of World War I associated with Archduke Ferdinand's assassination in Sarajevo more than eighty years earlier, neither the hatreds and divisions that opened the twentieth century from the Balkans nor those that closed them there were inevitable. Even with the war's devastation, the Bosnia I saw had not yet become "Islamicized"; that began later, no doubt a result of the world's collective failure to address the underlying injustices that led to the war and to believe that people could transcend their religious identities.[85] Before the war, Bosnia had been deeply secular with intermarriage and shared communities and with many cross-cutting cleavages in people's self-identification.[86] Even amid the devastation, in the weeks I was there I was reminded of this countless times: the interpreters for the small group I led, who were the products of different kinds of intermarriage; the members of the tiny but very old Jewish community in Sarajevo who felt as much Bosnian as they did Jewish and did not want to leave; the well-known "prison restaurant" in Tuzla where convicts of every religious and ethnic background worked side by side to cook and wait tables.

But I also heard political speeches and rallies filled with promises of reconstructing the decimated country on a foundation of rigid group identities, and it is an unfortunate truth that social injustice, coupled with the manipulation of public perceptions, spreads hatred like wildfire. Ideology is invariably fragile, and needs to be constantly fed. But it seems to take far longer to cultivate tolerance for diversity and respect for the equal humanity in others, than it does to ignite violent prejudice.

Nevertheless it is possible to counter those narratives based on hatreds, and to construct alternative narratives that are not based on reducing ourselves and our collective identities to one dimension. In 2014, almost twenty years after I was in Bosnia, during a workshop on HRBAs in the context of maternal health, I spent several days with activists from South Sudan during a brief respite from the barbaric violence that had erupted between the Dinka and Nuer tribes. The cruelty of the fighting represented the ultimate denial of humanity in the "other"—and later both sides were accused of committing crimes against humanity.

The Dinka and the Nuer were both pastoralists with no significant cultural differences. It was difficult to see how they could so easily stop seeing one another as human beings, slaughtering each other for little apparent reason other than the political machinations of their leaders.[87] South Sudan had struggled for decades under the tyranny of the North, an oppression that was as much based on economic exploitation as it was justified by racial and ethnic discrimination. But it was not the first time that the Dinka and the Nuer had fought each other either; indeed, the conflict has festered and recurred, with hatred passing from one generation to the next.[88]

It was at that workshop that one participant, Grace, suggested that women, who suffered the most from the horrific violence but did not engage in the killing, were the ones to lead a meaningful process of reconciliation based upon meeting everyone's needs, and to overcome the ingrained dehumanization of the other group that had been propagated by men. Women were best placed to change how children thought too. But, Grace noted, to lead a process to recognize the humanity in "the other group" in this society, where women were often treated as little more than chattel in customary law and practice, women first needed to understand they themselves had dignity and rights. "I as a woman should know that I am a human being, and I should know that as a human being that I have rights . . . and how unfair it is when I don't have them even though I should. . . . If I don't know I have rights, what can my life be? And what can my country be if others don't have the same rights?"[89]

In short, the principles of human rights do not neatly resolve debates within the public health and development fields as to which health inequalities are necessarily inequities; on the contrary, they call for fair processes to bring to the surface the contested theories of justice that lie beneath many critical health-related policy dilemmas. Further, interpreting formal and substantive equality guarantees relating to health and the organization of health systems requires us to engage in interdisciplinary discussions without hollow sloganeering. However, a human rights framework does establish that all people, by virtue of being human and regardless of their ethnic, religious, gender, or other attributes, have a right to live lives of dignity and to legal and institutional arrangements that demonstrate equal concern and respect from our governments. That simple concept can enable us to denaturalize some of the entrenched discrimination and violent hatred, as well as the vast economic inequalities, that pervade and corrode our societies and, as I discuss in the next chapter, our world.

Chapter 8

Our Place in the World:
Obligations Beyond Borders

> Power recalls the past not to remember but to sanctify; to justify
> the perpetuation of privilege. . . . Exoneration requires un-
> remembering. . . . To turn infamies into feats, the memory of the
> North is divorced from the memory of the South, accumulation is
> detached from despoliation, opulence has nothing to do with plunder.
> Broken memory leads us to believe that wealth is innocent of poverty.
> —Eduardo Galeano, *Upside Down: A Primer*
> *for the Looking-Glass World*

> The donors come with their music and the government dances its jig.
> —Tanzanian health rights activist

I was living in Tanzania when I first toured Temeke Hospital in early 2012. Temeke, which serves a large catchment area in a poor part of Dar es Salaam, has historically been the most dysfunctional of the city's district hospitals. Unlike the other districts, Temeke, which includes some peri-urban and semirural areas as well, has few private facilities and, at the time, the hospital was invariably overcrowded. On that first visit, the labor ward had three or four women to a bed and women delivering on the floor with just a *khanga* spread beneath them. The overworked staff appeared numb to the chaos, the smells of blood and other fluids they were walking through on the floor, and the constant low-level of groaning that filled the air.

Over decades of doing this work I have grown accustomed to the overcrowding, the filthy conditions, and the lack of basic supplies and running water of such labor wards, which typify but also seem to surpass the generalized unresponsiveness of many health systems. Indeed, there is often a Dante-esque quality to the very places where we ask women to come to bring life into the world, as though they were being condemned to suffer in some inner circle of Hell for the sin of having had sex, and for being women.[1] In response to a woman crying out during contractions, something to the effect of "You weren't complaining when you opened your legs the first time, were you?" is a refrain I've heard from facility staff more times than I can count. But perhaps the greatest evidence of misogyny is that governments and donors alike allow these conditions to persist.

On that first visit to Temeke, I encountered something I had not seen before: a dead woman was lying smack in the middle of the delivery room. Misriya had died the day before, having required more blood than the two bags allotted to her. She was still hooked up to the intravenous drip, her body rotting in the unbearably steamy February heat of Dar es Salaam—amid at least a dozen other women who were struggling to bring forth life. And on a shelf nearby was a small bundle wrapped in a *khanga* cloth. I thought at first it was the dead baby, but later I saw it was alive. The baby had not been given any formula or even sugar water since it had been born; the family was outside but had not been notified of either the baby's birth or Misriya's death.

When I related this story in a meeting with one of Tanzania's largest donors a few weeks later, there were generalized expressions of dismay about the depths of indifference shown by Tanzanian health workers. Yet I noted that the health workers themselves were horrifically overstretched. Indeed, had the one nurse on duty left the ward to take the woman to the morgue and find the family to notify them, she would have been abandoning multiple women in labor. Both Misriya's death and the treatment of her body immediately afterward stemmed from more systemic failures—for which they as donors were at least partly responsible.

It is difficult to live for long in Tanzania without coming to feel that the entire global development enterprise is an elaborate charade. Tanzania is a "donor darling." In the twenty-year period between 1990 and 2010, Tanzania received approximately USD 27 billion in aid from the United States alone. In 2010–2011, donors financed 28 percent of the national budget and more than 80 percent of the development budget.[2] In contrast to its East African neighbors, Tanzania has neither the deadly ethnic strife of Kenya, with its president and vice president indicted by the International Criminal Court, nor the autocratic and patently kleptocratic type of leader of Uganda. But Tanzania is far from a democracy. The same party has been in power since independence more than fifty years ago. Indeed the Chama Cha Mapinduzi (CCM) is effectively "the state"; the intelligence service infiltrates a great many civil society organizations, and critical reflection in the media remains extremely limited. Half a century after Julius Nyerere's promise of a socialist democracy in Africa, those hopes remain almost totally unfulfilled.

Nyerere's curious brand of socialism and his emphasis on "*Ujamaa*," or "familyhood," went far toward reducing tribal hatred.[3] But in its execution, if not its conception, it no doubt also contributed to a culture in which dissent and critical thought were undermined and had unintended perverse effects on the productive economy. Nevertheless, the reasons for the condition Tanzania is in today are many, and blaming it all on socialism, as is often done, is far too facile. There are, of course, the historical impacts of the slave trade, as well as colonialism under the Germans and then the British.[4] These combine with an educational system so broken it seems deliberately so; a one-party state saturated at every point with corruption; and an overwhelming aid dependency—which together have left the country with little capacity for meaningful democratic development.[5]

Nevertheless, apparently wanting to match China's ever-growing influence, the West continues to pour aid into Tanzania and to trumpet its "successes" in self-justification. Tanzania is often described in "development talk" in ways that are nearly unrecognizable to people who have lived there and which make a mockery of the individuals and institutions that are indeed trying to foster real democracy. At the MDG Summit in 2010, for example, President Barack Obama pledged that the United States would focus its development efforts "on countries like Tanzania that promote good governance and democracy; the rule of law and equal administration of justice; transparent institutions with strong civil societies; and respect for human rights."[6]

The Tanzanian government's "commitment" to health and development similarly are often hailed in international circles despite the lack of investment, implementation of programming, and meaningful results in practice. Indeed, the president during the time I lived there, Jakaya Kikwete, who was known internally for spending more time outside the country than within its borders, was named to co-chair the prestigious WHO Accountability Commission on Women's and Children's Health in 2011, signaling recognition of Tanzania's commitment to women's and children's health.[7] Yet the facts on the ground tell a very different story. Tanzania's maternal mortality ratio has remained stubbornly high, at 454 per 100,000 live births, according to the Tanzanian Demographic and Health Survey in 2010, and repeated promises to vastly increase contraceptive access have turned out to be hollow.[8] In terms of effort, it is telling that as a percentage of the total government budget, the amount dedicated to health fell from 10.5 percent in 2010/11 to 8.6 percent in 2011/12.[9] Corruption takes a bite as well; for example, a 2013 *Wall Street Journal* article reported that roughly 20 percent of U.S.-funded malaria medication is diverted and sold on the private market each year, with Tanzania being one of the biggest culprits.[10] But the thing about global development, which Tanzania reveals so dramatically, is that donors, aid contractors, and governments alike have vested interests in pretending the emperor has clothes.

Indeed, Tanzania illustrates an array of seemingly dichotomous ways of understanding approaches to global health and development, these ways are critical to analyze in order to promote meaningful human rights approaches to health. As discussed throughout this book, so much of people's possibilities to effectively enjoy their health and other rights in the global South are determined by global institutional arrangements, as well as by global development paradigms and practices. In this chapter, I briefly explore four questions regarding how we understand the purposes of development and its potential contributions, as well as its limitations, of applying a human rights framework to advance global health justice. First, how do we understand the tension between seeing development as a means to meeting basic human needs, and addressing underlying structural and institutional relations that establish systematic patterns of ill-health? Second, should development aid be seen as charity, or can we understand development in the context of accountability for international assistance and cooperation? Third, can we address immense human suffering in the world through a strongly statist model, or do we require a more cosmopolitan understanding of obligations across borders which stretches current thinking in human rights as well as development? Finally, how do we understand what being human means in a rights framework, and how does that shape our responses to suffering in the world which returns us to a fundamental theme of this book.

Meeting Basic Needs Versus Addressing Structural Power Relations

Throughout this book, I have discussed the need to think about the impacts of human rights frameworks on health more broadly than just in terms of outcomes. Applying human rights frameworks to health ultimately seeks to empower diverse women, children, and men to live lives of dignity. Thus, it calls for institutional, political, and legal changes that open new opportunity structures and allow people to subvert entrenched inequalities, as well as improved outcome indicators. Although some of these impacts need to be measured in law and policy, others require measuring shifts in public perceptions, or values, and still others require measuring outcomes.

In Chapter 2, I suggested that the MDGs had largely reverted to a "basic needs" approach to development, eschewing the more integrated and holistic view that had been reflected in many of the UN conference documents during the 1990s.[11] The MDGs also diverged from previous models of measuring development progress in not distinguishing between starting points for different countries, as had generally been done previously, which had distorting effects. Moreover, the reduction of the broad Millennium Declaration into a set of nested goals, targets, and indicators not only drove narrow funding and programming but came to instantiate how progress was defined.

The story of what happened to sexual and reproductive health rights (SRHR), in Tanzania and elsewhere, painfully illustrates the impacts of these changes. The only goal related to SRHR in the MDGs was MDG 5, which set a goal of improvement in maternal health and set a target of a 75 percent reduction in maternal mortality ratios (MMRs) from 1990 levels by 2015. The indicators used to measure MDG 5 were MMRs and the use of SBAs.[12] In 2005, another target, MDG 5B, relating to universal access to reproductive health was approved, in the face of substantial political opposition, and indicators for measuring MDG 5B were introduced as late as 2007, which in effect marginalized issues of access to contraception until a few years before the MDGs were set to expire.[13]

Narrow, Vertical Approaches Focused on Technological Solutions

The goals and targets selected for MDG 5, as well as other goals, encouraged implementation approaches that were conceptually narrow, vertically structured, and heavily dependent on technological solutions. The calls for social change and the need for strengthening national institutions, which had been highlighted by the ICPD and Beijing, were sidelined.[14] Under the MDGs, SRHR was by no means the only area in which this occurred. For example, the hunger target encouraged the pursuit of short-term, narrow improvements to remedy complex long-term goals. Feeding and nutritional supplement programs were chosen over expanding access to food and land, supporting sustainable agriculture, fostering food security through international trade, promoting gender equity, and other initiatives that were suggested in the broad approach of the 1996 World Food Summit.[15] The 1990s UN conference agendas were interconnected; for example, women's health was understood to be related not just to ICPD and Beijing but to the World Conference on Human Rights, the World Food Summit, the Education for All agenda, and others.[16]

In a country that is as deeply aid dependent as Tanzania, the framing of the development discourse has enormous effects. Approximately 40 percent of the entire Tanzanian health budget comes from foreign aid, and donor dollars make up an astounding 92 percent of the Ministry of Health and Social Welfare's (MoHSW) development budget, which funds programs and activities.[17] Thus it is not surprising that the MDG agenda became Tanzania's national agenda, displacing any other priorities it may have had previously. Health Sector Strategy Plans, as well as development engagement documents, were designed around meeting the MDG targets on the MDG schedule; indeed, Tanzania's Health Sector Strategic Plan III was specifically framed as "Partnerships for Delivering the MDGs."[18]

Despite the fact that the MDGs were originally intended as global goals, they quickly came to be used by donors and national governments alike as national planning targets, including in Tanzania.[19] That is, a reduction in MMRs by 75 percent *in global terms* has a very different meaning than a reduction by 75 percent in each country's MMR. Think of how different that challenge is for a country such as Chile, for example, than for Tanzania. Nevertheless, that is exactly how the MDGs came to be understood in Tanzania and elsewhere. Moreover, the government was to be held "accountable" to donors for meeting MDG targets—a chimera of accountability, which displaced more meaningful relationships of entitlement and obligation with its own citizens.

Once the targets were converted into national planning tools, there was an almost exclusive focus on the MDG indicators, including MMRs, to measure progress. However, for both statistical and practical reasons, MMRs are very poor measures of a health system's progress with respect to maternal health.[20] Maternal deaths are hard to count and verify and, even in countries of high prevalence, they are rare enough that "confidence intervals" make it difficult to discern results of policy and programming changes on trends. Tanzania's health system was particularly poorly suited to be able to calculate MMRs with any degree of certainty.[21]

Similarly, the use of SBAs, which was intended to compensate for some of the statistical issues with MMRs and provide process indicators to regularly assess health-system performance, was effectively made meaningless in Tanzania. In the Health Sector Strategy Plan III, for example, "Proportion of Births Attended by Trained Personnel in Health Facility" is measured as follows—Numerator: Number of Deliveries in Health Facilities; Denominator: Projected Number of Births."[22] Thus the use of SBAs became "institutional deliveries," which means almost nothing if there is not the capacity to save women's lives, and has perverse incentives that drive coercion of women to deliver in facilities. If a woman surveyed merely recalls that someone in a uniform attended her, anyone working in a facility, including a cleaner, is likely to be counted as a skilled attendant. For this reason, there is an enormous amount of what social scientists refer to as "uncertainty absorption" that "takes place when inferences are drawn from a body of evidence, and the inferences instead of the evidence itself, are then communicated."[23] The end result is that the numbers are not reliably comparable across country contexts, and they say little about progress over time. Yet both MMRs and the use of SBAs have driven funding and programming in Tanzania, largely as a result of donor priorities.

In part because of the MDGs and in part because of other vertical programming, such as the U.S. President's Emergency Program for AIDS Relief (PEPFAR), funding for HIV/AIDS programs saw exponential increases during the 2000s, from USD 2.56 billion in 2003 to USD 6.48 billion in 2010. Tanzania received a healthy share of this funding, USD 1.08 billion from 2009 through 2011.[24] But, with the exception of PMTCT initiatives, most HIV programs were built up almost entirely in parallel with the general health system. Temeke District Hospital painfully illustrates some of the results of such donor-driven health funding and programming: The newly constructed wings and state-of-the-art laboratories, as well as all of the staffing paid for through PEPFAR contractors and other vertical programs for HIV, contrasts sharply with the dilapidated remaining structures, the perpetually overstretched workers without basic supplies, and the patently inadequate single operating theater.

Examining the mechanisms for aid delivery reveals why this is the case. Although "there is much discussion among donors about increasing funds transferred to developing countries through general health-sector support,"[25] it is a very small part of development and health assistance in Tanzania, and has declined in recent years. "Basket funding," or a general form of sectoral budget support, does not allow donors to set priorities in the same way but is crucial for system strengthening—necessary to fund such pedestrian but essential items as washing powder and fuel for ambulances and generators. But in Tanzania, as well as in many other countries, this type of funding is currently outweighed by "nonbasket," or project-based, aid. The last year that basket funding exceeded nonbasket funding—TZS 1 billion (Tanzanian shillings) (USD 0.6 million) to TZS 60 million (USD 36,300)—was 2006/7. By 2010/11, nonbasket funding exceeded basket funding by TZS 2.1 billion (USD 1.27 million) to TZS 1.3 billion (USD 0.79 million). As noted in Tanzania's 2010/11 Health Sector Expenditure Review, "The dominance of non-basket foreign funding clearly indicates that development partners, notably the Global Fund and PEPFAR, are increasingly channeling their support to the health sector through projects. This trend poses challenges, especially regarding aid coordination and harmonization in health interventions."[26] Donors committed to an HRBA and to supporting the health system as a core institution may end up in effect subsidizing other donors' programs that are undermining the system.

Indeed, Tanzania is a laboratory for development ideas, including seemingly every variant of so-called "results-based financing," which in a general way attempts to compensate for what are seen as ineffective or corrupt governmental structures "by shifting the focus from inputs to results."[27] There is undoubtedly corruption throughout the Tanzanian government, including in the health sector.[28] Nevertheless, an HRBA to health and human rights frameworks more broadly, is inherently political and requires engagement with those political structures in ways that empower citizens to seek transformation and demand accountability. Siri Lange notes that the depoliticization of development approaches in Tanzania and elsewhere in Africa has produced so little change precisely because "parallel structures easily come into conflict with local government structures [and among other things] persons of authority [are] able to convince many citizens not to contribute cash or labour by suggesting that their money or efforts would be misused."[29] The circumvention of political processes and systems make the changes across the circle of accountability needed in an HRBA impossible.

Charity Versus Accountability for "International Assistance and Cooperation" and Extraterritorial Obligations

Under international human rights law, wealthy governments have not just moral but legal obligations relating to respecting, protecting, and fulfilling health and other rights through "international assistance and cooperation."[30] Yet in practice efforts to advance global health and development are generally treated as issues of beneficence.[31]

Aid Levels and Choices

It is unquestionably true that development assistance for improving health has expanded markedly in the past twenty years. Resources quadrupled between 1990 and 2007, and the rate of growth increased substantially after 2002.[32] Health aid rose from USD 4.1 billion to USD 5.3 billion from 2001 to 2006.

However, much of the influx of resources has not been from governments but from private philanthropy, as well as from foreign investment. In 2012 alone, the Bill and Melinda Gates Foundation awarded USD 2.5 billion in grants to global health-and-development programs, making it the third-largest international health-and-development donor in the world, behind only the United States and the United Kingdom.[33] Further, according to a comprehensive review published in the *Lancet* in 2009, although the scale-up of global health funding from the Gates Foundation is dramatic, the magnitude of resources mobilized from other private sources and, in particular, corporate drug and equipment donations, was greater.[34] Philanthropy of all kinds is of course subject to the vicissitudes of people's largesse. For example, if the Gates Foundation fails to support programs to facilitate safe abortion because of Melinda Gates's personal views on the matter, that is entirely within its discretion, as is whether it decides to change course and fund something totally different in coming years.

However, public sources have displayed the same kind of volatility. For the first time since monitoring began in 2003, the official development assistance (ODA) for maternal, newborn, and child health declined in 2009.

And despite the upturn in the global financial crisis, ODA continued to decline substantially as of 2012, below assistance given in 2008.[35] As budgets tighten, the global community—northern donors in particular—have begun to rethink their development commitments, as well as their domestic social policies—leaving a bigger role for the private sector. But as Linsey McGoey notes, "Philanthrocapitalists have helped to perpetuate a dubious belief: the idea that corporations and private entrepreneurs are subsidising gaps in development financing created by increasingly non-interventionist states. In reality, it is often governments subsidising the philanthrocapitalists."[36]

Moreover, even when governments maintain aid commitments, they tend to eschew language that would imply legal accountability. In arguing for the importance of conceptualizing health as a right in foreign policy, Flavia Bustreo and Curtis Doebbler note that "however laudable," financial contributions from donors without reference to the right to health "appear to be voluntary contributions rather than the fulfillment of a legal obligation."[37]

The CESCR has been clear: "It is particularly incumbent on States parties and other actors in a position to assist, to provide 'international assistance and cooperation, especially economic and technical' which enable developing countries to fulfill their core and other obligations."[38] Although the United Kingdom is, as of this writing, considering legislating an obligation of foreign assistance, aid figures as well as priorities tend to emerge from political negotiations and expediency, and respond little to a notion of international responsibility.

The extent of binding international obligations to provide resources, and the standards to which donor states should be held, have not been well-developed in international human rights law to date. The Paris Principles on Aid Effectiveness, for example, emphasize "harmonization" and "alignment" without binding commitments based on rights.[39] The Accra Agenda for Action, meant to follow on the Paris Principles, calls for assistance to be done "in ways consistent with their agreed international commitments on gender equality, human rights, disability and environmental sustainability."[40] However, this wording is not followed by the elaboration of specific obligations of support, which will be critical in the future.

A human rights framework does impose some circumscription on *how* a government goes about providing aid. For example, the U.S. government had required grantees to sign an "anti-prostitution pledge" that prohibited HIV funds from being used to support sex workers, which was challenged on the basis that it violated freedom of speech.[41] The U.S. Supreme Court held that the law, which required grantees to have a policy explicitly stating they oppose "prostitution," violated the First Amendment by compelling speech as a condition of receiving government funds.[42] For groups such as Sisi Kwa Sisi in Tanzania, which depends on U.S. funding to provide clinical services as well as condoms and lubricants to the beleaguered LGBT population, including sex workers, those policy differences translate into differences between life and death for their clients.

Beyond those situations in which courts in donor countries have jurisdiction to ensure compliance of government actions with their own laws, it has proven difficult to translate some human rights standards, and the principles of Paris and Accra into practice. In Tanzania, for example, the Development Partners Group (DPG) for Health includes a triumvirate of UN agencies, donors, and the government.[43] But this institutional convening platform has not proven adequate to streamline approaches to aid or to monitoring and evaluation frameworks. Many donors' approaches to health and other development are set in their capitals—in Washington, D.C., or Ottawa, for example—with almost no flexibility to adjust to the realities of local context, which is a prerequisite for the application of a meaningful human rights approach. With some notable exceptions, such as Danida, it is rare for international donors to attempt to align their funding with preexisting priorities, whether set by the government or by private grantees, or to adopt the grantees' own monitoring and evaluation frameworks.[44] One grantee in Tanzania noted that it was required to submit 126 separate reports that year, often tracking different indicators, for the different international donors. The proliferation of almost meaningless log frames, coupled with short-term targets designed more for the benefit of self-justification to taxpayers at home than for the people of Tanzania, undermine possibilities for transformative change.

The Obligation to "Do No Harm"

Donor countries also have obligations to refrain from direct interference and to *prevent* third-party interference from other actors. International treaty-monitoring bodies as well as domestic courts have been more willing to subject compliance with these obligations to "do no harm" to scrutiny, and these may well provide avenues for increased international accountability. As Paul Hunt, the first UN special rapporteur on health stated, "States are obliged to respect the enjoyment of the right to health in other jurisdictions, *to ensure that no international agreement or policy adversely impacts upon the right to health*, and that their representatives in international organizations take due account of the right to health, as well as the obligation of international assistance and cooperation, in all policy-making matters."[45]

For example, just looking within the health sector itself, wealthy countries have impaired and continue to decimate public health systems in countries across East Africa and the global South generally by attracting health-care workers away from low-paying poor conditions to meet shortages of health-care personnel in their own countries. In East Africa, health workers go to other countries in Africa as well, notably South Africa. Nevertheless, in the United States, for example, 1 in every 4 doctors is currently trained overseas, and the number will only increase as it is estimated that there will be a shortage of 200,000 doctors in the United States by 2022.[46]

If we care about global equity, freedom of movement for individuals needs to be balanced with a population's right to health. In 2013, Tanzania had a 1:30,000 doctor-to-population ratio (the WHO recommends 1:1,000), and yet 8.2 percent of Tanzanian doctors reside outside the country. Kilimanjaro Christian Medical University College Principal, Professor Egbert Kessy, estimates this number to be much higher, citing that roughly 60 percent of all locally trained medical experts turn down job offers to seek better pay and facilities outside the country[47]—and 35 percent of those are living in North America and Europe.[48] Moreover, many doctors who stay in Tanzania end up working for NGO contractors for international donors, which pay higher salaries and offer better benefits and per diem rates than any job in clinical practice.[49]

Donors only began taking serious action to address health-worker shortages in Tanzania in 2009, years after it had become an obvious structural problem in the health system. Although health-care workers often send back significant remittances, these are not nearly sufficient to compensate for the devastation of the health system as a core institution, or health as a public good. When there is evidence that a Northern government, or private entities sanctioned by a Northern government, has targeted health-care workers in specific countries, meaningful accountability might require some form of restitution in addition to the adoption of Codes of Conduct to make policies consistent with promotion of the right to health, as various individual governments, the Commonwealth Medical Association, and the World Health Assembly have already adopted.[50] Calculating the amount of restitution would, of course, be complex. Nevertheless, we could imagine a framework of accountability in which an obligation of restitution for such behavior, say taken as a percentage of taxes collected on salaries of immigrant doctors in the recipient countries or otherwise, was incorporated into restitution to the countries of origin for use in relation to health. The Commonwealth Code of Practice for the International Recruitment of Health Workers contains a provision on compensatory and reciprocation measures, including programs for reciprocations, the development of training programs, and arrangements to facilitate the return of recruits.[51] Yet a recent study found that provisions of the code are rarely monitored or enforced, and compensation is almost never paid.[52]

Investments beyond the health sector also have enormous potential impacts on social determinants of health. Taking seriously the obligation to prevent interference by private actors would require consideration of the impact on health and other rights of foreign investment and corporate activity. UN Treaty monitoring bodies are increasingly examining countries' extraterritorial obligations in this light.[53]

The obligation to do no harm requires consideration of the actions of multilateral institutions, which represent donor countries, in addition to corporations and other actors within the own borders. In 2002, I represented the CESR in a fact-finding delegation organized by Public Citizen's Water Rights Project, which was investigating the potential effects on water, health, and other rights stemming from the World Bank's plan to privatize Ghana's urban water supply system. The World Bank argued that investing in an inefficient government system was wasteful and would not expand water supply, and it therefore conditioned further loan assistance on privatization. Ghana developed a private-sector participation (PSP) proposal, in which urban water supply was separated from sanitation and sent out for bids from transnational corporations.

At the time, there was no doubt that the system for water provision and distribution in Ghana was seriously deficient and that everyone would not receive access to adequate amounts of piped water in the near future.[54] However, under the International Monetary Fund (IMF) and World Bank scheme, the government would be left with providing sanitation services, which are never profitable, while private corporations would be allowed to profit from people's water use. The private companies would be operating under an entirely different set of ground rules than the long-established rules of the underresourced Ghana Water Company. For example, the private multinationals were not responsible for expansion of the system—that is, progressive realization of universal access for all—under the terms of the PSP proposal. The touted "efficiency" apparently related to effectively metering and charging for water, rather than effectively meeting the public health needs of the population. The PSP called for full cost recovery with a "lifeline tariff provision" meant to address concerns about barriers to affordable access by the poor. But our fact-finding delegation noted, among other things, that indigent residents of the many multifamily compounds in urban Ghanaian slums would end up paying higher fees. Also, those people far from taps and forced to buy water from tankers would not benefit at all from the lifetime tariff under the PSP proposal.[55]

In a human rights framework, as stressed throughout this book, water is, among other things, a precondition to health and is not simply a commercial commodity that can be priced through contractual arrangements that value cost-recovery over equity. Applying the framework to Ghana, such a fundamental decision affecting the water rights of the public could not be adopted in a manner that demonstrated disregard for the voices of Ghanaian citizens and communities. Understanding the management and distribution of water as a basic rights issue changes how we evaluate both the actions of the government of Ghana and the donors. In this case, for example, in keeping with CESCR's General Comment 2, in any structural adjustment program or other loan program, international financial institutions have an obligation to ensure that (1) the right to water is protected in policies promoting or enabling the privatization of water services or the creation of water markets, (2) the human rights implications of such policies have been thoroughly considered and addressed through a broad process of consultation, and (3) necessary checks and balances have been put in place to protect the interests of the most vulnerable and indigent members of society.[56]

The requirements imposed by the IMF under its Poverty Reduction and Growth Facility Loan and the conditioning of a number of loans from the World Bank on PSP in the water sector were not consistent with obligations under international law, which subsequently have been developed more clearly.[57] The Ghanaian example is far from unique. Tanzania went through its own set of rigidly imposed structural adjustment programs. In the wake of the nationalization that occurred as part of Nyerere's socialist vision, IMF-sponsored structural adjustment brought a menu of fiscal and monetary policies and reprivatization beginning in the 1980s; land and other assets ended up being parceled out through political patronage, which did little to benefit poor Tanzanians.[58] And as recently as President Obama's 2013 trip to Tanzania, privatization of some water and power was being trumpeted as the natural solution to the perpetually inefficient government agencies, and as a key to Tanzania's development.[59]

The Role of Transnational Corporations

Privatization of water around the world illustrates acutely the inordinate power and role that transnational private actors are playing in development, with enormous consequences for the enjoyment of people's health and other rights. Three transnational corporations—Suez, Veolia, and RWE[60]—are responsible for the vast majority of privatized water provision and distribution in the world, which is on the rise. Moreover, transnational corporations also use enormous quantities of water for agricultural cultivation and manufacturing processes—sustaining and processing sugar cane crops, which can drain aquifers, for example—while the poor struggle to have enough water to survive.[61]

Tanzania has some of the largest aquifers in Africa. Yet, expanding corporate control of water in Tanzania is destroying areas of lands used by small-scale subsistence farmers. Small-scale farmers are uprooted and converted into landless laborers, who end up working on Unilever's tea plantations in Iringa, for example, or migrating to Dar es Salaam and other urban settings.

One major reason for the lack of significant poverty reduction, despite economic growth, in Tanzania is that the government has not succeeded in raising productivity in agriculture, which can barely keep up with population growth in rural areas, where 80 percent of the poor live.[62] Thus, from the perspective of the Tanzanian government, bringing in the private sector might seem to be the natural solution. And from the perspective of the corporations, shifting control of these natural resources from those engaged in creating subsistence livelihoods to property owners engaged in investing for profit increases economic output, and the concomitant shift of wages downward only increases profitability further. But the loss of livelihoods has enormous implications in terms of food, health, and other rights.[63]

From a human rights perspective, some efforts have been made to impose obligations on transnational private actors by national courts and supranational tribunals, as well as by treaty-monitoring committees.[64] A recent movement is underway to develop a treaty with respect to the rules governing transnational corporations.[65] Other efforts have focused on imposing extraterritorial obligations on states where the transnational corporations are based.[66]

There remains an enormous gap, however, in practice. When a state has problems providing public services, such as health care or water or electricity—it is usually in a poor position to exert sufficient regulatory power over the private sector to effectively protect health and other rights, especially when the private actor is a transnational corporation.[67] The SDGs imbue private actors and PPPs with enormous importance to development, so we will see how these conflicts get played out over the next fifteen years.

What an Unjust Global Architecture Means in Practice

Studies done by World Bank economist Branko Milanovic find that wealth inequalities between countries, expressed as an intercountry Gini coefficient, have been steadily growing over recent decades. Indeed, between-country inequality over the last fifty years grew at an even greater pace than within-country inequality.[68] In his 2012 report, Milanovic notes that in contrast to past centuries, in the current state of the world, "more than 80 per cent of global income differences is due to large gaps in mean incomes between countries, and unskilled workers' wages in rich and poor countries often differ by a factor of 10 to 1."[69] Other studies, such as that by Thomas Piketty, focusing on the rise in incomes among the top 1 percent, confirm the growth in global inequality.[70]

We could examine any of an array of legal and institutional arrangements that bolster the increasing inequity of the global architecture, from trade to intellectual property to labor regulations. Let's take one: the perpetuation of so-called illicit financial flows, including rules that foster commercial tax evasion. We have discussed the critical role that tax revenue plays in enabling a country to have the available resources to discharge its ESC rights obligations, including in relation to health. Commercial tax evasion and other illicit financial flows lead to an estimated tax loss of USD160 billion per year, which is approximately twice the total amount of annual development aid. For example, a recent report estimates that tax exemptions given to both transnational and domestic corporations in Tanzania amounted to USD 288 million between 2008 and 2011.[71]

Other kinds of illicit financial flows, stemming from such factors as exploration of Tanzania's recently discovered large natural gas reserves, create shortfalls between resources for development and the amount of revenues coming in. Despite being a "donor darling," Tanzania loses considerably more revenue to these illicit transfers and to deals that allow foreign (as well as some domestic) companies to avoid taxation than it receives in aid.[72] And the loss of revenues leads to greater aid dependency, which in turn leads to weaker positions in bargaining with transnational investors, creating a vicious circle of dependency. Although it is private corporations and actors that may benefit, it is the governments in the North that fail to protect health and other rights in countries such as Tanzania, through the global financial regulations they establish, which allow Northern-based corporations to benefit from wholesale evasion of taxes, mispricing of trade, secrecy jurisdictions, and the like.

The results of rigged global "rules of the game," including illicit financial flows, are devastating in terms of people's chances to live lives of dignity based on where in the world they were born. With an annual GDP per capita of USD 532 (2011) and a Human Development Index rank among the lowest 20 percent, Tanzania is one of the poorest fifteen nations in the world. More than two-thirds of the population live below the internationally recognized extreme poverty line of USD 1.25 a day and almost 90 percent live on less than two dollars a day.[73]

Tanzania is slated to become a "middle income country" by approximately 2025. Yet "middle income" in the case of Tanzania means something between USD 2 and USD 10 per capita per day, that is, abjectly poor by Western standards.[74] Further, if current trends persist, income inequality and unequal distribution of effective enjoyment of ESC rights will only deepen with economic growth, with all of the associated problems discussed in Chapter 7.

In addition, from the perspective of human rights, economic assessments of "development levels" tend to overvalue the significance of the availability of consumer durables, such as televisions and cell phones, which indeed have exponentially increased in Tanzania as a result of technological revolutions and drops in relative prices. For example, cell-phone subscriptions have increased from 2 percent to 57 percent of the population in the last ten years.[75] Internet users as well have increased eighteen times.[76] But, as Milanovic notes, "A cell phone does not a middle class make."[77] A cell phone without a functioning health system, education system, or rule of law, and without access to stable employment does not add up to a life of dignity.

How Can Applying Human Rights Frameworks Help to Address Global Inequality? Evolving Understandings of Global Justice in Rights Frameworks

Just as applying a human rights framework should help us make visible the power relations and human decisions at the national level that create suffering, so too should it enable us to see the noninevitability of the global institutional arrangements that perpetuate global inequality, deprivations of dignity, and misery. However, despite the intuitive appeal of slogans proclaiming that we are all "citizens of the world," in political philosophy and constitutional theory, rights have historically been conceived of in terms of social contracts between individuals and their governments. Under international law, the primary duty-bearer is the state; conversely, the state bears a primary duty to the subjects within its own territories.

What of reinforcing the broader obligations to do no harm and to redress the inequities in the global architecture? Current efforts underway to remedy deficiencies in the global health architecture include a Framework Convention on Global Health (FCGH), for which the raison d'être is largely to establish meaningful accountability by states' parties for meeting obligations beyond borders as well as at home.[78] Supranational judicial mechanisms would hold states accountable for maintaining agreements and fulfilling the right to health through the FCGH. Similarly, proposals were made in 2013 by the Lancet–University of Oslo Commission on Global Governance for Health to enhance accountability by using the international justice system, which the commission called "an important backstop for national systems [that] could offer a useful mechanism for strengthened transnational accountability."[79] In 2014, in the wake of Argentina's default caused by holdout bond-holders extorting interest on its foreign debt, the UN Human Rights Council issued a declaration calling foreign debt a human rights issue and an independent expert on foreign debt was named.[80] Concluding observations from UN treaty monitoring bodies and some judgments from domestic courts are increasingly on extraterritorial obligations as well.[81]

If we are to rewrite the social contracts we have in the light of the increasing globalization of the world, we will need to strike new balances between domestic and extraterritorial legal obligations. For example, if a country provides agricultural subsidies or tariff protections, respect for human rights might require that the benefits to domestic farmers and manufacturers be weighed against the detrimental impact on local farmers, and in turn on food, health, and other ESC rights provoked in other countries. Or if the Affordable Care Act draws more foreign doctors and other health-care workers to the United States, perhaps there are obligations of restitution so that it does not increase health inequities in other countries.[82]

Moreover, many decisions that have a bearing on health and other rights in the global South will necessarily involve collective obligations of the international community. For example, maintaining stable national and economic financial systems requires collective efforts from the international community, including macroeconomic policy coordination and equity and stabilization of international commodity prices for food staples.[83] Think of the devastation that might have been avoided were price and trade schemes for food in place before the crisis of 2009, which led to starvation and malnutrition in poor countries unable to subsidize imported foodstuffs.[84] A 2010 nonbinding report of the UN High Level Task Force of the Working Group on the Right to Development suggested that there should be some form of balance between domestic and extraterritorial concerns and efforts to address such collective decisions and, as noted, there are recent attempts to impose some constraints on both powerful national governments and international organizations.[85] However, there is still much normative grounding, as well as political consciousness change, required before human rights legal obligations can consistently impose meaningful restraints on globally exercised power.

Concluding Reflections

When Julius Nyerere came to power as the first president in the newly independent Tanganyika in 1961, he sought to create a country that was united and stood independently from the colonial powers.[86] His vision for Tanzania incorporated ideas of equitable economic production and distribution, as well as self-reliance and nonexploitative development.[87] He sought to unite Tanzania by breaking down tribal identities and building a national identity through the Swahili language, among other things. Nevertheless, as noted earlier, Nyerere's utopian vision has largely not come to pass. This is not just because of the deep-seated corruption and ineptitude of the governments that followed his but also because of problems in the original scheme, and the illusory hope that a small East African country would be able to stand outside the very biased world order for very long.

Our Place in the World   225

During the years I lived in Tanzania, Temeke Hospital, perhaps because of its reputation as being the "worst" of the district hospitals in Dar es Salaam, became the target for immense donor investment, which included the construction of a new maternity ward in an attempt to improve quality and stem some of the overcrowding. Moreover, a new two-hundred-bed Baobab Maternity Hospital, also funded with donor monies, is currently slated to open in late 2015 to address the ever-burgeoning number of births in Dar es Salaam. At the same time, donors to Tanzania are increasingly concerned that the country's high fertility rates not only fuel poor maternal and child health outcomes but also threaten its "sustainable development."

Global recognition of the need for environmental as well as social and economic sustainability was the impetus behind the idea of SDGs, which will become the blueprint for development for the next generation.[88] And nowhere will the importance of understanding what we want out of "sustainable development" be greater than in countries such as Tanzania. It is likely that the effects of climate change will be felt as or more acutely on Africa than on any other continent, where food supplies and livelihoods will be threatened with an increase in droughts, floods, heat waves, sea-level rises, and harsher storms.[89]

But what is at stake in how we define sustainable development is related to the measuring of outcomes versus changes in political processes and institutions more broadly, as discussed earlier. But even more fundamentally, it is related to how we think of being human, which has been a theme running through this book.

On a first level, sustainable development needs to be concerned with sustainability of consumption.[90] Surely development cannot mean enjoying the same rights to environmental degradation as people in the North have for too long taken for granted.[91]

On a second level, however, as emphasized throughout these pages, human beings are far more than merely consumers of health goods and services or of energy and products that degrade the environment. We are citizens who inhabit various communities and identities. Therefore, development in a human rights framework is more than about the lifestyle changes necessary in our relation to consumption. Referring to an influential 1987 report by a commission headed by the former director general of the WHO, Gro Brundtland, Amartya Sen argues that the call to do more than "leave the world as you found it" but to ensure that future generations can meet their needs, including their health needs., is a critical addition to thinking through what sustainable development means beyond consumption patterns.[92] Together with the emphasis on intragenerational equity across the world in meeting those needs, this understanding of what we mean by sustainable development incorporates more of what we would care about in a human rights or human capabilities framework.

Nevertheless, in a rights framework, as well as in Sen's capabilities perspective, human beings are also more than just "people with needs." As I have emphasized throughout these chapters, in a human rights framework, humans are "agents of change who can—given the opportunity—think, assess, evaluate, resolve, inspire, agitate, and, through these means, reshape the world."[93] When development adopts a view that reduces human beings to being some kind of "patients" who are dependent on largesse of beneficent governments and donors, it ends up focusing on on basic needs and short-term outcomes—as opposed to transformative processes that enable people to exercise greater choice in their lives.

This raises lessons explored in earlier chapters, such as that if the *ends* of development are to foster greater freedom, we also need to treat people not as passive beneficiaries but as active agents in the *process* of development. As discussed previously, people need to be empowered to meaningfully participate in deciding how the diverse needs they define will be met and prioritized, through legitimate processes as well as through background conditions that account for power asymmetries in practice.[94] In addition, we again need to acknowledge that the simple expressions of needs may not be sufficient in a world where people internalize domination, practice self-denigration that reifies the injustices they experience from others, and lower expectations about how they should be treated. As Sen notes, "People who are used to living in a persistent state of undernourishment, illiteracy and lack of basic healthcare may come to think of nourishment or school education or medical attention as a luxury, rather than as a 'need,' so that even if we go by their own self-perception of needs, we may take an unjustly limited view of their deprivation."[95]

Thus much is at stake in terms of how sustainable development is defined and who defines it. Our understanding of what sustainability can and should be will no doubt encode institutional arrangements for a generation or more to come, and in turn it will shape power relations between and within countries. But part of the message of this book is that how we see the plasticity of global institutional arrangements—and the noninevitability of patterns of poverty and inequality in the world—will in turn depend on how we understand what it means to be human.

A few years after I was in Temeke Hospital for the first time, I thought about this again. On International Women's Day—March 8—in 2015, I was in south Texas at a rally of the Nuestro Texas campaign for access to sexual and reproductive health and rights in the lower Rio Grande Valley. It was an unusually cold day, and rainy, but the marchers were unfazed and the speakers impassioned: "The rain will not stop us; nothing will stop us, the people united will never be defeated." These were women whose possibilities for escaping grinding poverty and accessing essential reproductive health care had been repeatedly constrained by federal legislation differentiating access to entitlements on the basis of qualifying immigration status, and state laws limiting funding for health services as well as state targeting of abortion services in particular. Yet, as Lucy Felix, one of the inspirational leaders, declared, "We are not victims; we are strong women, . . . and we are agents for change." The Nuestro Texas Campaign was explicitly using human rights tools—connecting grassroots mobilization through the National Latina Health Network, among other groups, and legal advocacy at state, national and international levels, through the Center for Reproductive Rights, to raise awareness and create both political and legal leverage for change.[96]

These are the women whose suffering was not counted in the MDGs because they are poor but live in a rich country. And these are the women, just as do many others in this book, who defy the understanding of being human that conventional approaches to sustainable development imply. They are not just interested in packages of care; they want to have their voices heard and their dignity respected, they want to be treated as equal members of the society to which they contribute, with equal dignity.

One of the greatest critiques of the MDGs was that they focused on development for poor countries, largely ignoring inequalities within countries and poverty in the global North. The SDGs, by contrast were supposed to set out a universal development agenda, and pay attention to these inequalities. We have yet to see what that will mean in practice for women like those in the Nuestro Texas campaign and whether human rights tools and strategies more broadly, can be meaningfully applied in the SDG agenda to advance global justice.

At the same time, efforts to articulate extraterritorial and collective obligations show an important evolution in human rights thinking and practice, but historically the construction of public international law has been aimed at limiting the accountability of states. And both conceptually and in practice, the international human rights framework has at times sat very comfortably with global capitalism.

For human rights to remain a powerful mobilizing and insurrectional discourse, there will need to be some adaptation in terms of the way social contracts within states are written to enable extraterritorial obligations, as well as the institutions and procedures through which they can be held individually and collectively accountable. In the end, human rights tools and frameworks are useful insofar as they meaningfully regulate power in ways that advance human dignity and equality—righting the egregious imbalances of economic as well as political power, whether those imbalances occur across borders or within them.

Conclusion: Another World Is Possible

> Too much sanity may be madness and the maddest of all, to see life as it is and not as it should be.
>
> —Miguel de Cervantes Saavedra, *Don Quixote de la Mancha*

> Compassion is an unstable emotion. It needs to be translated into action, or it withers.
>
> —Susan Sontag, *Regarding the Pain of Others*

One of my favorite "stories" by the Argentine fiction writer Jorge Luis Borges is "Pierre Menard: Author of the *Quixote*." In this very short piece, Borges writes a literary critique of a French author—Pierre Menard—and his version of *Don Quixote* is word for word, line for line, identical to the original Cervantes story. But Borges says the story is not just a crude copy. It is actually infinitely richer than the original version because it has all the advantages of three hundred years of allusion to be read into it: "To compose the *Quixote* at the beginning of the seventeenth century was a reasonable undertaking, necessary and perhaps even unavoidable; at the beginning of the twentieth, it is almost impossible. It is not in vain that the three hundred years have gone by, filled with exceedingly complex events. Among them, to mention only one, is the *Quixote* itself."[1]

I thought about this piece differently when I was in Argentina in 2003 on a human rights delegation for the group that is now called Disability Rights International (DRI). As is widely known, Argentina went through an economic crisis at the end of 2001 and the economy completely toppled in 2002. The currency collapsed; Argentina defaulted on its foreign debt as it did again in 2014; a run on the banks resulted in the government imposing restrictions on how much money people could take out of their accounts and converting dollar holdings into peso holdings in the famous *"pesificación."*[2] Pensioners' savings were wiped out; there was massive unemployment; and more than half of the Argentine population was thrust into poverty.[3] But what is less well known is that people were often medically treated in response to the massive psychosocial distress, and those without adequate social support networks were even sometimes placed in psychiatric hospitals, particularly in urban centers.

With the DRI delegation, I was in Argentina in 2003 to examine conditions in psychiatric hospitals, including the Hospital Tobar García, which is a psychiatric institution for children in Buenos Aires. We had almost finished the tour of the facility and were on the top floor in a locked ward for adolescent boys. Just the day before, a melee had erupted and the boys had accused the orderlies of using excessive force in restraining them. While my colleagues were sorting out what happened, my eye was drawn to a boy who looked much younger than the others. He was probably fourteen or fifteen, but he looked to be no more than about eleven years old. I went over and introduced myself, and I asked if I could see his room.

In his room, Daniel took out a book and asked if I had read it. Much to my surprise, it was Charles Dickens's *Oliver Twist.* I replied that I had, and after a moment of caressing the cover, Daniel asked me earnestly, "How is it possible that an English man writing hundreds of years ago could so perfectly imagine and describe what goes on in Buenos Aires today?"

It turned out that Daniel's life in many ways resembled the life of young Oliver Twist, who in the story was born into a workhouse in London and had various misadventures on the streets of London with gangs. Daniel had lived with his mother and his younger sister. He didn't know who his father was. His mother had been left unemployed in the economic crisis and as a result they had lost their apartment. They had been living with a series of men who were reportedly abusive or alcoholic or both. Daniel had dropped out of school and was selling chewing gum and little things on the street, or just begging. He was clearly a sensitive boy and had become overwhelmed— developing anxiety and depression, in clinical terms. And, because his mother couldn't take care of him, she had decided to put him in this psychiatric hospital.

Daniel assured me, "She is going to come and get me as soon as she can, to take me home. She collects the bus money. Whenever she's able to collect the bus money, she comes to visit me." After some more minutes of talking about his life and *Oliver Twist*, Daniel said, "You know, I'm writing a story, too. And my story is about a world in which children get to live with their parents. They get to stay in school, and they don't get hurt. And someday the world that I am writing about is going to come true, too." He showed me his journal, with painstakingly neat handwriting, in which he was indeed creating a world in which he and the other children could live safe, happy lives in loving families. When the rest of my delegation came to get me, it was hard to tear myself away from this extraordinary young man.

I think it would be easy to dismiss Daniel's story as just a neurotic fantasy, as quixotic—as, in fact, Don Quixote's imagination could be taken to be just the rantings of a crazy old man. But we should resist that temptation. Think about this young man—having faced a lifetime's worth of hardship by the time he was a teenager, trapped day in and day out in a bleak institutional setting, and yet still able to conjure an image of another, more just, world. I have argued throughout this book that applying a human rights framework to health calls on us to do just that, to imagine a different world.

As Borges illustrated in "Pierre Menard," we humans ineluctably allegorize our world. And one message of this book is that we can choose how we collectively do so. Why should we accept the manufactured realities fed to us on television every day or marketed by companies telling us we can find happiness in a bottle of soda? Why is it severe poverty that brings shame to people rather than wealth extracted from the exploitation of others? Why are adolescent girls who become pregnant stigmatized when our cultures perpetually tell them their value lies in being sexual objects? Why do we allow so many of our religious and political leaders to tell loving, gay men that they are "sick" while the abusiveness by so many heterosexual men is condoned and normalized?

In life, we all more or less end up accepting our own stories; to not do so is to go crazy. But in a world so torn by injustice, what lies does that require us to internalize in our personal and societal narratives? As I have argued throughout these pages, applying human rights to health in an empowering way calls on us to reorient our thoughts, as well as our politics, so that we are not inevitably "presupposing and reproducing" the injustices in the contexts in which we live, which prevent diverse people from living with dignity, rights, and well-being.[4] It calls on us to challenge the shaping power of the narratives that we take for granted every day in our religious and cultural practices, in the orthodoxies of both public health and human rights fields, and in the hegemonic economic models for organizing our societies and our world.

My starting place was to say that applying a human rights framework to health requires us to reframe the way we understand our own suffering and that of others. All suffering is not a reflection of injustice. So much of the sorrow and tragedy we feel in life relates to our health and to matters of life and death: the teenager suddenly struck by a rare degenerative disease, the vibrant young mother diagnosed with cancer, the loving husband paralyzed in a hit and run, the freak accident that leaves a child in a coma. And then there is simply the inherent loss wrought by the passage of time, which inevitably expresses itself in our physical and emotional well-being—deaths of loved ones and friends, the crumbling of friendships that held our lives together, the bottomless ache of love affairs that don't end like fairy tales, the deadening of passions that had once animated our souls. In addition to the immense joy life brings, pain is part of the human condition. And spiritual as well as philosophical traditions have much to teach us about how we navigate this vale of tears.

I have argued that we need to distinguish those forms of suffering from the suffering that is a product of arbitrary or discriminatory laws and policies; of institutional arrangements at national and global levels that systematically disadvantage certain people; of systemic neglect and abuse committed with impunity, whether in public or private; or of social, cultural, and religious norms that inhibit some people from understanding themselves as full human beings with equal claims to respect and inclusion in society. I have asserted that indifference to this latter kind of suffering of fellow human beings—born of social injustice and political failure that places an unnecessary burden of infirmity and indignity on so many—demeans all of our humanity.

That so many of the stories in this book have related to maternal mortality is not a coincidence. As I noted in the introduction, I have spent much of my professional life working on maternal health and SRH issues. However, that is not a coincidence. I came to public health from a perspective of social justice. No global health issue may more acutely capture the culmination of conspiring inequities within, as well as between, countries than maternal mortality. And it is likely that no global health issue more graphically illustrates the role of health systems, their potential both for promoting greater democracy and for reinforcing exclusion and discrimination along gender, class, racial, and ethnic lines, which further marginalizes certain groups. Maternal morbidity and mortality are overwhelmingly preventable; we have known for decades what causes them. Yet across the world we continue to see technocratic approaches, which, even when successful in averting a percentage of deaths, do little to transform the health systems or the social and political determinants that deprive women of the ability to live their lives as equal members of society, rather than as subordinated second-class citizens or instruments of reproduction.

I have argued in these pages that applying a human rights framework to health makes visible the "manifest injustice" of maternal mortality—and other conditions.[5] Human rights frameworks also present those who are most affected, together with those of us who stand in "pragmatic solidarity," as Paul Farmer says, with strategies and tools to hold duty-bearers accountable for taking the appropriate steps to address the inequity that gets reflected in health patterns.

Throughout this book, I have suggested that in many ways health is the most radical of subjects for rights precisely because it challenges what we consider to be *natural*. If health is a matter of rights, then it cannot just be a matter of divine or genetic fate. For example, if there is a right to be free of avoidable maternal mortality, then we cannot accept that the women's deaths recounted in this book and beyond are simply "God's will." On the contrary, we have to grapple with what is avoidable; what is preventable under different sets of circumstances; and with the role that legal frameworks, budgetary decisions, and social practices play in circumscribing the possibilities for individual choices that affect our well-being.

A right to health does not equalize the enjoyment of health, but it does mean that the state has some responsibility for evening out the opportunities we have to enjoy health and for ensuring a fair distribution of access to care, as well as to preconditions of health, such as potable water and sanitation. Moreover, the right to health is interdependent with and indivisible from many other rights, including CP rights, in a human rights framework. Thus, applying a transformative human rights framework to health calls on us to rethink the underlying causes of substantive inequalities among different people and groups with respect to social determinants and the right to health per se. It also causes us to rethink the nature of power and how it is exercised in concrete contexts to maintain domination over certain people with ensuing effects on health. Ultimately, I have argued, it causes us to rethink what it means to be human, in a world where people are too often reduced to consumers or targets of programs.

Applying Human Rights Frameworks to Health: Starting Points

The right to be treated as a human being, whose dignity matters, is the foundational concept of human rights and calls for tectonic shifts in how we structure both individual and social behavior. In Chapter 1, I argued that the concept of human dignity—as it is understood across many philosophical and religious traditions—includes an element of connection to equality with other human beings. In Kant's formulation, having dignity means that human beings should be treated as ends and not means; we cannot reduce human beings to instruments in ways that fail to recognize their independent agency. Thus, as has been recognized in many traditions, living a life of dignity requires not only respect for ourselves as agents with the capacity for self-government but also respect for the dignity in others. There is no subject more than health that shows how inexorably interdependent our societies, and world, really are. And there is no application of a human rights framework that demonstrates more vividly that respect for the dignity of others requires understanding the connections between collective choices about the set of *rights* reflected in laws and our institutional arrangements and practices.

Thus, for example, the power over one's life that is required to live life with dignity calls for rights to protect against affronts on people's bodily or moral integrity, whether in the public or the private sphere. It calls for freedom from torture and cruel, inhuman, and degrading treatment, whether committed by security forces, as in the Quijano case in Mexico City, or by personnel in health facilities. People's rights to be free from such abuse by the state apply to acts of omission as well as commission, from active denial of certain services, such as abortion, to laws, regulations, and policies that fail to provide for the most basic pain relief. In Chapter 1, I went on to argue that understanding the conditions necessary to live with dignity also requires challenging ways in which domination can become internalized, making it impossible for many children, and especially girls in many parts of the world, to develop a sense of themselves as full human beings with equal dignity and agency over their lives.

In Chapter 2, we further expanded the understanding of the conditions necessary for exercising some power over one's life and, in turn, for a life of dignity. When people, such as the impoverished indigenous woman Pilar in Mexico, are reduced to extreme poverty, they in effect cannot make independent choices about their lives. Historically, liberal notions of the state were accompanied by liberal notions of human rights as CP rights and were essentially conceived of as shields from intrusion by the state. This dichotomy was always misleading, as both CP rights and ESC rights entail various dimensions of obligations on the part of states—respecting, protecting, and fulfilling rights—and all rights require progressive realization as well as resources. Tremendous normative evolution has taken place with respect to health and other ESC rights, as rights that entail some equalization of entitlements by the state, and the application of human rights principles and frameworks to health. Moreover, there has been a recognition, in international as well as in some domestic jurisprudence, that welfare states bear responsibilities to the worst off in society and have legal, not just moral, obligations to provide minimum essential levels of health and other rights.

Nevertheless, a fundamental challenge to meaningfully using human rights is that the prevailing liberal narrative about rights as freedoms from state intrusion, which is deeply tied to the neoliberal organization of economies at national and global levels, continues to pervade much public discourse as well as practice. It is crucial to develop empowering HRBAs to health that can challenge the sophistry that underlies restricting the application of human rights norms to a thin slice of questions about civil and political freedoms, which fails to challenge the distribution of resources in society.

In Chapter 3 using an example from India, I went on to assert that applying a human rights framework to health can and should also challenge us to rethink mainstream medical and public health practice. The biomedical vision of health is also based on a certain individualism, a notion of autonomous people floating free from social constraints. But, as the WHO definition of health reflected more than sixty years ago, people do not live that way. Scientifically sound and evidence-based policies and programs are essential to a rights-based approach to health. However, we also need to recognize that both patterns of health and disease, as well as the meaning we ascribe to our experiences of suffering, inherently vary with the contexts in which we live our lives.

Despite the abundant evidence regarding the impact of social determinants stemming from power relations in society on patterns of population health, most public health and medical efforts focus on narrow technical interventions. Applying a human rights perspective calls for a focus on these *unnatural* and non-inevitable social determinants that shape patterns of ill-health. However, what applying a human rights framework distinctively adds to other approaches to health focused on equity and social determinants is an emphasis on accountability, through which problems are transformed into claims. This changes the relationship between citizens and the state.

I argued in Chapter 4 that a health system, conceived as a core social institution, lies at the center of both the right to health and the application of human rights principles to health. Referring to the context of Colombia, I argued that the health system enshrines and communicates values in the overall society and is not merely a technical apparatus for the delivery of goods and services.[6] Moreover, a health system can contribute toward greater equity and inclusion in the overall society. For example, a universal system of entitlements—in which all users feel they have a claim on the system as an asset of citizenship—plays a very different role in society than a public system designed to provide minimal care for the poor while the well-off turn to the private market. Priority-setting processes, including those engaged in taking decisions toward achieving universal health coverage, also encode norms and values regarding equality and rights. In a human rights framework, priority setting should be done through a legitimate and transparent process, which publicly acknowledges competing interests in the allocation of inevitably limited resources and where decisions can be justified, claimed by beneficiaries, and reviewed in the light of new evidence.

Because some have argued that theories of change are too often left implicit in HRBAs, and human rights more broadly, I explicitly argue that transforming a health system in an HRBA requires changing decisions at each stage of the policy cycle, which calls for shifts in institutions, processes, and outcomes.[7] At the same time, it requires changing relationships between parliamentarians and policy makers, policy makers and program implementers, program implementers and providers, providers and patients, and those citizens who use the health system and their elected representatives.[8] I also noted the importance of connecting how we think about health and suffering with actions and stressed that law, and legal narratives, can create and shape social meaning.

Applying Human Rights Frameworks to Health: Elements

The second part of this book presents the central elements of a human rights framework, or an HRBA—how those elements should be understood, how they relate to one another, and how they might be applied in practice. As discussed in Chapter 5, the central value of applying human rights frameworks to health may lie in establishing tools and mechanisms for accountability, which places limits on the untrammeled exercise of power. In a society with greater accountability, there is less need for charity. Imagine a society—and a world—where the rights to housing, food, and health were publicly and privately recognized and claimed as entitlements and were universally enforced as such. There would be no need to rely on the compassion of a particular sheriff who finds evictions distasteful, no need to demonstrate low actuarial risk to obtain health coverage or "normality" to receive certain sexual and reproductive goods and services, and no need to secure pity to receive food donations from a global philanthropy.

In Chapter 5, I asserted that transformative accountability requires us to go beyond "naming and shaming" health workers such as Rebecca in Sierra Leone to identify systemic responsibilities for policy and programming failures that deprive people such as Yerie Marah of health rights. The goal in an HRBA cannot be just to punish, and certainly not to scapegoat, frontline health workers; remedies can be used more broadly to reform systems and institutions. Although accountability in a human rights framework requires answerability from multiple actors throughout the policy cycle to be meaningful, I have argued that courts have a central role to play in balancing the discretion of the political organs of government. Emerging structural approaches to litigation may foster greater social learning around health as a topic of rights and may enable some disentrenchment of powerful interests within and beyond health sectors.

I went on to unpack what obligations we should be especially concerned about in applying a human rights framework to health. Normative obligations under international human rights law to "take appropriate steps and measures" with respect to the right to health must be linked to the best evidence from public health; and both clinical and cost effectiveness are relevant concerns. With respect to obligations to progressively realize health and related rights within a state's maximum available resources, I argued that it is also essential to establish accountability for the effort shown by the state in implementation of policies and programs, and for the extent of resources a government is devoting to progressive realization. Finally, in a human rights framework a state is answerable for the process through which it seeks to promote health rights, including equality and meaningful participation. And I stressed that even in a situation as daunting as Sierra

Leone, there are ways to approach enhancing accountability at different points in the circle.

In Chapter 6, I returned to the question of how we understand the forms of power that prevent people from living lives of dignity and how we can challenge those power asymmetries and transform people's opportunity structures. Just as we need to expand our understanding of rights from those narrowly conceived in a liberal paradigm, so too do we need to expand our understanding of how power relations structure subordination in societies, with ensuing health impacts. This view would challenge facile approaches to participation, based on assumptions about where power resides in the liberal state, which lead to creating spaces where participation is managed and controlled by the state and other private actors. By contrast, creating transformative change calls for inherently messy—and political—struggles for power, and making visible how agendas for what gets to be decided within decision-making forums can suppress conflict and the potential for real change in relation to health, as well as other issues. Understanding that "participatory forums" can mask inequalities in power should also make us wary of forums and processes, including for priority setting in health, which are set against backdrops of extreme inequality in which meaningful participation may not be possible.

Finally, internalization of low expectations and inferiority may mean that the preferences that systematically disadvantaged women and men express regarding their health and lives should not be taken at face value. Thus, developing critical consciousness among children, youths, and the disempowered is necessary for meaningfully empowering participation that changes opportunity structures in practice, and is part of a long-term effort to promote a culture of human rights, including in relation to health. Using the example of Peru, I noted that not only transforming consciousness but creating networks and institutions to promote change takes time.

In Chapter 7, in the context of South Africa, I explored the concepts of nondiscrimination and equality, which are fundamental principles in human rights law and in applying human rights to health. Equality has two dimensions in human rights. The first is formal equality, which requires that the state be impartial and treat similarly suited people equally without any arbitrary differentiation based on gender, race, caste, sexual orientation, disability, or other prohibited ground. Formal equality is crucial to promoting the notion that all people are equal in dignity and is closely related to the idea that people with the same conditions should have access to the same entitlements within a health system.

However, formal equality is desperately inadequate to ensure equal enjoyment of health and other rights for people such as Nomkhosi. Substantive equality under many national constitutions of modern welfare states, as well as under international law, recognizes that people who are in very different situations in practice require different measures to achieve equal enjoyment of their rights. Thus, women require services that men do not; populations suffering historic disadvantage require affirmative measures to be able to enjoy their health and other rights; disabled people may require certain provisions to be made in order to be able to enjoy their health rights.

Moreover, although traditionally the human rights community has eschewed the implications of human rights for economic policy, I argued that we can indeed determine some parameters for social equality that would stem from a state's obligations to show equal concern and respect for all citizens. Furthermore, doing so is crucial for the relevance of human rights frameworks to perhaps the most serious deprivations of human dignity that face large portions of humanity across the globe.

Finally, beginning with a story from Tanzania, in Chapter 8, I suggested that in devising empowering human rights frameworks to apply to health, we must come to grips with the extent to which people's health in the global South is determined through decisions taken elsewhere and by a global order that is fundamentally unfair. Although it is critical to hold national states accountable under human rights law, we must also hold donor states accountable for their decisions bilaterally and collectively, which influence the possibilities of health. I reviewed some of the evolving advocacy for new arrangements of global governance, based at least in part on shifting understandings of what social contracts are required in a globalized world. But I also noted limitations to grounding expanded extraterritorial legal obligations in a human rights framework and the need for further normative innovation.

In *Inventing Human Rights*, Lynn Hunt argues that through reading novels, Westerners in the eighteenth century were able to empathize with the suffering of others and this in turn gave rise to the notion that everyone should have rights, including, for example, the right to be free from torture.[9] Regardless of whether one agrees with Hunt's analysis of the origins of modern human rights, I have argued that the goal of enabling—or demanding— that we take the suffering of other human beings seriously remains centrally relevant.

In practice, though, we are still far short of the solidarity within countries or across borders necessary to ensure that health and other human rights are truly universal. Mapping the pain of the world needs to go beyond congratulating ourselves for feeling others' sorrow or our generous humanitarianism, to fostering greater understanding of our shared responsibilities for the social and institutional arrangements that perpetuate it. Moreover, if human rights is to remain a common language for collective human aspirations to dignity, it must not only incorporate an account of the suffering and indignity produced by socioeconomic inequality, as well as the myriad international forces that drive inequality between nations. It must also overcome entrenched apathy and mobilize collective action within countries and across borders in the North and South.

Applying Human Rights Frameworks to Health: From Analysis to Action

Although it can be difficult to know where to begin to disentangle all the different factors that are integral to creating a social order in which everyone can realize their health and other rights, I have repeatedly argued that analysis must not paralyze action. As Amartya Sen writes in *The Idea of Justice*: "Rather than concentrating on the long-distance search for the perfectly just society," we should concentrate on giving priority to the removal of manifest injustice and inequality that wrack the world and have such devastating health impacts today.[10] Thus, at the same time as I have suggested that if human rights (and HRBAs) are to remain relevant in the twenty-first century and to offer meaningful strategies to address the suffering of so many people around the world, we will need to transform certain limited understandings and approaches to rights, and we will also need to take concrete actions to shift norms, transform institutions and systems, and open meaningful opportunities for mobilization from the ground up. Throughout this book, I have discussed different ways to do so.

Applying human rights frameworks to health demands multiple strategies and will necessarily involve multiple actors—for example, diverse NGOs, policy makers, service providers, and courts—playing different roles. Social change requires networks of actors—and it requires time. Using human rights in meaningfully empowering ways will invariably challenge entrenched interests and therefore will entail political struggles among actors within health systems and beyond. And choices regarding timing and building synergies among different strategies—from policy operationalization to litigation to law reform to social mobilization—depend on the opportunity structures in specific contexts and cannot be dictated from the top down.

The implications of operationalizing human rights frameworks, and HRBAs to health, are now far better understood than previously. The UN "Technical Guidance" and other "guidelines" indicate to policy makers, as well as to other actors, how decisions can and should be changed at every step of the policy cycle, in contrast to a conventional approach. Further, as discussed in Chapter 4, the UN "Technical Guidance," while aimed at SRH, sets out a "circle of accountability" framework that is more broadly applicable to health policy making and implementation. In my view, it is important that such operational guidance regarding HRBAs not become another formula or checklist dispensed to policy makers and civil society advocates alike in "operational manuals" that depoliticize the inherent struggles involved in applying human rights frameworks to health.[11] On the contrary, the point of such operational guidance is to make explicit for the multiple actors involved in how a shift to a rights framework changes specific decisions in the light of different understandings of a health issue and its causes, the enabling environments and situational assessments required, the kinds of accountability to be promoted in the health system and beyond, and the monitoring and evaluation frameworks needed.

I have also signaled the importance of litigation in cases where there is an evident lack of political will to comply with human rights obligations relating to health. Litigation, although too often slow and limited, is being used effectively in cases around the globe to establish rights to freedoms as well as entitlements regarding health, at both national and international levels. For instance, in the groundbreaking case of *Alyne da Silva Pimentel v. Brazil*, discussed throughout this book, the CEDAW Committee established the obligation of states to guarantee women access to timely, nondiscriminatory, and appropriate maternal health care and the obligation of the government of Brazil to pay at least partial reparations and acknowledge that it had committed a violation of human rights.[12] Courts, although relatively weak actors (and often lacking in capacity or independence) can be essential in putting checks on the untrammeled discretion of political bodies. They can also play a pivotal role in creating new narratives of issues, such as abortion or same-sex union, that allow people to claim their full citizenship within social contexts.

In many countries, we saw that law reform, which has sometimes been triggered by litigation or structural judicial decisions, as in Colombia and

India, is also critical to enabling conditions for enjoyment of health and related rights. Law reform at the international level is also important for reframing obligations of states and for advancing the contours of norms relating to health and other rights—and the international and national levels are inextricably related through recursive feedback links. For example, CESCR's General Comment 14, which elucidated the content of the right to health under the ICESCR, has had repercussions on the development of national standards, from a Statutory Law on Health in Colombia to the Kenyan Constitution of 2010. In 2008, I was in Kenya shortly after the elections and would not have dreamed it possible that such a progressive constitution could emerge from the hideous ethnic violence that had been manufactured by certain political interests. Nevertheless, the Constitution of 2010 adopted verbatim some of the language of General Comment 14 in Article 43. In 2014, I interviewed plaintiffs in a collective suit along with Kenyan colleagues who were actively using litigation to enforce the principles enshrined in the constitution, and in 2015, I was named to the Oversight Committee of the Commission on the Implementation of the Constitution in its efforts to translate into practice the constitution's guarantee regarding the right to health. These processes are far from linear, but we need to be aware of the iterative and recursive processes that are necessary for social change.

Raising awareness of the legal enforceability of health rights and training of both practicing lawyers and sitting judges promotes the effectiveness and potential equity in impact of litigation, such as that being brought in Kenya. At Harvard's FXB Center for Health and Human Rights, we have both organized and participated in just such trainings to foster thinking on the part of legal practitioners about the equity and justice implications of bringing different kinds of health-rights litigation, as well as arguments for the enforceability of health-related rights.[13] These courses, together with other regional networks on health-rights litigation and judicial colloquia, some of which Harvard FXB has also been involved in, have led to cross-fertilization across contexts, enabled participants to go on to conduct further trainings of judges and lawyers in their own countries, as well as to bring successful litigations.[14]

As important as the law is, it is imperative that accountability move beyond the legal domain to encompass social mobilization and accountability and to change the culture to one of justification. Local initiatives, such as the one I described in Chapter 6, demonstrate how social accountability can be put into action and demonstrate that using human rights frameworks can effect both material change in people's lives and changes in social narratives of citizenship and rights. I also mentioned successful examples of social accountability in other countries. For example, the Social Accountability Monitoring (SAM) carried out by Sikika in Tanzania in conjunction with local communities in several districts uncovered inconsistencies between allocated budgets and actual implementation of health projects, and citizens are now demanding justifications for spending.[15] As I have stressed throughout this book, this change in the way people relate to each other—citizens and elected officials, patients and providers, and others—is essential to a circle of accountability and to applying human rights frameworks to health, and small changes can be made even in the most desperate of situations.

Effectively moving from analysis to action in deploying human rights strategies requires efforts to educate different actors involved at all stages of the policy cycle "circle of accountability" and across these multiple relationships. We have seen in examples throughout this book that education and awareness-raising initiatives, from Latin America to Africa, can and indeed must take many shapes, including critical consciousness and popular education about rights, sensitization of health professionals, dialogues among health-system users and with other actors in health systems; and public education for citizens and legislators alike regarding health as a rights issue. Applying human rights to health requires changes not only in policy but also in politics in order to produce social transformation.

Finally, sustaining change on the ground will require a shift in the understanding of the impact and the evidence of the impact regarding HRBAs and applying human rights tools in general.[16] If indicators are not used to measure what we care about from a human rights perspective, human rights will be reduced to little more than preambulatory language in policy and programming documents. Governments, donors, and NGOs, which claim to be adopting HRBAs, need to use monitoring and evaluation frameworks that are aligned with rights-based concerns. And some indeed are. As discussed in Chapter 8, some donors align their monitoring and evaluation frameworks to grantees' own frameworks, which minimizes both distortions in incentives and displacement of accountability to health system users.[17] Other donors and national governments, as well as NGOs and UN agencies, are also avidly developing rights-based indicators or mainstreaming rights concerns into their monitoring and evaluation frameworks. Nevertheless, further developing our understandings of evidence of impact—which entail profound questions about explicitly defining elements of human rights frameworks, standards of evidence, and the nature of the impact we are interested in—as well as refining our methodological approaches to measurement, are imperative to make application of human rights to health meaningful in practice.

Applying Human Rights Frameworks to Health: Revisiting the "So What" Question

At the same time as I have discussed successful and promising applications of human rights in practice, I have also noted that there are enormous challenges for advancing health and social justice in the world today and that human rights do not afford simple, "magic bullet" solutions. Thus, perhaps the central challenge for this book—and this field—is not just considering how an HRBA, or the adoption of a human rights framework to health, might differ from conventional approaches but determining why we should care about human rights at all. Why should we accept the inherently incremental approach of a human rights approach to health if what we really want to do is change the world? I believe the responses to this aspect of the "so what" question are centrally tied to how we see society and power and, ultimately, human beings.

For example, human rights presents a sharp contrast to the impulse to change the egregious inequities we face in the world through violent national revolution. Indeed, Samuel Moyn argues that the historical emergence of human rights as "the last utopia"—despite being about "slow and piecemeal reform," occurred only because other visions based on revolutionary nationalism "imploded."[18] I agree with Moyn with respect to the disenchantment with revolutions in practice, yet I also believe revolutions can encode different approaches to transforming power, and that it is precisely the fragmented approach of human rights that may in the end enable it to respond better to the inherent contestation and flux needed to preserve diverse people's dignity.

When I was growing up, the oligarchic control of much of Latin America and the connection between economic and social inequality and political repression were painfully evident; the Montoneros in Argentina and some of the other guerilla groups in Latin America seemed to be fighting on the side of justice.[19] Of course, different guerrilla movements are indeed different, and ex-fighters have gone on to become prominent proponents of democracy, as in the case of Pepe Mujica, who became the president of Uruguay. But the practical reality of revolutionary nationalism in Latin America has been quite dismal. It is generally the marginalized in society who have suffered the most in practice in the wake of guerrilla movements' promises to bring "New Democracy" and social justice to Latin America and elsewhere.[20]

Unlikely images can reveal enormous truths about our social aspirations as well as realities, and life is filled with them if only we look. For example, in the district of Azángaro in the north of the department of Puno in Peru, there is an extraordinary church called Tintiri. Tintiri is a replica of a Gothic cathedral that the son of a landowner had seen on his travels to Spain in the nineteenth century and ordered re-created in the middle of the *Altiplano*. It is a perfect replica, complete even with flying buttresses when it was constructed, but built completely of adobe.

Azángaro is one of the districts where we worked with the CARE health promoters, described in Chapter 6—and when passing by Tintiri, I have often thought about the workers who dedicated years of their lives to constructing this church at the beginning of the new Peruvian republic. The republic had promised rights for all and, in fact, the battle of Azángaro was the last battle for Peruvian independence.[21] Yet the peasants who risked their lives for the cause of independence and were the same men who toiled away essentially as slaves on the construction of Tintiri never saw the social emancipation they had been promised. Indeed, they were never even permitted to congregate in the church they had erected.

Later, in the 1980s, Azángaro became a "red zone" controlled by the Shining Path rebels (Sendero Luminoso) and Tintiri was converted into a barracks and storehouse for weapons. The Catholic saints and icons were stripped away and destroyed. But thirty years later, whatever hopes for creating a "dictatorship of the proletariat" Tintiri had contained during the years it was used by Sendero Luminoso, had long since evaporated.[22] Tintiri now stands shuttered and abandoned, apart from the usual sheep and llamas being herded by a few indigenous *campesinos*, whose lives have changed all too little since its construction.

Tintiri is a symbol of these different narratives of emancipation, and a physical reminder that, as Crane Brinton has written, revolutions too often lead to little meaningful change.[23] There is a tendency to romanticize revolution, proclaiming that it "marks a new era" or "ends forever the abuses of the old regime." In his now-classic book, *The Anatomy of Revolution*, Brinton traced the various and consistent stages of four successful revolutions, from breakdown of the old order through the "Thermidorian reaction." And as Mark Perry notes, "Brinton's narrative describes precisely the kinds of movements that became the Arab Spring"; that is, a symbolic event that took place in societies governed by inequitable and morally, as well as sometimes economically, bankrupt governments and was fueled by disaffected youth, led to protest, which was met with violence, and eventually produced the overthrow of the regimes.[24]

Brinton concludes that the revolutions he studied actually achieved very little in terms of social justice and, in particular, a lack of day-to-day change in social relations, such as those between men and women. The same might come to be true of appraisals of the Arab Spring. Brinton writes, "It is in the social arrangements that most intimately and immediately touch the average man [sic] that the actual changes effected by our revolutions seem slightest."[25] But, as I have described throughout this book, those are precisely the arrangements and relations that most affect diverse women's and men's capacity to live life with dignity.

Thus, as Indian legal philosopher Upendra Baxi writes, "For those who take people's suffering seriously, there is no rejoicing; even revolutions provide transient occasions of celebration."[26] If we imagine power as a block, the revolution acts as a sledgehammer and smashes it to pieces. However, the dissolution that results from this revolution is temporary, as the power block inevitably seems to get glued back together in another configuration. In practice, corrupt politicians sell out their ideals and clamp down on dissent and CP rights. Power is rarely spread throughout society to create more dignity, equality, and social justice, to enable diverse citizens to have greater choices over their private and public lives. This kind of rearrangement of power, which I witnessed in various countries in Latin America, is not the transformation we wish to see in the world.

Think again of Article 28 of the Universal Declaration, which states: "Everyone is entitled to a social and international order in which the rights and freedoms set forth in this Declaration can be fully realized."[27] Power in such a social order is fluid and contestable and is in inherent flux through constant processes of social negotiation, which occur through the appropriation of health and other rights. Thus, individuals are freer to interact with one another as individuals who possess equal dignity "rather than as placeholders in the system of class, communal, role, or gender contrasts," as Roberto Unger puts it.[28]

As I have also argued in this book, the goals of a transformative human rights approach to health should include destabilizing solidified expectations of institutions that are insulated from political change, within and beyond the health sector, and not merely palliative reform.[29] I have tried to show how applying a rights framework to health can facilitate seeing one another as full human beings who possess equal dignity, rather than as mere "placeholders." But this radical potential is only possible when we understand the multiple ways in which power is exercised to keep people from living with health and dignity, and the ensuing implications for constructing sets of rights obligations. If HRBAs are reduced to being top-down formalistic legal tools anchored by fixed understandings of norms or, even worse, "pleas for human rights to be conferred by the state," they will cease to be meaningful options for social transformation to the very people they purport to help.[30]

However, the "wholesale substitution of one institutional order by another" through revolution is not necessarily the path to meaningful social transformation either.[31] Indeed, the dichotomy between incrementalist measures and totalizing revolution is unduly Manichaean. As Unger writes, "We always need a way of thinking through our presuppositions—not all the way through, but just through to the next step."[32] Indeed, as we have discussed at various points, that in a human rights framework human beings are endowed with agency demands an incremental *process* by which they can express their diverse views. Such incrementalism is also often necessary to ensure that fundamental freedoms and other safeguards remain in place and that social choices taken on the path to changing some institutional arrangements do not congeal other forms of tyranny.[33] And incremental and disorganized change need not mean we lose a fundamental commitment to transformation, to true diffusion of power.

In short, the answer to the "so what" question is that, on the one hand, rights represent—or can represent—a distinctive domain for institutional reconstruction, which allows power to be simultaneously diffused and appropriated across both public and private spheres and which is unlikely to be achieved simply through political revolution. Applying a rights framework to health encodes an understanding of human agency that reflects the value of dignity in our lives, but also requires a process that enables diverse people to participate in defining and achieving the changes they want to see in society and the world.[34]

Concluding Reflection

I have been profoundly inspired by the stories I have heard from people I interviewed—including Daniel—in every country where I have worked. These are the people who have shown me the meaning of human suffering and dignity. I have also been profoundly inspired by the people with whom I have worked, not least of all in Uganda. One colleague there had been kidnapped by the Lord's Resistance Army (LRA) as part of a group of women who were forced into sexual slavery by the forces of the LRA's sociopathic megalomaniac leader, Joseph Kony; she later dedicated her professional life to women's reproductive and sexual rights in her country. Another colleague, who was orphaned early in life and bereft of family support, took on perhaps the most challenging social issue in Uganda: LGBT rights. Facing harassment and repudiation, he has gone into exile more than once because of his activism. Yet another colleague who founded an NGO committed to using the rights-based strategies I have discussed through these pages—social mobilization, media, network-building, law reform, and litigation—to transform Ugandan society, bringing, among other things, a groundbreaking case calling for access to maternal health care.[35] And there was David, who litigated that maternal health case and was as passionate an advocate as there ever was for the most disempowered women and children across the country.

David grew up in absolute destitution, in an orphanage in central Uganda, in a region where many Rwandans fleeing the genocide had settled. The priest who ran the orphanage was by all accounts an exceptional man who managed to inculcate great hopes, and even greater expectations, into the children he oversaw. A number of the children became professionals, lawyers, and businessmen. After the priest died, the orphanage fell into disrepair and was largely abandoned until David and some of his former fellow residents took on the management of the institution where they had once lived and created a vocational school.

Today the orphanage is run more like a boarding school for the most destitute of families than the typical charity-warehouse model of orphanage. And "Our Lady Technical and Vocational School," which includes among its core values both nondiscrimination and "changing the world," serves primarily adolescent girls who have been chased out of their homes and discarded by their communities for having abortions or for some other transgression. The school offers training in skills that include clothing design and construction, cosmetology and hairdressing, catering, journalism, and computer literacy. But from what I've seen, what these girls—and some boys—gain most is a sense of themselves as human beings with dignity and life plans that matter.

David is a man of deep faith, whose coherence and compassion I have come to respect immensely. Outraged that the capacities and dignity of

Uganda's most vulnerable citizens are systematically ignored and suppressed in his country, he sees very clearly the suffering caused by human agency, discrimination, and indifference. In discussing abortion one day, he said, "Why should [those who make laws criminalizing abortion] see themselves as God? Why should they decide who lives and dies?" And it is perhaps because he feels so keenly that he has felt the grace of God that David wants other impoverished children to experience it as well. When I asked him why he thinks he was able to achieve so much in his own life, David said, "I didn't know that I didn't have a right to dream of big things, to have great expectations for my life—so I did."

Ultimately, applying a meaningfully empowering human rights framework to health calls on us to create difference in the world, to make a different world, and to make ourselves different in the process.[36] Imagine how Uganda, and the world, would be transformed if everyone had expectations for living a life of dignity, for having the chance to be somebody. Imagine if both the privileged and the oppressed understood at a visceral level that the realities of our tangled lives—in our homes, in our communities, in our societies, and on our planet—need not and *must not* always be the way they are now, even if we are unsure of what they will be when they are no longer what they are.

Notes

Introduction

Citation for the first epigraph: Blue Mountain Arts Collection, *Believe: The Words and Inspiration of Desmond Tutu* (Auckland: P. Q. Blackwell Limited, 2007)..

1. Richard Stahler-Sholk, "Globalization and Social Movement Resistance: The Zapatista Rebellion in Chiapas, Mexico," *New Political Science* 23 (2001): 493–516.

2. Heidi Moksnes, "Factionalism and Counterinsurgency in Chiapas: Contextualizing the Acteal Massacre," *Revista Europea de Estudios Latinoamericanos y del Caribe*, 76 (2004): 109–17.

3. Alicia Ely Yamin, Thomas S. Crane, and Victor B. Penchaszadeh, *Health Care Held Hostage: Human Rights Violations and Violations of Medical Neutrality in Chiapas, Mexico* (Boston: Physicians for Human Rights, 1999).

4. Chinua Achebe, *Things Fall Apart* (New York: Anchor Books, 1994): 135.

5. Richard Horton. "Offline: Who Cares About Human Rights Anyway?" Comment in www.thelancet.com 382, October 26, 2013.

6. UN General Assembly, "Universal Declaration of Human Rights," UNGA Res. 217 A (III) (1948). Available at www.un.org/Overview/rights.html.

7. World Health Organization, "Children: Reducing Mortality. Fact sheet No 178," WHO, 2012, www.who.int/mediacentre/factsheets/fs178/en/index.html#.

8. Amartya Sen, *The Idea of Justice* (Cambridge, Mass.: Harvard University Press, 2009).

9. Peter Uvin, *Human Rights and Development* (Bloomfield, Conn.: Kumarian, 2004): 9–13; Philip Alston and Mary Robinson, "The Challenges of Ensuring the Mutuality of Human Rights and Development Endeavors," in *Human Rights and Development: Towards Mutual Reinforcement*, ed. Philip Alston and Mary Robinson (New York: Oxford University Press, 2005): 1–18.

10. "The Human Rights–Based Approach: Advancing Human Rights," United Nations Population Fund (UNFPA), www.unfpa.org/rights/approaches.htm.

11. See United Nations Development Group, "The Human Rights Based Approach to Development Cooperation Towards a Common Understanding Among UN Agencies," HRBA Portal (2003), http://hrbaportal.org/the-human-rights-based-approach-to-development-cooperation-towards-a-common-understanding-among-un-agencies.

12. Paul Farmer, *Pathologies of Power, Health, Human Rights and the New War on the Poor* (Berkeley: University of California Press, 2003).

13. Alicia Ely Yamin, "Toward Transformative Accountability: A Proposal for Rights-Based Approaches to Fulfilling Maternal Health Obligations," *Sur: An International Journal* 7, no. 12 (2010): 95–122.

14. Ebenezer Durojaye et al., eds., *Litigating the Right to Health in Africa: Challenges and Opportunities* (London: Ashgate, 2015); Laura Clérico et al., eds., *Salud: Sobre (des) Igualdades y Derechos* (Buenos Aires: Editorial Abelardo Perrot, 2013); Andrew Clapham, Mary Robinson, Claire Mahon, and Scott Jerbi, eds., *Realizing the Right to Health,* Swiss Human Rights Series (Zurich: Ruffer and Rub, 2009); Lawrence O. Gostin, *Global Health Law* (Cambridge, Mass.: Harvard University Press, 2014); and Jonathan Wolff, *The Human Right to Health,* Amnesty International Global Ethics Series (New York: Norton, 2012).

15. Flavia Bustreo et al., *Women's and Children's Health: Evidence of Impact of Human Rights* (Geneva: World Health Organization Press, 2013).

16. Ibid.

17. Jonathan Gottschall, *The Storytelling Animal: How Stories Make Us Human* (New York: Houghton Mifflin Harcourt, 2012). 272 pages.

18. Alasdair MacIntyre, *After Virtue: A Study in Moral Theory* (Notre Dame, Ind.: University of Notre Dame Press, 1984): 212.

19. Maya Unnithan-Kumar, "Reproduction, Health, Rights," in *Human Rights in Global Perspective: Anthropological Studies of Rights, Claims and Entitlements,* ed. John Mitchell and Richard Wilson (New York: Routledge, 2003): 183–208.

20. Paul H. Lewis, *Guerrillas and Generals: The "Dirty War" in Argentina* (Westport, Conn.: Praeger, 2002).

21. *NML Capital, Ltd. v. Republic of Argentina,* No. 03–cv–8845 (S.D.N.Y. Dec. 14, 2011), ECF No. 452; *EM Ltd. v. Republic of Argentina,* 695 F.3d 201 (2d Cir. 2012); *Republic of Argentina v. NML Capital,* 573 U.S. (2014).

22. The Center for Legal and Social Studies and the Center for Economic and Social Rights, "CESR Joins CELS in Challenging Human Rights Impacts of Vulture Funds," www.cesr.org /article.php?id=1620; UN Human Rights Council, "Effects of Foreign Debt and Other Related International Financial Obligations of States on the Full Enjoyment of All Human Rights, Particularly Economic, Social and Cultural Rights: The Activities of Vulture Funds," UN Doc. A/HRC/27/L.26 (2014).

23. Paul Farmer, "Challenging Orthodoxies: The Road Ahead for Health and Human Rights," *Health and Human Rights: An International Journal* 10, no.1 (2008): 5–19.

24. Lynn P. Freedman, "Achieving the MDGs: Health Systems as Core Social Institutions," *Development* 48, no. 1 (2005): 19–24; Lynn P. Freedman et al., "Who's Got the Power? Transforming Health Systems for Women and Children," UN Millennium Project Task Force on Child Health and Maternal Health (2005): 11.

25. See UN Human Rights Council, "Technical Guidance on the Application of a Human-Rights Based Approach to the Implementation of Policies and Programmes to Reduce Preventable Maternal Morbidity and Mortality," UN Doc. A/HRC/21/22 (2012).

26. Michael Neocosmos, "Civil Society, Citizenship and the Politics of the Impossible: Rethinking Militancy in Africa Today," *Interface: A Journal for and About Social Movements* 1, no. 2 (209): 278.

27. Christopher Jencks, *The Homeless* (Cambridge, Mass.: Harvard University Press, 1994): 39.

28. Barbara Kingsolver, *Flight Behavior* (New York: HarperCollins, 2012): 29.

29. "Ebola Survivor Dr. Kent Brantly's Full Remarks: 'God Saved My Life'," *NBC News*, August 21, 2014, www.nbcnews.com/storyline/ebola-virus-outbreak/ebola-survivor-dr-kent-brantlys-full-remarks-god-saved-my-n185956.

30. See, for example, Bas de Gaay Fortman, *Political Economy of Human Rights: Rights, Realities and Realization*, Routledge Frontiers of Political Economy (London: Routledge, 2011); Susan R. Holman, *Beholden: Religion, Global Health, and Human Rights* (New York: Oxford University Press, 2015); and Katherine Marshall, *Global Institutions of Religion: Ancient Movers, Modern Shakers*, Routledge Global Institutions Series (New York: Routledge, 2013).

Chapter 1. Dignity and Suffering

1. The Echoing Green Fellowship provides funding and technical assistance over two years for early-stage social entrepreneurs' work on global social change. For more information on the fellowship, see www.echoinggreen.org/fellowship.

2. Tim Golden, "Mexico's Human Rights Agency Urges Arrest of 13 Police Officers," *New York Times*, April 1, 1992.

3. Elaine Scarry, *The Body in Pain: The Making and Unmaking of the World* (Oxford: Oxford University Press, 1985).

4. Ibid., 34.

5. Ibid., 47.

6. Jacobo Timerman, *Prisoner Without a Name, Cell Without a Number*, trans. from the Spanish by Toby Talbot (Madison: University of Wisconsin Press, 1981): 148.

7. Charles Taylor, "To Follow a Rule," in *Philosophical Arguments* (Cambridge, Mass.: Harvard University Press, 1995): 168, 170, 178, cited in Kwame Anthony Appiah, *The Ethics of Identity* (Princeton, N.J.: Princeton University Press, 2005): 54.

8. UN General Assembly, "Universal Declaration of Human Rights," UNGA Res. 217 A (III), (1948), preamble.

9. Immanuel Kant, *Grounding for the Metaphysics of Morals*, trans. J. W. Wellington (Cambridge, Mass.: Hackett Publishing, 1785/1981): 434.

10. See, e.g., Christopher McCrudden, "Human Dignity and the Judicial Protection of Human Rights," *European Journal of International Law* 19 (2008): 655.

11. Martin Buber, *I and Thou* (New York: Charles Scribner's Sons, 1937).

12. Mahabharata Brihaspati, Anusansana Parva, Section CXIII, Verse 8.

13. Desmond Tutu, *No Future Without Forgiveness* (New York: Doubleday, 1999).

14. Timothy Murithi, "Practical Peacemaking: Wisdom from Africa: Reflections on Ubuntu," *Journal of Pan African Studies* 1, no. 4 (2006): 28.

15. Tutu, *No Future*, 34–35.

16. Kwame Anthony Appiah, *The Ethics of Identity* (Princeton, N.J.: Princeton University Press, 2010): 269.

17. Ibid.

18. Peter Singer, *Animal Liberation: A New Ethics for Our Treatment of Animals* (New York: Random House, 1975).

19. Alice Miller, "Sexual but Not Reproductive: Exploring the Junction and Disjunction of Sexual and Reproductive Rights," *Health and Human Rights* 2, no. 4 (2000): 95.

20. Roberto Mangabeira Unger, *False Necessity: Anti-Necessitarian Social Theory in the Service of Radical Democracy* (Cambridge: Cambridge University Press): 1988.

21. Kant, *Grounding for the Metaphysics of Morals*, 434.

22. Case No. 12.502, Inter-Am. CHR Series C No. 239 (February 24, 2012).

23. Charles Taylor, "The Politics of Recognition," in *Multiculturalism and the Politics of Recognition: An Essay* (Princeton, N.J.: Princeton University Press. 1992): 34.

24. Miller, "Sexual but Not Reproductive," 90.

25. *Soobramoney v. Minister of Health (KwaZulu-Natal)* 1998 (1) SA 765 (CC) (S.Afr.) [Concurring Opinion], Albie Sachs (S. Afr.): para. 54.

26. Ronald Dworkin, *Justice for Hedgehogs* (Cambridge, Mass.: Harvard University Press, 2011): 337.

27. Erving Goffman, *Asylums: Essays on the Social Situation of Mental Patients and Other Inmates*, with an introduction by William B. Helmreich Vol. 277 (New York: Anchor Books, 1961).

28. Ervin Staub, "The Psychology and Culture of Torture and Torturers," in *Psychology and Torture*, ed. Peter Suedfeld (New York: Hemisphere, 1990): 49–76.

29. "The Constitution of the United States," Art. 1, Sec. 2, Para. 3.

30. See the Institute of Medicine's full report: Brian Smedley, Adrienne Stith, and Alan Nelson, eds. *Unequal Treatment: Confronting Racial and Ethnic Disparities in Health Care* (Washington, D.C.: National Academies Press, 2003).

31. Patricia J. Williams, "Alchemical Notes: Reconstructing Ideals from Deconstructed Rights," in *Feminist Legal Theory: Foundations*, ed. D. Kelly Weisberg (Philadelphia: Temple University Press, 1993): 504.

32. Bartolomé de las Casas, *A Short Account of the Destruction of the Indies*, trans. Herma Briffault (Baltimore: Johns Hopkins University Press, 1992).

33. María Emma Mannarelli, *Limpias y modernas: género, higiene y cultura en la Lima del novecientos* (Lima: Ediciones Flora Tristán, 1999).

34. See Joanna Bourke, *What It Means to Be Human* (London: Virago, 2011).

35. Betty Friedan, "Address Before the First National Conference on Abortion Laws. Abortion: A Women's Civil Right (speech, Chicago, February 1969). Reprinted in Linda Greenhouse and Reva Siegel, eds., *Before Roe v Wade: Voices That Shaped the Abortion Debate Before the Supreme Court's Ruling* (New York: Kaplan, 2010): 38; cited in Rebecca Cook et al. eds., *Abortion Law in Transnational Perspectives* (Philadelphia: University of Pennsylvania Press, 2014): 19.

36. Women's Link Worldwide and R. J. Cook, "Excerpts of the Constitutional Court's Ruling That Liberalized Abortion in Colombia," *Reproductive Health Matters* (2007), 160–162.

37. Tribunal Federal Supremo de Argentina. FAL case (2012).

38. Felicity Callard et al., *Mental Illness, Discrimination and the Law: Fighting for Social Justice* (Oxford: John Wiley & Sons, 2012); and Jan Branson and Don Miller, *Damned for Their Difference: The Cultural Construction of Deaf People as Disabled* (Washington, D.C.: Gallaudet University Press, 2002).

39. Susan Sontag, *Regarding the Pain of Others* (New York: Farrar, Straus and Giroux, 2003): 102.

40. See Dworkin, *Justice*, 272, discussing Kant's maxim as applied to aid.

41. Sontag, *Regarding the Pain*, 42.

42. Jonathan M. Mann et al., "Health and Human Rights," *Health and Human Rights* 1, no. 1 (1994): 7–23.

43. UN General Assembly, "Convention Against Torture and Other Cruel, Inhuman or Degrading Treatment or Punishment," December 10, 1984, United Nations, Treaty Series, vol. 1465, art. 1.

44. Physicians for Human Rights and Human Rights First, "Leave No Marks: Enhanced Interrogation Techniques and the Risk of Criminality," *Physicians for Human Rights and Human Rights First* (2007), www.humanrightsfirst.org/wp-content/uploads/pdf/07801-etn-leave-no -marks.pdf.

45. Leonard S. Rubenstein, "Dual Loyalty and Human Rights," *Journal of Ambulatory Care Management* 26, no. 3 (2003): 270–72.

46. Physicians for Human Rights, "Broken Laws, Broken Lives: Medical Evidence of Torture by U.S. Personnel and Its Impact" (2008).

47. UN Economic and Social Council, "Siracusa Principles on the Limitation and Derogation Provisions in the International Covenant on Civil and Political Rights," UN Doc. E/CN.4/1985/4 (1985).

48. See James Howard Jones, "The Tuskegee Syphilis Experiment," in *The Oxford Textbook of Clinical Research Ethics*, ed. Ezekiel J. Emanuel et al. (New York: Oxford University Press, 2008): 86–96.

49. Jonathan Mann, *Hastings Center Report*, 27, no. 3 (May–June 1997): 9.

50. Jones, "Tuskegee," 86.

51. See Center for Reproductive Rights and Poradna pre obcianske a ludské práva, "Body and Soul: Forced Sterilization and Other Assaults on Roma Reproductive Freedom in Slovakia" (2003), http://reproductiverights.org/en/document/body-and-soul-forced-sterilization-and-other -assaults-on-roma-reproductive-freedom; and Cladem, "Mamerita Mestanza Case, Peru (Forced Sterilization)," *Cladem Online* (2010).

52. UN Committee on the Elimination of Discrimination Against Women (CEDAW), "CEDAW General Recommendation No. 24: Article 12 of the Convention (Women and Health)," UN Doc. A/54/38/Rev. 1 (1999).

53. Center for Reproductive Rights, "*KL v. Peru* (United Nations Human Rights Committee)" (2008), http://reproductiverights.org/en/case/kl-v-peru-united-nations-human-rights -committee.

54. Ibid.

55. Center for Reproductive Rights, "Reproductive Rights Violations as Torture and Cruel, Inhuman, or Degrading Treatment or Punishment: A Critical Human Rights Analysis" (2010).

56. UN Human Rights Council, "Report of the Special Rapporteur on Torture."

57. *Garrua* is the fine mist of equatorial Peru. For reference, see Frederick Alexander Kirkpatrick, *South America and the War* (Cambridge: Cambridge University Press, 1918): 3.

58. See *The Scream* by Edvard Munch, one of the most iconic and recognized images in art history.

59. Indeed, there is a Stop Torture in Health Care Campaign supported by the Open Society Foundations, which includes advocacy by Human Rights Watch and many other organizations on access to palliative pain relief as well as other forms of torture and cruel and inhuman treatment in health care settings.

60. Françoise Girard, "Stop Torture in Health Care," *Open Society Foundation* (March 29, 2011), www.opensocietyfoundations.org/voices/stop-torture-health-care-0.

61. Roberto Mangabeira Unger, *The Critical Legal Studies Movement* (Cambridge, Mass.: Harvard University Press, 1983): 36.

62. UN General Assembly, "Convention on the Rights of the Child," UN Doc. A/RES/44/25 (1989): art. 3.

63. UNICEF and Centers for Disease Control and Prevention (CDC), "Violence Against Children in Tanzania: Findings from a National Survey 2009," United Republic of Tanzania (2011): 27, www.unicef.org/media/files/violence_against_children_in_tanzania_report.pdf.

64. Ibid, 10.

65. Steve Eder and Pat Borzi, "NFL Rocked Again as Adrian Peterson Faces a Child Abuse Charge," *New York Times*, September 12, 2014.

66. UN General Assembly, "Convention on the Elimination of All Forms of Discrimination Against Women," UN Doc. A/RES/4/180 (1979), art. 5; and UN General Assembly, "Convention on the Rights of the Child."

67. Council of Europe, "Convention on Preventing and Combating Violence Against Women and Domestic Violence (Istanbul Convention): The Convention in Brief" (2004), www.coe.int/t /dghl/standardsetting/convention-violence/brief_en.asp.

68. Rangita de Silva de Alwis and Jeni Klugman, "From Violence and the Law: A Global Perspective in Light of the Chinese Domestic Violence Law," *East Asia Law Review,* in press Winter 2015.

69. Ann L. Coker et al., "Physical Health Consequences of Physical and Psychological Intimate Partner Violence," *Archives of Family Medicine* 9, no. 5 (2000): 451–57.

70. World Health Organization, "Global and Regional Estimates of Violence Against Women: Prevalence and Health Effects of Intimate Partner Violence and Non-Partner Sexual Violence" (2013). Accessed at: http://apps.who.int/iris/bitstream/10665/85239/1/9789241564625_eng.pdf ?ua=1.

71. World Health Organization, "WHO Multi-Country Study on Women's Health and Domestic Violence Against Women" (2005). Accessed at: http://apps.who.int/iris/bitstream/10665 /43310/1/9241593512_eng.pdf?ua=1.

72. De Silva de Alwis and Klugman, "From Violence and the Law." Sarah Twigg, Jennifer McCleary-Sills, Tazeen Hasan, and Juliet Andrea Santamaria, "Voice and Agency: Empowering Women and Girls for Shared Prosperity," World Bank Group, 2014.

73. Appiah, *Ethics*, 20.

74. Martha Nussbaum and Jonathan Glover, eds., *Women, Culture, and Development: A Study of Human Capabilities* (Oxford: Clarendon Press, 1995), cited in Steven Lukes, *Power: A Radical View*, Second Edition (London: Palgrave Macmillan, 2005): 119.

75. Committee Against Torture, "Consideration of Reports Submitted by States Parties Under Article 19 of the Convention: Supplementary Reports of States Parties Due in 1992," UN Doc. CAT/C/17/Add.3 (1992) (Summary record), www.univie.ac.at/bimtor/dateien/mexico_cat_1992 _report.pdf.

76. Alicia Ely Yamin, *Justice Corrupted, Justice Denied: Unmasking the Untouchables of the Mexican Federal Judicial Police* (New York: World Policy Institute, 1992).

Chapter 2. The Powerlessness of Extreme Poverty

Epigraphs: Nelson Mandela, BBC News, February 3, 2005; Thomas Pogge, *Freedom from Poverty as a Human Right: Who Owes What to the Very Poor?* (New York: Oxford University Press, 2007), 4.

1. Lázaro Cárdenas, the president of Mexico from 1934 to 1940, is remembered as a great social reformer. The land-reform policies that were enacted under him are widely recognized as having helped relieve poverty, particularly in the agrarian peasant population. See

Michael W. Foley, "Privatizing the Countryside: The Mexican Peasant Movement and Neoliberal Reform," *Latin American Perspectives* 22, no. 1 (1995): 59–76.

2. Katherine Boo, *Behind the Beautiful Forevers* (New York: Random House, 2012), xx.

3. The expression "Sophie's choice" is adapted from the title of William Styron's 1979 book, in which a mother is forced to decide which of her children will die at a concentration camp in Nazi Germany.

4. Alicia Ely Yamin, "Health and Human Rights in Latin America: A Lawyer's Experience with Public Health Internationalism," in *Comrades in Health: U.S. Health Internationalists, Abroad and at Home,* ed. Anne-Emanuelle Birn and Theodore M. Brown (New Brunswick. N.J.: Rutgers University Press, 2012).

5. Minnesota Advocates for Human Rights, *Civilians at Risk: Military and Police Abuse in the Mexican Countryside* (Minneapolis: Minnesota Advocates for Human Rights, 1993), www .theadvocatesforhumanrights.org/uploads/civilians_at_risk_-_military_and_police_abuses _in_the_mexican_countryside_2.pdf.

6. Yamin, "Health and Human Rights in Latin America," 238.

7. Deepa Narayan et al., *Voices of the Poor: Crying Out for Change* (New York: Published for the World Bank, Oxford University Press, 2000): 36.

8. Pogge, *Freedom From Poverty as a Human Right,* 3–4.

9. UN General Assembly, "Universal Declaration of Human Rights," UNGA Res. 217 A (III), (1948), preamble.

10. UN Committee on Economic, Social and Cultural Rights (CESCR), "General Comment No. 14, The Right to the Highest Attainable Standard of Health," UN Doc. No. E/C.12/2000/4 (2000).

11. UN General Assembly, "International Covenant on Economic, Social and Cultural Rights (ICESCR)," UN GA Res. 2200, UN Doc. No. A/6316 (1966): art. 12.

12. U.S. Government, *Statement at the U.N. Commission on Human Rights,* 59th Sess., Comment on the Working Group on the Right to Development (February 10, 2003).

13. International Foundation for Electoral Systems and United Nations Development Program, "Getting to the CORE: A Global Survey on the Cost of Registration and Elections" (2006), http://content.undp.org/go/cms-service/stream/asset/?asset_id=472992.

14. Mamta Badkar, "Eight Incredible Facts About India's Massive Elections," *Business Insiders,* April 8, 2014.

15. "India Cuts Healthcare Spending by 10% in 2014–15 Government Budget," *HIS,* February 18, 2014.

16. UN General Assembly, "Vienna Declaration and Programme of Action," July 12, 1993, UN Doc. A/CONF.157/23 (1993): sec. 5.

17. For one of the first articulations of this tripartite understanding of state obligations, see "Report on the Right to Food as a Human Right," UN Doc. E/CN.4/Sub.2/1987/23 (1987). See also CESCR, "General Comment No. 14, The Right to the Highest Attainable Standard of Health."

18. CESCR, "General Comment No. 14, The Right to the Highest Attainable Standard of Health," UN Doc. No. E/C.12/2000/4 (2000).

19. Amartya Sen, "Elements of a Theory of Human Rights," *Philosophy and Public Affairs* 32 (2004): 329.

20. Committee on Social Determinants of Health, "Closing the Gap in a Generation: Health Equity Through Action on the Social Determinants of Health. Final Report of the Commission on Social Determinants of Health" World Health Organization (2008); and Bjorn Hallerod and

Jan-Eric Gustafsson, "A Longitudinal Analysis of the Relationship Between Changes in Socio-Economic Status and Changes in Health," *Social Sciences & Medicine* 72 (2011): 116–23.

21. Norman Daniels, *Just Health* (Cambridge: Cambridge University Press, 1985); and Martha Nussbaum and Amartya Sen, *The Quality of Life* (Oxford: Oxford University Press, 1993).

22. Jonathan M. Mann et al., "Health and Human Rights," *Health and Human Rights* 1, no 1 (2004): 6–23.

23. UN General Assembly, "International Covenant on Economic, Social and Cultural Rights (ICESCR)," art. 12.

24. Robert E. Black, "Where and Why Are 10 Million Children Dying," *Lancet* 361 (2003): 2226–34.

25. Li Liu et al., "Global, Regional, and National Causes of Child Mortality: An Updated Systematic Analysis for 2010 with Time Trends Since 2000," *Lancet* 379 (2012): 2151–61.

26. CESCR, "General Comment No. 14, The Right to the Highest Attainable Standard of Health" "UN Doc. No. E/C.12/2000/4 (2000); CESCR, "General Comment No. 3, The Nature of States Parties' Obligations," UN Doc. E/1991/23 (1991); CESCR, "General Comment No. 7, The Right of Everyone to Benefit from the Protection of the Moral and Material Interests Resulting from any Scientific, Literary or Artistic Production of Which He or She Is the Author," UN Doc. E/C.12/GC/17 (2006); and CESCR, "General Comment No. 19: The Right to Social Security," UN Doc. E/C.12/GC/19 (2008).

27. CESCR, "General Comment No. 14, The Right to the Highest Attainable Standard of Health," UN Doc. No. E/C.12/2000/4 (2000).

28. Katharine G. Young, "The Minimum Core of Economic and Social Rights: A Conception in Search of Content," *Yale Journal of International Law* 33 (2008): 113, 114.

29. WHO Health and Human Rights Team, "Health and Human Rights," World Health Organization (2012).

30. CESCR, "General Comment No. 14, The Right to the Highest Attainable Standard of Health" UN Doc. No. E/C.12/2000/4 (2000); UN Committee on the Elimination of Discrimination Against Women (CEDAW), "CEDAW General Recommendation No. 24: Article 12 of the Convention (Women and Health)," UN Doc. A/54/38/Rev.1 (1999): chap. I; UN Committee on the Rights of the Child (CRC), "CRC General Comment No. 4: Adolescent Health and Development in the Context of the Convention on the Rights of the Child," UN Doc. CRC/GC/2003/4 (2003); and CRC, "General Comment No. 15 on the Right of the Child to the Enjoyment of the Highest Attainable Standard of Health (Art. 24)," UN Doc. CRC/C/GC/15 (2013).

31. UN Human Rights Council, "Technical Guidance on the Application of a Human-Rights Based Approach to the Implementation of Policies and Programmes to Reduce Preventable Maternal Morbidity and Mortality," UN Doc. A/HRC/21/22 (2012).

32. Flavia Bustreo et al., "Women's and Children's Health: Evidence of Impact of Human Rights," World Health Organization (2013).

33. Alicia Ely Yamin and Siri Gloppen, eds., *Litigating the Right to Health: Can Courts Bring More Justice to Health?* (Cambridge, Mass.: Harvard University Press, 2011).

34. Judgment T-760, Corte Constitucional [C.C.] [Constitutional Court], July 31, 2008, Sentencia T-760/08 (Colom.); and *Minister of Health and Others v Treatment Action Campaign and Others* 2002 (2) SA 8/02 (CC) ZACC 15 (S.Afr.).

35. *Nada personal: reporte de derechos humanos sobre la aplicación de la anticoncepción quirúgica en el Perú 1996–1998* [Nothing Personal: Human Rights Report on the Use of Surgical

Contraception in Perú 1996–1998] (Lima: Latin American and Caribbean Committee for the Defense of Women's Rights, 1999).

36. See Defensoría del Pueblo, *Informe Defensorial No. 7. La Aplicación de la anticoncepción quirúrgica y los derechos reproductivos I: casos investigados por la Defensoría del Pueblo* (Lima: Defensoría del Pueblo, 1998); Defensoría del Pueblo, *Informe Defensorial No. 27. La Aplicación de la anticoncepción quirúrgica y los derechos reproductivos II: casos investigados por la Defensoría del Pueblo* (Lima: Defensoría del Pueblo, 1999); Kenyan National Commission on Human Rights, *Realising Sexual and Reproductive Health Rights in Kenya: A Myth or Reality? A Report of the Public Inquiry into Violations of Sexual and Reproductive Health Rights in Kenya* (Nairobi: Kenyan National Commission on Human Rights, 2012), www.knchr.org/Portals/0/EcosocReports /Reproductive_health_report.pdf.

37. Claudio Munoz, "Human Rights: Stand Up for Your Rights," *Economist*. March 22, 2007.

38. See Kenneth Roth, "Defending Economic, Social and Cultural Rights: Practical Issues Faced by an International Human Rights Organization," *Human Rights Quarterly* 26 (2004): 63–73.

39. UN General Assembly, "Universal Declaration of Human Rights."

40. Case No. 2009-43-01 On Compliance of the First Part of Section 3 of State Pensions and State Allowance Disbursement in 2009–2012 insofar as It Applies to State Old-Age Pension with Article 1, Article 91, Article 105, and Article 109 of the Satversme (Constitution) of the Republic of Latvia, Constitutional Court of the Republic of Latvia; and CESCR, "General Comment No. 19: The Right to Social Security."

41. Ronald Dworkin, *Justice for Hedgehogs* (Cambridge, Mass.: Harvard University Press, 2011): 2.

42. Ibid., 2–3.

43. Cass Sunstein, *The Second Bill of Rights: FDR'S Unfinished Revolution and Why We Need It More Than Ever* (New York: Basic Books, 2004): 23.

44. Judgment C-1064, Corte Constitucional [C.C.] [Constitutional Court], October 10, 2001, Sentencia C-1064/01 (Colom.).

45. *Soobramoney v. Minister of Health (KwaZulu-Natal)* 1998 (1) SA 765 (CC) (S. Afr.), P Chaskalson, para 8.

46. *Chandra Bhavan Boarding & Lodging v. State of Mysore* (1970) 2 S.C.R. 600, 612 (India) (Hegde, J.).

47. *Government of the Republic of South Africa and Others v. Grootboom and Others* 2011 (1) SA 46 (CC) (S. Afr.).

48. Statement of the United States of America delivered by Richard Wall, "Item 10: Economic, Social and Cultural Rights" at the 59th Session of the United Nations Commission on Human Rights, April 7, 2003, www.us-mission.ch/humanrights/statements/0407Item10.htm.

49. The emphasis on privacy has meant that poor women who cannot afford abortions do not have meaningful rights to them. In *Harris v. McRae*, 448 U.S. 297 (1980), the Court held that States that participated in Medicaid (a federally funded program to provide health care to people living in poverty) were not required to fund medically necessary abortions for which federal reimbursement was unavailable as a result of a recent federal law (the Hyde Amendment), which restricted the use of federal funds for abortion.

50. *Planned Parenthood v. Casey*, 505 U.S. 833 (1992).

51. See S. 142, 113th Congress: Hyde Amendment Codification Act (2013).

52. Lynn P. Freedman, "Human Rights and the Politics of Risk and Blame: Lessons from the International Reproductive Rights Movement," *Journal of the American Women's Association* 54 (1997): 165–73; Susana Chiarotti, "Mujeres y derechos humanos: convergencias y tensiones entre dos movimientos sociales" in *Los derechos económicos, sociales y culturales en América Latina: Del invento a la herramienta [Economic, Social and Cultural Rights in Latin America: From Ideals to Tools]*, ed. Alicia Ely Yamin (Mexico City: Plaza y Valdés Editores, 2006).

53. Pogge, *Freedom*, 6.

54. Andy Sumner, "Where Will the World's Poor Live? An Update on Global Poverty and the New Bottom Billion," *Center for Global Development Working Paper* (2012).

55. Patrick J. McGowan and Dale L. Smith, "Economic Dependency in Black Africa: An Analysis of Competing Theories," *International Organization* 32, no 1 (1978): 179–235.

56. Amartya Sen, *Development as Freedom* (Oxford: Oxford University Press, 1999): 86–87.

57. UN Committee on Economic, Social and Cultural Rights, "Substantive Issues Arising in the Implementation of the International Covenant on Economic, Social and Cultural Rights: Poverty and the International Covenant on Economic, Social and Cultural Rights," UN Doc. E/C.12/2001/10 (2001): para. 17 (noting also that "in accordance with General Comment No. 14, it is particularly incumbent on all those who can assist, to help developing countries respect this international minimum threshold. If a national or international anti-poverty strategy does not reflect this minimum threshold, it is inconsistent with the legally binding obligations of the State party").

58. Alicia Ely Yamin and Vanessa M. Boulanger, "Embedding Sexual and Reproductive Health and Rights in a Transformational Development Framework: Lessons Learned from the MDG Targets and Indicators," *Reproductive Health Matters* 21, no 42 (2013): 74–85.

59. Fukuda-Parr, Sakiko, Alicia Ely Yamin, and Joshua Greenstein, "The Power of Numbers: A Critical Review of Millennium Development Goal Targets for Human Development and Human Rights," *Journal of Human Development and Capabilities* 15.2–3 (2014): 105–117.

60. Sakiko Fukuda-Parr and Alicia Ely Yamin, "The Power of Numbers: A Critical Review of MDG Targets for Human Development and Human Rights," *Development* 56, no.1 (2013): 58–65.

61. Felicia Marie Knaul et al., "The Quest for Universal Health Coverage: Achieving Social Protection for all in Mexico," *Lancet* 380 (2012): 1259–79.

62. Lia Fernald et al., "Ten-Year Effect of Oportunidades, Mexico's Conditional Cash Transfer Programme, on Child Growth, Cognition, Language, and Behavior: A Longitudinal Follow-Up Study," *Lancet* 374 (2009): 1997–2005.

63. Julio Frenk et al., "Comprehensive Reform to Improve Health System Performance in Mexico," *Lancet* 368 (2006): 1527.

64. Susan Sontag, *Regarding the Pain of Others* (New York: Farrar, Straus and Giroux, 2003): 79.

Chapter 3. Redefining Health

1. Kabliji Hospital and Rural Health Centre (2014), www.kablijihospital.com/.

2. Jim Yardley, "India Eyes Muslims Left Behind by Quota System," *New York Times*, March 9, 2012.

3. Lydia Polgreen, "Scaling Caste Walls with Capitalism's Ladders in India," *New York Times*, December 21, 2011.

4. Lisa Berkman and Ichiro Kawachi, eds., *Social Epidemiology* (New York: Oxford University Press, 2000); Michael Marmot and Richard Wilkinson, eds., *Social Determinants of Health*

(Oxford: Oxford University Press, 1999); and Débora Tajer, "Latin American Social Medicine: Roots, Development During the 1990s and Current Challenges," *American Journal of Public Health* 93, no. 12 (2003): 2023–27.

5. Rudolf Virchow, "Der Armenarzt," *Medicinske Reform* 1848; 18: 125–27.

6. Ichiro Kawachi and Bruce Kennedy, *The Health of Nations: Why Inequality Is Harmful to Your Health* (New York: New Press, 2002); Berkman and Kawachi, *Social Epidemiology*; and Marmot and Wilkinson, *Social Determinants*.

7. WHO Commission on Social Determinants of Health. *Closing the Gap in a Generation: Health Equity Through Action on the Social Determinants of Health: Commission on Social Determinants of Health Final Report.* Ed. World Health Organization. World Health Organization, 2008.

8. World Health Organization, "Constitution of the World Health Organization as adopted by the International Health Conference," (1946), preamble.

9. Ibid.

10. John Tobin, *The Right to Health in International Law* (Oxford: Oxford University Press, 2012).

11. Amnesty International, "Deadly Delivery: The Maternal Health Care Crisis in the USA" (2010), www.amnestyusa.org/sites/default/files/pdfs/deadlydelivery.pdf.

12. Bruce G. Link and Jo Phelan, "Social Conditions as Fundamental Causes of Disease," *Journal of Health and Social Behavior*, Extra Issue 35 (1995): 80–94.

13. Anahad O'Connor, "Weight Loss Surgery May Not Combat Diabetes Long-Term," *New York Times*, November 28, 2012; Nicholas Bakalar, "Risks: More Red Meat, More Mortality," *New York Times*, March 12, 2012; Cathryn M. Delude, "Unlocking the Diabetes-Heart-Disease Connection," *New York Times*, January 10, 2006; Mike Stobbe, "Diabetes Rates Rocket in Oklahoma, South," *Boston Globe*, November 15, 2012; and Lindsey Tanner, "Obesity-Related Diabetes Found Riskiest in Children," *Boston Globe*, July 26, 2006.

14. Lawrence Wallack, "The Role of Mass Media in Creating Social Capital: A New Direction for Public Health," in *Health and Social Justice: Politics, Ideology, and Inequity in the Distribution of Disease*, ed. Richard Hofrichter (San Francisco: Jossey-Bass, 2003): 594–626.

15. Jennifer Prah Ruger, "Toward a Theory of the Right to Health: Capabilities and Incompletely Theorized Agreements," *Yale Journal of Law and the Humanities* 18 (2006): 314.

16. Alicia Ely Yamin, "Embodying Shadows: Tracing the Contours of Women's Rights to Health," in *From the Margin of Globalization: Critical Perspectives on Human Rights*, ed. Neve Gordon (New York: Lexington Books, 2004): 223–57; Lynn Freedman, "Reflections on Emerging Frameworks of Health and Human Rights," *Health and Human Rights* 1, no. 4 (1994): 314–49, at 323.

17. Anne Fadiman's *The Spirit Catches You and You Fall Down: A Hmong Child, Her American Doctors, and the Collision of Two Cultures* (New York: Farrar, Straus and Giroux, 1997) is a powerful book that provides unique insight into this subject. See also K. S. Jacob, Dinesh Bhugra, Keith Lloyd, and Anthony Mann, "Common Mental Disorders, Explanatory Models and Consultation Behavior Among Indian Women Living in the UK," *Journal of the Royal Society of Medicine* 91, no. 2 (1998): 66–71.

18. See Arthur Kleinman, *Culture and Healing in Asian Societies: Anthropological Psychiatric and Public Health Studies* (Boston: G. K. Hall, 1978).

19. Elizabeth Fee and Nancy Krieger, "Understanding AIDS: Historical Interpretations and the Limits of Biomedical Individualism," *American Journal of Public Health* 83, no. 10 (1993): 1477–86.

20. For a seminal example of writing in the bioethics tradition, see Ezekiel Emanuel and Linda Emanuel, "Four Models of the Physician-Patient Relationship," *Journal of the American Medical Association* 267 (1992): 2221–23.

21. Michel Foucault, *Madness and Civilization: A History of Insanity in the Age of Reason* (New York: Random House, 1965).

22. Chiku Ali and Agnete Strom, "It Is Important to Know That Before, There Was No La-walawa: Working to Stop Female Genital Mutilation in Tanzania," *Reproductive Health Matters* 20, no. 40 (2012): 69.

23. Ibid, 70.

24. Richard Epstein, *Mortal Peril* (New York: Addison-Wesley, 1997): 2–3.

25. Jonathan Mann, "Human Rights and the New Public Health," *Health and Human Rights* 1, no. 3 (1995): 229.

26. Nancy Krieger, "Proximal, Distal, and the Politics of Causation: What's Level Got to Do with It?" *American Journal of Public Health* 98, no. 2 (2008): 221–30, at 223.

27. World Health Organization, "Childhood Lead Poisoning" (2010). Accessed at: http://apps .who.int/iris/bitstream/10665/136571/1/9789241500333_eng.pdf?ua=1&ua=1.

28. See Section 8 of the Housing Act of 1937, 42 U.S. Code § 1437f, as repeatedly amended, www.law.cornell.edu/uscode/text/42/1437f.

29. WHO Commission on Social Determinants of Health, *Closing the Gap in a Generation: Health Equity Through Action on the Social Determinants of Health: Commission on Social Determinants of Health Final Report*. World Health Organization, 2008.

30. Steven H. Woolf et al., "Giving Everyone the Health of the Educated: An Examination of Whether Social Change Would Save More Lives Than Medical Advances," *American Journal of Public Health* 97, no. 4 (2007): 679–83.

31. Ibid, 679.

32. WHO Commission on Social Determinants of Health. *Closing the Gap in a Generation,* 179.

33. Ole Petter Ottersen et al., "The Political Origins of Health Inequity: Prospects for Change," *Lancet*. 383 (9917) (2014): 630–667.

34. Susan Fawcus, "Maternal Mortality and Unsafe Abortion," *Best Practice and Research Clinical Obstetrics and Gynaecology* 22, no. 3 (2008): 533–48.

35. Peter Uvin, *Human Rights and Development* (West Hartford, Conn.: Kumarian Press, 2004): 191.

36. *William García Alvarez v. Caja Costarricense de Seguro Social*, Judgment 5934 Sala Constitucional de la Corte Suprema de Justicia, [Sup. Ct. Const. Ch.] Exp. 5778-V-97 N. 5934-97 (1997).

37. Ibid.

38. *Minister of Health and Others v. Treatment Action Campaign and Others* 2002 (1) SA 9 ZACC 16 (CC) (S. Afr.).

39. See, for instance, Jim Yardley, "A Village Rape Shatters a Family, and India's Traditional Silence," *New York Times*, October 27, 2012.

40. United Nations Populations Fund (UNFPA), "International Conference on Population and Development (ICPD) Programme of Action," UN Doc. A/CONF.171/13/Rev.1 (1995).

41. Ibid.

42. Laura Reichenbach and Mindy Jane Roseman, eds., *Reproductive Health and Human Rights: The Way Forward* (Philadelphia: University of Pennsylvania Press, 2009).

43. United Nations, "Beijing Declaration and Platform of Action," adopted at the Fourth World Conference on Women, October 27, 1995, UN Doc. A/CONF.177/20 (1995).

44. UN Committee on the Elimination of Discrimination Against Women (CEDAW), "Views of the Committee on the Elimination of Discrimination Against Women Under Article 7, Paragraph 3, of the Optional Protocol to the Convention on the Elimination of All Forms of Discrimination Against Women Concerning Communication No. 17/2008," UN Doc. CEDAW/C/49/D/17/2008 (2011). Alyne da Silva case.

45. Ingrid Vik, Anne Stensvold, and Christian Moe, "Lobbying for Faith and Family: A Study of Religious NGOs at the United Nations," *Norwegian Agency for Development Cooperation* (2013), www.norad.no/no/resultater/publikasjoner/norads-rapportserie/publikasjon?key=401801.

46. High-Level Task Force for ICPD, "Policy Recommendations for the ICPD Beyond 2014: Sexual and Reproductive Health & Rights for All," *International Conference on Population and Development* (2013): 1.

47. *United States v. Windsor*, 570 U.S. 12 (2013).

48. *National Legal Services Authority v. Union of India and Others*, Writ Petition (Civil) No. 604 of 2013 (India), http://supremecourtofindia.nic.in/outtoday/wc40012.pdf.

49. The Anti-Homosexuality Act, Uganda (2014), http://wp.patheos.com.s3.amazonaws.com/blogs/warrenthrockmorton/files/2014/02/Anti-Homosexuality-Act-2014.pdf.

50. *Prof. J. Oloka-Onyango & 9 Ors v. Attorney General* [2014] UGCC 14 (1 August 2014) (Uganda).

51. Erving Goffman, *Stigma: Notes on the Management of Spoiled Identity* (New York: Simon & Schuster, 1963).

52. Fistula Foundation, "Kupona Foundation Spotlight on Obstetric Fistula: Giving Women Another Chance," 2013, www.fistulafoundation.org/kupona-foundation-spotlight-on-obstetric-fistula-giving-women-another-chance/.

Chapter 4. Health Systems as "Core Social Institutions"

Epigraph: Lynn P. Freedman, "Achieving the MDGs: Health Systems as Core Social Institutions," *Development* 48 (2005): 19–24.

1. Gabriel García Márquez, *One Hundred Years of Solitude* (Buenos Aires: Editorial Sudamericans, 1967).

2. In magical realist texts, "the supernatural is not a simple or obvious matter, but it *is* an ordinary matter, an everyday occurrence—admitted, accepted, and integrated into the rationality and materiality of literary realism. Magic is no longer quixotic madness, but normative and normalizing." See Wendy B. Faris and Lois Parkinson Zamora, "Introduction: Daiquiri Birds and Flaubertian Parrot(ie)s" in *Magical Realism: Theory, History, Community*, ed. Wendy B. Faris and Lois Parkinson Zamora (Durham, N.C.: Duke University Press, 1995): 3. For a commonly used example of the genre, see Márquez, *One Hundred Years of Solitude*.

3. Fernando Botero is a Colombian artist whose art is known for depicting oversized figures and heads. See Mariana Hanstein, *Botero* (Cologne, Germany: Taschen, 2003).

4. Mieke Wouters, "Ethnic Rights Under Threat: The Black Peasant Movement Against Armed Groups' Pressure in the Chocó, Colombia," *Bulletin of Latin American Research* 20, no. 4 (2001): 498–519.

5. UN Human Rights Council, "Report of the Special Rapporteur on the Situation of Human Rights and Fundamental Freedoms of Indigenous People, Mr. James Anaya—Addendum—The Situation of Indigenous Peoples in Colombia: Follow-Up to the Recommendations Made by the Previous Special Rapporteur," UN Doc. A/HRC/15/37/Add.3 (2010).

6. Arturo Escobar, "Displacement, Development, and Modernity in the Colombian Pacific," *International Social Science Journal* 175 (2003): 157–67.

7. Giselle Lopez, "The Colombian Civil War: Potential for Justice in a Culture of Violence," *Jackson School of International Studies Policy Brief* 2, no. 1 (2013).

8. World Bank, "GDP per Capita (Current US$)," http://data.worldbank.org/indicator/NY .GDP.PCAP.CD.

9. Jesús López-Rodríguez and María Cecilia Acevedo, "Second Nature Geography and Regional Income Disparities in Colombia," *Documento de Trabajo CEDE* (2008): 2008–9.

10. Marjorie Andrea Gonzalez Ramirez, "In the Colombian Chocó: Hunger Amongst Richness," *The Prism*, April 24, 2012, www.theprisma.co.uk/2012/04/24/in-the-colombian-choco -hunger-amongst-richness/.

11. Miriam Wells, "UN Documents Inequality Suffered by Afro-Colombians," *Colombia Reports*, November 22, 2011, http://colombiareports.co/un-documents-the-inequality-suffered-by -afro-colombians/.

12. Lynn P. Freedman et al., *Who's Got the Power? Transforming Health Systems for Women and Children,* UN Millennium Project Task Force on Child Health and Maternal Health (London: Earthscan, 2005): 97. http://www.unmillenniumproject.org/documents/maternalchild -complete.pdf.

13. UN Human Rights Council, "Technical Guidance on the Application of a Human-Rights Based Approach to the Implementation of Policies and Programmes to Reduce Preventable Maternal Morbidity and Mortality," UN Doc. A/HRC/21/22 (2012).

14. World Health Organization, "Everybody's Business: Strengthening Health Systems to Improve Health Outcomes, WHO's Framework for Action" (2007), www.who.int/healthsystems /strategy/everybodys_business.pdf.

15. Freedman et al., *Who's Got the Power?*

16. Ibid., 16.

17. UN Human Rights Council, "Report of the Special Rapporteur on the Right of Everyone to the Enjoyment of the Highest Attainable Standard of Physical and Mental Health, Paul Hunt," UN Doc. A/HRC/4/28 (2007).

18. Alicia Ely Yamin and Ole Frithjof Norheim, "Taking Equality Seriously: Applying Human Rights Frameworks to Priority Setting in Health," *Human Rights Quarterly* 36 (2014): 296–324.

19. Freedman et al., *Who's Got the Power?*

20. Henriette Sinding et al., eds., *Juridification and Social Citizenship in the Welfare State* (Cheltenham, UK: Edward Elgar, 2014).

21. Freedman et al., *Who's Got the Power?* 31.

22. This section draws heavily from Alicia Ely Yamin et al., *Deadly Delays: Maternal Mortality in Perú: A Rights-Based Approach to Safe Motherhood* (Cambridge, Mass.: Physicians for Human Rights, 2007); and Alicia Ely Yamin, "Maternal Mortality," in *The Right to Health,* ed. Gunilla Backman (Stockholm: Studentlitteratur, 2012).

23. UN Committee on Economic, Social and Cultural Rights (CESCR), "General Comment No. 14, the Right to the Highest Attainable Standard of Health," UN Doc. No. E/C.12/2000/4 (2000): para. 12.

24. Deborah Maine, *Safe Motherhood Programs: Options and Issues* (New York: Center for Population and Family Health, 1991).

25. Dr. Mahmoud Fathalla is professor of obstetrics and gynaecology, former president of FIGO (International Federation of Gynecologists and Obstetricians); former dean of the medical school at Assiut University, Egypt; and chair of the World Health Organization Advisory Committee on Health Research. See Amnesty International, "Maternal Health Is a Human Right," www.amnestyusa.org/our-work/campaigns/demand-dignity/maternal-health-is-a-human-right.

26. Yamin, "Maternal Mortality."

27. UN Committee on Economic, Social and Cultural Rights (CESCR): para 12(a); UN Human Rights Council, "Report of the Special Rapporteur on the Right of Everyone to the Enjoyment of the Highest Attainable Standard of Physical and Mental Health": para. 68.

28. Maine, *Safe Motherhood Programs.*

29. WHO, UNICEF, UNFPA, "Guidelines for Monitoring the Availability and Use of Obstetric Services" (1997): para. 25; World Health Organization, "Monitoring Emergency Obstetric Care: A Handbook" (2009), www.who.int/reproductivehealth/publications/monitoring/9789241547734/en/.

30. CESCR, Comment No. 14, the Right to the Highest Attainable Standard of Health, paras. 12(c) and 27; UN Human Rights Council, "Report of the Special Rapporteur on the Right of Everyone to the Enjoyment of the Highest Attainable Standard of Physical and Mental Health," para. 74.

31. UN Committee on the Elimination of Discrimination Against Women (CEDAW Committee), "CEDAW General Recommendation No. 24: Article 12 of the Convention (Women and Health)," UN Doc. A/54/38/Rev.1 (1999): para. 22.

32. CESCR, "Comment No. 14, the Right to the Highest Attainable Standard of Health,",para. 12(d); UN Human Rights Council, "Report of the Special Rapporteur on the Right of Everyone to the Enjoyment of the Highest Attainable Standard of Physical and Mental Health," para. 75.

33. Diana Bowser and Kathleen Hill, USAID-TRAction Project, *Exploring Evidence for Disrespect and Abuse in Facility-Based Childbirth* (Boston: Harvard School of Public Health, 2010).

34. Human Rights Council, "Technical Guidance,"

35. See Alicia Ely Yamin and Rebecca Cantor, "Between Insurrectional Discourse and Operational Guidance: Challenges and Dilemmas in Implementing Human Rights–Based Approaches to Health," *Journal of Human Rights Practice* 6, no. 3 (2014): 451–465.

36. Human Rights Council, "Technical Guidance," para. 53.

37. Ibid.; Alicia Ely Yamin and Kathryn Falb, "Counting What We Know: Knowing What to Count: Sexual and Reproductive Rights, Maternal Health, and the Millennium Development Goals," *Nordic Journal on Human Rights* 30, no. 3 (2012): 350–71.

38. Human Rights Council, "Technical Guidance," para. 77.

39. UN General Assembly, "Resolution Adopted by the General Assembly on 27 July 2012: 66/288 The Future We Want," UN Doc. A/RES/66/288 (2012).

40. World Health Organization, "Health Systems Financing: The Path to Universal Coverage" (2010).

41. WHO, "Universal Coverage: Three Dimensions," www.who.int/health_financing/strategy/dimensions/en/.

42. Pan American Health Organization, 53rd Directing Council, 66th Session of the Regional Committee of WHO for the Americas, "Resolution: Strategy for Universal Access to Health and Universal Health Coverage," CD53.R14 (2014).

43. Norman Daniels, *Just Health: Meeting Health Needs Fairly* (New York: Cambridge University Press, 2008); and Keith Syrett, *Law, Legitimacy, and the Rationing of Health Care: A Contextual and Comparative Perspective* (Cambridge: Cambridge University Press, 2007).

44. Ibid.

45. Yamin and Norheim, "Taking Equality Seriously."

46. *Soobramoney v. Minister of Health (KwaZulu-Natal)* 1998 (1) SA 765 (CC) (S. Afr.) [Concurring Opinion], Albie Sachs (S. Afr.): para 52.

47. Syrett, *Law.*

48. Human Rights Council, "Technical Guidance."

49. Syrett, *Law*, 89.

50. Trygve Ottersen et al., "Making Fair Choices on the Path to Universal Health Coverage: Final Report of the WHO Consultative Group on Equity and Universal Health Coverage," World Health Organization (2014).

51. Eugene B. Brody, *Biomedical Technology and Human Rights* (UNESCO, 1993), cited in *Soobramoney v. Minister of Health (KwaZulu-Natal)*, CCT 32/97, South African Constitutional Court (1998), J Sachs, concurrence at para. 54.

52. Yamin and Norheim, "Taking Equality Seriously."

53. Robert Lin, Rozalyn Levine, and Brian Scanlan, "Evolution of End-of-Life Care at United States Hospitals in the New Millennium," *Journal of Palliative Medicine* 15, no. 5 (2012).

54. Yamin and Norheim, "Taking Equality Seriously."

55. Federal Interagency Forum on Aging-Related Statistics, "Population. Indicator 1: Number of Older Americans," www.agingstats.gov/Main_Site/Data/2012_Documents/Population .aspx.

56. *Soobramoney v. Minister of Health (KwaZulu-Natal)*, 1998 (1) SA 765 (CC) (S. Afr.) [Concurring Opinion], Albie Sachs (S.Afr.): para. 57.

57. WHO, "Cancer Fact Sheet," www.who.int/mediacentre/factsheets/fs297/en/.

58. Daniels, *Just Health.*

59. Simon Ellis et al., *Grading Evidence and Recommendations for Public Health Interventions: Developing and Piloting a Framework* (London: Health Development Agency, 2005).

60. Jaime Sepulveda et al., "Improvement of Child Survival in Mexico: The Diagonal Approach," *Lancet* 368 (2006): 2017–27; Felicia Marie Knaul et al., "Evidence Is Good for Your Health System: Policy Reform to Remedy Catastrophic and Impoverishing Health Spending in Mexico," *Lancet* 368 (2008): 1828–41; Emmanuela Gakidou et al., "Assessing the Effect of the 2001–06 Mexican Health Reform: An Interim Report Card," *Lancet* 368 (2006): 1920–35; Eduardo Gonzalez-Pier et al., "Priority Setting for Health Interventions in Mexico's System of Social Protection in Health," *Lancet* 368 (2006): 1608–18; Julio Frenk et al., "Comprehensive Reform to Improve Health System Performance in Mexico," *Lancet* 368 (2006): 1524–34; and Rafael Lozano et al., "Benchmarking of Performance of Mexican States with Effective Coverage," *Lancet* 368 (2006): 1729–41.

61. Daniels, *Just Health*, 118–19.

62. Ibid.

63. Ibid.

64. Ibid.

65. El Tiempo Casa Editoral, "Hasta el Omeprazol lo niegan," www.eltiempo.com/Multimedia /infografia/tutelassalud/, cited in *Defensoria del Pueblo*, "La tutela y el derecho a la Salud 2012."

66. Judgment T-760, Corte Constitucional [C.C.] [Constitutional Court], July 31, 2008, Sentencia T-760/08 (Colom.).

67. Procuraduria General de la Nación (PGN/Attorney General's Office) and Centro de Estudios de Derecho, Justicia y Sociedad (DeJusticia), "El derecho a la salud en perspectiva de Derechos Humanos y el Sistema de Inspección, Vigilancia y Control del Estado Colombiano en Materia de Quejas en Salud" (2008).

68. Judgment T-760.

69. Ibid.

70. Syrett, *Law*; CESCR, "Comment No. 14, the Right to the Highest Attainable Standard of Health," UN Doc. No. E/C.12/2000/4 (2000).

71. Roberto Gargarella, "Dialogic Justice in the Enforcement of Social Rights," in *Litigating Health Rights: Can Courts Bring More Justice to Health?* ed. Alicia Ely Yamin and Siri Gloppen (Cambridge, Mass.: Harvard Human Rights Program Series, Harvard University Press, 2011).

72. César Rodríguez-Garavito, "Beyond the Courtroom: The Impact of Judicial Activism on Socioeconomic Rights in Latin America," *Texas Law Review* 89, no. 7 (2011): 1669–98.

73. Judgment T-760, Corte Constitucional [C.C.] [Constitutional Court], July 31, 2008, Sentencia T-760/08, Aclaración de voto a la Sentencia T-760/08 [Concurring Opionion], Manuel José Cepeda Espinosa (Colom.).

74. Tina Rosenberg, "The Human Incubator," *New York Times*, December 13, 2010, http://opinionator.blogs.nytimes.com/2010/12/13/the-human-incubator/?_r=0.

Chapter 5. Beyond Charity

Epigraphs: St. Augustine, as quoted in Sydney J. Harris, *Majority of One* (Boston: Houghton Mifflin, 1957), 283. Desmond Tutu on the *Today* show, January 9, 1985.

1. Amnesty International, "Demand Dignity," www.amnestyusa.org/our-work/campaigns /demand-dignity.

2. Stephen Hopgood, *Keepers of the Flame: Understanding Amnesty International* (Ithaca, N.Y.: Cornell University Press, 2006).

3. Ergometrine is an oxytocic used to prevent postpartum hemorrhage. See Susan J. McDonald et al., "Prophylactic Ergometrine-Oxytocin Versus Oxytocin for the Third Stage of Labour," *Cochrane Database of Systematic Reviews* 1 (2004).

4. Malcolm Langford, *Claiming the Millennium Development Goals: A Human Rights Approach* (New York: United Nations, 2008): 15.

5. UN Office of the High Commissioner for Human Rights (OHCHR)/Center for Economic and Social Rights (CESR), "Who Will Be Accountable? Human Rights and the Post-2015 Development Agenda," UN Doc. No. HR/PUB/13/1 (2013).

6. World Health Organization, "World Health Statistics 2013" (2013), http://apps.who.int/iris /bitstream/10665/81965/1/9789241564588_eng.pdf?ua=1.

7. Leslie London, "What Is a Human-Rights Based Approach to Health and Does It Matter?" *Health and Human Rights* 10 (2008): 72.

8. Ibid., 73.

9. Lynn Freedman, "Human Rights, Constructive Accountability and Maternal Mortality in the Dominican Republic," *International Journal of Gynecology and Obstetrics* 82 (2003): 112.

10. Ibid.

11. See, e.g., Rebecca J. Cook, Mónica Arango Olaya, and Bernard M. Dickens, "Healthcare Responsibilities and Conscientious Objection," *International Journal of Gynecology and Obstet-*

rics 104 (2009): 249–52; and Center for Reproductive Rights (CRR), *"P. and S. v. Poland:* Poland's Obligations to Provide Legal Abortion Services to Adolescents" (2013).

12. UN Human Rights Council, "Technical Guidance on the Application of a Human-Rights Based Approach to the Implementation of Policies and Programmes to Reduce Preventable Maternal Morbidity and Mortality," UN Doc. A/HRC/21/22 (2012).

13. UN Committee on the Elimination of Discrimination Against Women (CEDAW Committee), "Views of the Committee on the Elimination of Discrimination Against Women Under Article 7, Paragraph 3, of the Optional Protocol to the Convention on the Elimination of All Forms of Discrimination Against Women Concerning Communication No. 17/2008," UN Doc. CEDAW/C/49/D/17/2008 (2011). Alyne da Silva case.

14. The World We Want, "Final Report of the Global Thematic Consultation on Governance and the Post-2015 Development Framework" (2014).

15. See, for example, Peter Houtzager, Anuradha Joshi, and Adrian Gurza-Lavalle, "State Reform and Social Accountability," IDS Bulletin 38, no. 6 (2008).

16. For more information, see Right to Food Campaign, www.righttofoodindia.org/campaign /campaign.html.

17. For a discussion of how this was the case in Peru, see Christina Ewig, "Gender Equity and Neoliberal Social Policy: Health Sector Reform in Peru" (Ph.D. diss., University of North Carolina at Chapel Hill, 2008).

18. See, for example, Peter Houtzager et al., "State Reform."

19. See, for example, Siri Gloppen, "Public Interest Litigation, Social Rights, and Social Policy," in *Inclusive States,* ed. Anis A. Dani and Arjan De Haan (Washington, D.C.: World Bank, 2008): 343–68.

20. Lisa Forman, "'Rights' and Wrongs: What Utility for the Right to Health in Reforming Trade Rules on Medicines?" *Health and Human Rights* 10, no. 2 (2008): 37–52.

21. *People's Union for Civil Liberties v. Union of India and Others,* Writ Petition (Civil) No. 196 of 2001 (India).

22. For more information, see Right to Food Campaign, www.righttofoodindia.org/campaign /campaign.html.

23. Siri Gloppen, "Litigation as a Strategy to Hold Governments Accountable for Implementing the Right to Health," *Health and Human Rights* 10, no. 2 (2008): 21–36; }See also Daniel Brinks and Varun Gauri, "A New Policy Landscape: Legalizing Social and Economic Rights in the Developing World," in *Courting Social Justice: Judicial Enforcement of Social and Economic Rights in the Developing World,* ed. Varun Gauri and Daniel Brinks (New York: Cambridge University Press, 2008): 303–52.

24. Roberto Gargarella, Pilar Domingo, and Theunis Roux, eds., *Courts and Social Transformation in New Democracies: An Institutional Voice for the Poor?* (Burlington, Vt.: Ashgate, 2006).

25. See Gauri and Brinks, *Courting Social Justice.*

26. Alicia Ely Yamin and Siri Gloppen, eds., *Litigating Health Rights: Can Courts Bring More Justice to Health?* (Cambridge, Mass.: Harvard Human Rights Series, Harvard University Press, 2011).

27. Colleen M. Flood and Aeyal Gross, eds., *The Right to Health at the Public/Private Divide: A Global Health Comparative Study* (New York: Cambridge University Press, 2014).

28. *Soobramoney v. Minister of Health (KwaZulu-Natal)* 1998 (1) SA 765 (CC) (S. Afr.) Chaskalson (S. Afr.): para. 29; and Center for Health, Human Rights and Development (CEHURD) & *3 Ors v. Attorney General,* Constitutional Petition No. 16 of 2011 (Uganda).

29. Bruce Porter, "Justiciability of ESC Rights and the Right to Effective Remedies: Historic Challenges and New Opportunities," in *Economic, Social and Cultural Rights and the Optional Protocol to the ICESCR* (Beijing: Chinese Academy of Social Sciences, 2008).

30. Corte Suprema de Justicia [SCJN] [Supreme Court], July 8, 2006, "Mendoza Beatriz Silvia y Otros C/ Estado Nacional y Otros s/Daños y Perjuicios" (Arg.).

31. Marcela Valente, "River Restoration Remains Out of Reach," *Global Issues,* February 12, 2013, www.globalissues.org/news/2013/02/12/15843.

32. See Mark Tushnet, *Weak Courts, Strong Rights: Judicial Review and Social Welfare Rights in Comparative Constitutional Law* (Princeton, N.J.: Princeton University Press, 2008).

33. See Rosalind Dixon, "Creating Dialogue About Socioeconomic Rights: Strong-Form versus Weak-Form Judicial Review Revisited," *International Journal of Constitutional Law* 5 (2007): 112–47; Charles Sabel and William Simon, "Destabilization Rights: How Public Law Litigation Succeeds," *Harvard Law Review* 117 (2004): 1015–101.

34. César Rodriguez-Garavito, "Assessing the Impact and Promoting the Implementation of Structural Judgments: A Comparative Case Study of ESCR Rulings in Colombia" (2009), www.escr-net.org/usr_doc/Rodriguez_-_Colombia.pdf.

35. Defensoría del Pueblo, "Serie Informes Defensoriales 27: Casos investigados por la Defensoría del Pueblo" (1999); and Defensoría del Pueblo, "Informe Defensorial No. 90: Supervisión a los Servicios de Planificación Familiar IV, Casos investigados por la Defensoría del Pueblo" (2005).

36. See National Human Rights Commission and Jan Swasthya Abhiyan, "Recommendations of National Action Plan to Operationalize the Right to Health Care," National Public Hearing on Right to Health Care, December 16–17, 2004, New Delhi (2004); Defensor del Pueblo de la Nación, Republica Argentina, www.dpn.gob.ar/; and Winfred O. Lichuma, "Realising Sexual and Reproductive Health Rights in Kenya: A Myth or Reality? A Report of the Public Inquiry into Violations of Sexual and Reproductive Health Rights in Kenya." Nairobi: Kenya National Commission on Human Rights (2012), accessed at http://www.knchr.org/portals/0/reports/reproductive_health_report.pdf.

37. Freedman, "Human Rights," 111–14.

38. UN General Assembly, "Vienna Declaration and Programme of Action," UN Doc. A/CONF.157/23 (1993).

39. UN Human Rights Committee, "CCPR General Comment No. 6: Article 6 (Right to Life)," UN Doc. HRI/GEN/1/Rev.9 (Vol. 1) (1982): para. 5.

40. Varun Guari and Daniel Brinks, "Introduction: The Elements of Legalization and the Triangular Shape of Social and Economic Rights," in *Courting Social Justice: Judicial Enforcement of Social and Economic Rights in the Developing World*, ed. Varun Gauri and Daniel Brinks (New York: Cambridge University Press, 2008): 1–35.

41. *Francis Coralie Mullin v. Union Territory of Delhi* (1981) 2 SCR 516, in *Litigating Health Rights: Can Courts Bring More Justice to Health?* ed. Alicia Ely Yamin and Siri Gloppen (Cambridge, Mass.: Harvard Human Rights Series, Harvard University Press, 2011): 165.

42. For one of the first articulations of the three dimensions of state obligations to respect, to protect, and to fulfill rights, see Asbjørn Eide et al., eds., *Food as a Human Right* (Tokyo: United Nations University, 1984).

43. UN General Assembly, "International Covenant on Economic, Social and Cultural Rights (ICESCR)," UN GA Res. 2200, UN Doc. No. A/6316 (1966).

44. Ibid.

45. UN Committee on Economic, Social and Cultural Rights (CESCR), "General Comment No. 14, the Right to the Highest Attainable Standard of Health," UN Doc. No. E/C.12/2000/4 (2000): para. 43.

46. See Allison Corkery, Sally-Anne Way, and Victoria Wisniewski Otero, "The OPERA Framework: Assessing Compliance with the Obligation to Fulfill Economic, Social and Cultural Rights," *Center for Economic and Social Rights* (2012), www.cesr.org/downloads/the.opera.framework.pdf.

47. UN General Assembly, "International Covenant on Economic, Social and Cultural Rights, (ICESCR)," UNGA Res. 2200, UN Doc. No. A/6316 (1966).

48. CEDAW Committee, "CEDAW General Recommendation No. 24: Article 12 of the Convention (Women and Health)," UN Doc. A/54/38/Rev.1 (1999): para. 26.

49. CESCR, para 43; UN General Assembly, "Note by the Secretary-General Transmitting the Report of the Special Rapporteur on the Right of Everyone to the Enjoyment of the Highest Standard of Physical and Mental Health," UN Doc. No. A/61/338 (2006): para. 29.

50. Alicia Ely Yamin et al., *Deadly Delays: Maternal Mortality in Perú: A Rights-Based Approach to Safe Motherhood* (Cambridge, Mass.: Physicians for Human Rights, 2007).

51. *Minister of Health v. Treatment Action Campaign (TAC)*, 5 SA 721 (CC) South African Constitutional Court, 2002.

52. Paul Farmer and Jim Yong Kim, "Community Based Approaches to the Control of Multidrug Resistant Tuberculosis: Introducing 'DOTS-plus,'" *British Medical Journal* 317 (1998): 671–74.

53. Trygve Ottersen et al., "Making Fair Choices on the Path to Universal Health Coverage: Final Report of the WHO Consultative Group on Equity and Universal Health Coverage," World Health Organization (2014).

54. *Minister of Health and Others v. Treatment Action Campaign and Others* 2002 (1) SA 9 ZACC 16 (CC) (S. Afr.).

55. UN General Assembly, "International Covenant on Economic, Social and Cultural Rights (ICESCR)," UN GA Res. 2200, UN Doc. No. A/6316 (1966): art. 12.

56. Agence France-Presse, "Sierra Leone Loses Track of Millions in Ebola Funds," *New York Times,* February 14, 2015.

57. See, e.g., Kenneth Roth, "Defending Economic, Social and Cultural Rights: Practical Issues Faced by an International Human Rights Organization," *Human Rights Quarterly* 26, no. 1 (2004): 63–73.

58. For example, International Budget Partnership, www.internationalbudget.org. ESCR-Net also has a working group on budget monitoring.

59. See, generally, Daniela Díaz Echeverría et al., *Muerte Materna y Presupuesto Publico* (Mexico City: Fundar, 2006). Sikika, "CSO Call for Government to Reduce Unnecessary Spending" (2009), www.emjee.biz/resources/Documents/case-study-Sikika-budget-allocation-2-dec.pdf.

60. See United Nations Development Programme (UNDP), "Human Development Report 2007/2008" (2007), http://hdr.undp.org/sites/default/files/reports/268/hdr_20072008_en_complete.pdf.

61. UN Human Rights Council, "Statement by Professor Philip Alston, Special Rapporteur on Extrajudicial, Summary or Arbitrary Executions to the Human Rights Council 27 March 2007" (2007).

62. Peter S. Heller, "Fiscal Space: What Is It and How to Get It?" *Finance and Development: A Quarterly Magazine of the International Monetary Fund* 2 (2005): 2.

63. CESCR, "General Comment No. 14, the Right to the Highest Attainable Standard of Health," UN Doc. No. E/C.12/2000/4 (2000).

64. CESCR, "An Evaluation of the Obligation to Take Steps to the 'Maximum of Available Resources' Under an Optional Protocol to the Covenant.'"

65. Judgment C-251, Corte Constitucional [C.C.] [Constitutional Court], May 28, 1997, Sentencia C-251/97 (Colom.).

66. Judgment C-1165, Corte Constitucional [C.C.] [Constitutional Court], September 6, 2000, Sentencia C-1165/00 (Colom.); and Judgment C-040, Corte Constitucional [C.C.] [Constitutional Court], January 27, 2004, Sentencia C-040/04 (Colom.).

67. CESCR, "General Comment No. 14, The Right to the Highest Attainable Standard of Health," UN Doc. No. E/C.12/2000/4 (2000): para. 17; United Nations Population Fund, "International Conference on Population and Development (ICPD) Programme of Action," UN Doc. A/CONF.171/13/Rev.1 (1995): para. 4; UN General Assembly, "Convention on the Rights of the Child," UN Doc. A/RES/44/25 (1989): art. 23; International Labour Organization (ILO), "Convention Concerning Indigenous and Tribal Peoples in Independent Countries," ILO Conv. 169, ILO 76th Session, reprinted in 28 ILM 1382 (1989): art. 25; and UN General Assembly, "Convention on the Rights of Persons with Disabilities," UN Doc. A/RE/ 61/106 (2007).

68. This is especially evident in the language of the Children's Convention and Article 1 of the UN Convention on the Rights of Persons with Disabilities: UN General Assembly, "Convention on the Rights of Persons with Disabilities," UN Doc. A/RE/ 61/106 (2007).

69. UN Human Rights Council, "Technical Guidance," para. 6.

70. Ibid., paras. 48, 74b.

71. Keith Syrett, Law, Legitimacy and the Rationing of Health Care: A Contextual and Comparative Perspective (Cambridge: Cambridge University Press, 2007): 231.

72. Center for Reproductive Rights and Poradňa pre občiankske a ludské práva, "Body and Soul: Forced Sterilization and Other Assaults on Roma Reproductive Freedom in Slovakia" (2003).

73. Defensoría del Pueblo, "Informe Defensorial No. 90: Supervisión a los Servicios de Planificación Familiar IV, Casos investigados por la Defensoría del Pueblo" (2005).

74. Yamin et al., Deadly Delays.

75. Augusto Portocarrero Grados, "La Equidad en la Asignación Regional del Financiamiento del Sector Público de Salud 2000–2005," Consorcio de Investigación Económica y Social (CIES) (2006).

76. See Encuesta Nacional de Hogares (ENAHO) 2003-IV, in Enrique Vásquez, ¿Los niños . . . primero? Volumen III: Niveles de vida y gasto público orientada a la infancia en el Perú 2004–2005 (Lima: Centro de Investigación de la Universidad del Pacífico, 2005): 51.

77. Debra Stevenson, Charles Kinyeki, and Mark Wheeler, "Evaluation of DFID Support to Healthcare Workers Salaries in Sierra Leone," Department for International Development (DFID) and UKAid (2012).

78. Amnesty International, "At a Crossroads: Sierra Leone's Free Health Care Policy" (2011); Realizing Rights, "Sierra Leone's Model for Improving Maternal Health and Women's Rights" (2010); and John Donnelly, "How Did Sierra Leone Provide Free Health Care?" Lancet 377 (2011): 1393–96.

79. Marlise Simons and J. David Goodman, "Ex-Liberian Leader Gets 50 Years for War Crimes," New York Times, May 30 2012, www.nytimes.com/2012/05/31/world/africa/charles-taylor-sentenced-to-50-years-for-war-crimes.html?pagewanted=all.

80. The Special Court for Sierra Leone, "Cases," www.rscsl.org/.

81. Ibid; and World Bank, "Poverty and Equity Data," http://data.worldbank.org/topic /poverty#boxes-box-topic_cust_sec.

82. Alicia Ely Yamin, "Ebola, Human Rights, and Poverty Making the Links," Inter Press News Agency, October 27, 2014.

83. Nancy Gibbs, "Time Magazine Person of the Year," *Time*, December 10, 2014.

Chapter 6. Power and Participation

Epigraphs: Cited in H. Potts, *Participation and the Right to the Highest Attainable Standard of Health* (Essex: University of Essex Human Rights Centre, 2008), 8. Magdalena Sepúlveda, Statement by the Special Rapporteur on Extreme Poverty and Human Rights at the 23rd Session of the Human Rights Council, A/HRC/23/36 (2013). Accessed at: http://www.ohchr.org/EN /NewsEvents/Pages/DisplayNews.aspx?NewsID=13407&LangID=E.

1. Alicia Ely Yamin et al., *Deadly Delays: Maternal Mortality in Peru: A Rights-Based Approach to Safe Motherhood* (Cambridge, Mass.: Physicians for Human Rights, 2007).

2. The Andean Plateau lies mostly within Bolivia and Peru and parts of Chile and Argentina. The famous Lake Titicaca lies at the Bolivia–Peru border on this plateau.

3. The program directed by the Movimiento Manuela Ramos, ReproSalud, had worked with many of the women previously. ReproSalud focused on social barriers to accessing reproductive health and rights and targeted the poorest, hardest-to-reach, Peruvian women in areas with underused health-care services. The project emphasized community education and mobilization as a way of empowering individuals and communities to improve women's sexual and reproductive health. For more information, see Cecila Moya, "ReproSalud: Nationwide Community Participation in Perú," *Transitions: Community Participation* 14, no. 3 (2002). See also Alicia Ely Yamin and Ariel Frisancho, "Human-Rights–Based Approaches to Health in Latin America," *Lancet* (2014), doi: 10.1016/S0140-6736(14)61280-0.

4. This project emerged out of a joint investigation between CARE Peru and Physicians for Human Rights (PHR), which I directed. See Yamin et al., *Deadly Delays*.

5. A *mestizo* is a man of mixed race. See *Oxford Dictionary Online*, s.v. "Mestizo" [Def. 1], http://oxforddictionaries.com/definition/american_english/mestizo.

6. Yamin and Frisancho, "Human Rights," 170–71.

7. Rosana Vargas V., "Sistematización de la iniciativa de vigilancia ciudadana de la calidad de lose servicios de salud en las provincias de Ayaviri y Azángaro—Puno," Serie: Fortaleciendo la Disponibilidad y la Capacidad de Respuesta del Personal de Salud (Lima: CARE Peru and Foro Salud, 2013); and Yamin and Frisancho, "Human Rights."

8. Steven Lukes, *Power: A Radical View*, second edition (London: Palgrave Macmillan, 2005): 114.

9. Ibid.

10. Ronald Dworkin, *Justice in Robes* (Cambridge, Mass.: Harvard University Press, 2008): 55.

11. Jean Drèze and Amartya Sen, *Hunger and Public Action*, Wider Studies in Development Economics (New York: Oxford University Press, 1991), and reprinted in *The Amartya Sen and Jean Drèze Omnibus* (New York: Oxford University Press, 1999).

12. Drèze and Sen, *Hunger*, 212.

13. Ibid., 210.

14. Robert Dahl, "The Concept of Power," *Behavioral Science* 2 (1957): 201–5.

15. See, e.g., Lukes, *Power*, 117.

16. Jonathan M. Mann et al., "Health and Human Rights," *Health and Human Rights* 1, no 1 (1994): 7–23.

17. Helen Potts and Paul H. Hunt, "Participation and the Right to the Highest Attainable Standard of Health," Project Report, Human Rights Centre, Colchester, Essex, 2008, 19. Accessed at http://repository.essex.ac.uk/9714/.

18. World Health Organization, "Development of Indicators for Monitoring Progress Toward Health for All by the Year 2000" (1981).

19. Yamin and Frisancho, "Human Rights"; Luiz Odorico Monterio de Andrade et al., "Social Determinants of Health, Universal Health Coverage, and Sustainable Development: Case Studies from Latin American Countries," *Lancet* (2014), doi: 10.1016/S0140-6736(14)61494-X; and Rifat Atun et al., "Health System Reform and Universal Health Coverage in Latin America," *Lancet* (2014), doi: 10.1016/S0140-6736(14)61646-9.

20. Alliance for Health Policy and Systems Research, "Strengthening Health Systems: The Role and Promise of Policy and Systems Research," *Global Forum for Health Research and World Health Organization* (2004), www.who.int/alliance-hpsr/resources/Strengthening_complet.pdf.

21. Walter Flores, Ana Lorena Ruano, and Denise Phe Funchal, "Social Participation Within a Context of Political Violence: Implications for the Promotion and Exercise of the Right to Health in Guatemala," *Health and Human Rights* 11, no. 1 (2009): 43.

22. Armando Arredondo and Emanuel Orozco, "Effects of Health Decentralization, Financing and Governance in Mexico," *Revista de Saúde Pública* 40, no. 1 (2006): 152–60.

23. Robert Dahl, *On Political Equality* (New Haven, Conn.: Yale University Press, 2006): 61.

24. See, for example, Bill Cooke and Uma Kothari, eds., *Participation: The New Tyranny?* (London: Zed Books, 2001).

25. Bill Cooke, "Rules of Thumb for Participatory Change Agents," in *Participation: From Tyranny to Transformation? Exploring New Approaches to Participation in Development*, ed. Samuel Hickey and Gils Mohan (London: Zed Books, 2004): 42.

26. Elmer E. Schattschneider, *The Semi-Sovereign People: A Realist's View of Democracy in America* (New York: Holt, Rinehart and Winston, 1960): 71, cited in Lukes, *Power,* 20. See also Peter Bachrach and Morton Baratz, *Power and Poverty: Theory and Practice* (Oxford: Oxford University Press, 1970).

27. The proposed bills are Conyers HR 676, Sanders S 703, and McDermott HR 1200, cited in National Economics and Social Rights Initiative (NESRI) and National Health Law Program (NHeLP), "A Human Rights Assessment of Single Payer Plans: Toward the Human Right to Healthcare: The Contributions of Single Payer Plans," www.nesri.org/Single_Payer_Human _Rights_Analysis.pdf: 2.

28. House Committee on Education and Labor, *Examining the Single-Payer Health Care Option: Hearing Before the Subcommittee on Health, Employment, Labor and Pensions, Committee on Education and Labor, House of Representatives* (2009), www.gpo.gov/fdsys/pkg/CHRG -111hhrg50116/pdf/CHRG-111hhrg50116.pdf; and Senate Committee on Finance, *High Health Care Costs: A State Perspective: Hearing Before the Committee on Finance, Senate* (2008), www.finance .senate.gov/hearings/.

29. CBS/New York Times Poll, "American Public Opinion: Today vs. 30 Years Ago," *CBS News*, January 11–15, 2009, 4, www.cbsnews.com/htdocs/pdf/SunMo_poll_0209.pdf.

30. Nancy Fraser, "Rethinking the Public Sphere: A Contribution to the Critique of Actually Existing Democracy," *Social Text* 25–26 (1990): 66.

31. Alicia Ely Yamin and Vanessa M. Boulanger, "Embedding Sexual and Reproductive Health and Rights in a Transformational Development Framework: Lessons Learned from the MDG Targets and Indicators," *Reproductive Health Matters* 21, no. 42 (2013): 74–85; and Paula Tibandebage and Maureen Mackintosh, "Maternal Mortality in Africa: A Gendered Lens on Health System Failure," *Socialist Register* 46 (2010).

32. Kent Buse and Andrew M. Harmer, "Seven Habits of Highly Effective Global Public–Private Health Partnerships: Practice and Potential," *Social Science & Medicine* 64 (2007): 259–71; Kent Buse and Gill Walt, "Global Public–Private Partnerships: Part II—What Are the Health Issues for Global Governance?," *Bulletin of World Health Organization* 78, no. 5 (2000): 699–709; Shahra Razavi, "World Development Report 2012: Gender Equality and Development: An Opportunity Both Welcome and Missed (An Extended Commentary)," *United Nations Research Institute for Social Development* (UNRISD) (2011); and Tibandebage and Mackintosh, "Maternal Mortality."

33. Matthew A. Crenson, *The Unpolitics of Air Pollution: A Study of Non-Decision Making in the Cities* (Baltimore: Johns Hopkins University Press, 1971): 69–70, cited in Lukes, *Power*, 45.

34. Mario Rios Barrientos and Henry Armas Alvarado, "Participacion y vigilancia ciudadana en la actividad minera: Implicaciones en el derecho a la salud. Estudio de caso de la comunidad campesina San Pedro de Tongos y la empresa minera Los Quenuales S.A., [Participation and Social Accountability in Mining Activity: Implications for the Right to Health. Case Study of the Campesino Community San Pedro de Tongos and the Mining Company Los Quenuales]," *Consorcio de Investigación Económica y Social (CIES) Observatorio del Derecho a la Salud/Universidad Peruana Cayetano Heredia* (2006).

35. *Criollo* refers to a person from southern Spain or Central America, particularly a person of purely Spanish descent. See *Oxford Dictionary Online,* s.v. "Criollo" [Def. 1], http://oxforddictionaries.com/definition/american_english/criollo.

36. Lynn P. Freedman, "Using Human Rights in Maternal Mortality Programs: From Analysis to Strategy," *International Journal of Gynecology and Obstetrics* 75 (2001): 51.

37. Worse still, specific techniques of participation can be selected by those in power and then judged as successful on their own terms even though the participation of the " 'development beneficiaries' [who] are deemed to have shifted from objects to empowered subjects" was really as carefully choreographed as a kabuki dance. Glyn Williams, "Toward a Repoliticization of Participatory Development: Political Capabilities and Spaces of Empowerment," in *Participation: From Tyranny to Transformation? Exploring New Approaches to Participation in Development,* ed. Samuel Hickey and Gils Mohan (London: Zed Books, 2004): 93.

38. Flores et al., "Social Participation."

39. Michael Neocosmos, "Civil Society, Citizenship and the Politics of the Impossible: Rethinking Militancy in Africa Today," *Interface: A Journal for and About Social Movements* 1, no. 2 (2009): 263–334.

40. Andrea Cornwall, "Making Spaces, Changing Places: Situating Participation in Development," *Institute of Development Studies Working Paper* 170 (2002): 24. See also Ranjani K. Murthy et al., "Sexual and Reproductive Rights in Service Accountability and Community Participation," *Women's Health Project, South Africa* (2003) [paper prepared for the Initiative for Sexual and Reproductive Rights in Health Reforms (April 2003)].

41. Andrea Cornwall, "Beneficiary, Consumer, Citizen: Perspectives on Participation for Poverty Reduction," *Swedish International Development Agency [SIDA] Study No. 2* (2000). See also Murthy et al., "Sexual and Reproductive Rights."

42. See Rosemary McGee et al., "Legal Frameworks for Citizen Participation: Synthesis Report," Logolink Research Report, Institute of Development Studies (2003).

43. See David Mosse, "'People's Knowledge,' Participation and Patronage: Operations and Representations in Rural Development," in *Participation: The New Tyranny?*, ed. Bill Cooke and Uma Kothari (London: Zed Books, 2001): 16–35.

44. Uma Kothari, "Power Knowledge and Social Control in Participatory Development," in *Participation: The New Tyranny?*, ed. Bill Cooke and Uma Kothari (London: Zed Books, 2001): 143.

45. Potts, "Participation and the Right to the Highest Attainable Standard of Health," 26.

46. Antonio Ugalde, "Ideological Dimensions of Community Participation in Latin American Health Programs," *Social Science and Medicine* 2 (1985): 41–53.

47. Ghazala Mansuri and Vijayendra Rao, "Localizing Development: Does Participation Work? A World Bank Policy Research Report," World Bank (2013).

48. UN Committee on Economic, Social and Cultural Rights (CESCR), "General Comment No. 14, the Right to the Highest Attainable Standard of Health," UN Doc. No. E/C.12/2000/4 (2000): para. 11.

49. Haile Mariam Kahssay and Peter Oakley, eds., *Community Involvement in Health Development: A Review of the Concept and Practice* (Geneva: World Health Organization, 1999).

50. *Ley No. 29124: Ley que establece la cogestión y participación ciudadana para el primer nivel de atención en los establecimientos de salud del Ministerio de Salud y de las Regiones*, Concordancias: D.S. No. 017-2008-SA (Reglamento), October 30, 2007 [Peru].

51. Williams, "Toward a Repoliticization of Participatory Development," 93.

52. Ranjani K. Murthy and Barbara Klugman, "Service Accountability and Community Participation in the Context of Health Sector Reforms in Asia: Implications for Sexual and Reproductive Health Services," *Health Policy and Planning* 19 (Suppl. 1) (2004): i78–i86.

53. See Bill Cooke, "The Social Psychological Limits of Participation," in *Participation: The New Tyranny?*, ed. Bill Cooke and Uma Kothari (London: Zed Books, 2001): 102–21.

54. Giorgio Cometto et al., "A Global Fund for the Health MDGs?" *Lancet* 373 no. 9674 (2009): 1500–1502; and Nicoli Nattrass, "Millennium Development Goal 6: AIDS and the International Health Agenda," *Journal of Human Development and Capabilities* 15, nos. 2–3 (2014): 232–46.

55. Lukes, *Power*, 28.

56. Raewyn Connell, "Gender, Health and Theory: Conceptualizing the Issue, in Local and World Perspective," *Social Science and Medicine*, 74 (2012): 1675–83.

57. See Frantz Fanon, *Black Skin, White Masks* (New York: Grove Press, 2008); and Frantz Fanon, *The Wretched of the Earth* (New York: Grove Press, 2004).

58. Martha Nussbaum, *Women and Human Development: The Capabilities Approach* (New York: Cambridge University Press, 2000): 114, cited in Lukes, *Power*.

59. In ethics, this is referred to as the problem of "adaptive preferences," in which the more difficult it is to imagine changing roles, the more likely it is for people to change their preferences so that they desire only things that are consistent with those roles.

60. See Nussbaum, *Women*, 43

61. See, for example, Physicians for Human Rights, "Epidemic of Inequality: Women's Rights and HIV/AIDS in Botswana and Swaziland" (2007); and the National Institute of Statistics and Informatics (INEI), *Perú: encuesta demografica y de salud familiar (Population and Family Health) (ENDES Continua 2004)* (Lima: Departamento de Puno, 2005): para. 158–71, cited in Yamin et al., *Deadly Delays*.

62. See Roberto Mangabeira Unger, *False Necessity: Anti-Necessitarian Social Theory in the Service of Radical Democracy* (Cambridge: Cambridge University Press, 1988).

63. Judgment C-180, Corte Constitucional [C.C.] [Constitutional Court], April 14, 1994, Sentencia C-180/94 (slip op.)(Colom.).

64. Paulo Freire, *Pedagogy of the Oppressed*, rev. thirtieth anniversary edition (New York: Continuum, 2002).

65. ActionAid, "Reflect," www.reflect-action.org/.

66. International Budget Partnership, "Centro Cultural Luiz Freire (CCLF)," www.inter nationalbudget.org/.

67. Freire, *Pedagogy*, 44.

68. See, for example, Susan B. Rifkin, "Paradigms Lost: Toward a New Understanding of Community Participation in Health Programs," *Acata Tropica* 61 (1996): 79–92.

69. Comité de América Latina y el Caribe para la Defensa de los Derechos de la Mujer (CLADEM) and Centro Legal para Derechoes Reproductivos y Politicas Públicas (CRLP), "Silencio y complicidad: violencia contra las mujeres en los servicios públicos de la salud en el Perú" (1998); Defensoría del Pueblo, "Anticoncepción quirúgica voluntaria II: Casos investigados por la Defensoría del Pueblo," Serie Informes Defensoriales No. 7 (1998), www.corteidh.or.cr/tablas /10636a.pdf; and Defensoría del Pueblo, "La Aplicación de la anticoncepción quirúgica y los derechos reproductivos II: Casos investigados por la Defensoría del Pueblo," Serie Informes Defensoriales No. 27 (1999), www.perusupportgroup.org.uk/files/fckUserFiles/file/Key%20Issues /Defensoria%20informe%2027%20%5Bsterilisations%5D.pdf.

70. CLADEM Perú, Movimiento Manuela Ramos, Flora Tristan, Movimiento el Pozo, Estudio para la Defensa de los Derechos de la Mujer (DEMUS), Asociación Pro Derechos Humanos (APRODEH), and Federación Internacional de Derechos Humanos (FIDH), "For Justice and Reparation Free of All Forms of Discrimination Against Women in Relation to Sexual Health and Sexual Violence During the Armed Conflict: Alternative Report on the Implementation of the UN Convention on the Elimination of All Forms of Discrimination Against Women (CEDAW) by Perú," *CLADEM Perú* (2007), www.refworld.org/pdfid/46f146a12.pdf.

71. Case No. 12.191, Inter-Am. C.H.R. 71/2003 [*María Mamerita Mestanza Chávez v. Perú*].

72. J. Jaime Miranda and Alicia Ely Yamin, "Políticas de Salud y Salud Politizada? Un análisis de las políticas de salud sexual y reproductiva desde la perspectiva de la ética médica, la calidad de atención y los derechos humanos (Health Policies and Politicized Health?: An Analysis of Reproductive and Sexual Health Policies in Perú from the Perspectives of Medical Ethics, Quality of Care and Human Rights)," *Cadernos de Saúde Pública* 24, no. 1 (2008): 7–15.

Chapter 7. Shades of Dignity

Epigraphs: Anatole France, *Le Lys Rouge* (Ann Arbor: University of Michigan Library, 1909), 87; United Nations, Report of the Committee on the Elimination of Discrimination Against Women (2004), p. 79.

1. Rupert Taylor, "Justice Denied: Political Violence in KwaZulu-Natal After 1994," *Violence and Transition Series* 6 (2002).

2. Gérard Labuschagne, "Features and Investigative Implications of Muti Murder in South Africa," *Journal of Investigative Psychology and Offender Profiling* 1, no. 3 (2004): 191–206. A *muti* killing is a ritual killing often to obtain body parts for incorporation into medicine and other concoctions.

3. Center for Reproductive Rights (CRR), "Forced Out: Mandatory Pregnancy Testing and the Expulsion of Pregnant Students in Tanzanian Schools" (2013), http://reproductiverights.org/en/document/tanzania-report-forced-out-mandatory-pregnancy-testing-expulsion.

4. Lisa Jones et al., "Prevalence and Risk of Violence Against Children with Disabilities: A Systematic Review and Meta-Analysis of Observational Studies," *Lancet* 380, no. 9845 (2012): 899–907.

5. Landon Myer and Abigail Harrison, "Why Do Women Seek Antenatal Care Late? Perspectives from Rural South Africa," *Journal of Midwifery and Women's Health* 48, no. 4 (2003): 268–72.

6. Agnes Odhiambo, "'stop Making Excuses': Accountability for Maternal Health Care in South Africa," *Human Rights Watch* (2011).

7. Australian Government, Department of Foreign Affairs and Trade, "'Nothing About Us Without Us': People with Disability Take the Lead in Tanzania," *Australia Africa Community Engagement Scheme (AACES) Annual Report, 2012–13* (March 18, 2014), http://aid.dfat.gov.au/Publications/web/aaces-annual-report-2012-13/Pages/story-people-with-disability-take-the-lead-in-tanzania.aspx.

8. A thromboembolic event occurs when a blood vessel is obstructed as a result of a blood clot that has become detached and traveled through the blood stream.

9. See Amartya Sen, *Inequality Reexamined* (New York: Oxford University Press, 1992).

10. World Bank, "Gini Index," http://data.worldbank.org/indicator/SI.POV.GINI.

11. *Government of the Republic of South Africa and Others v. Grootboom and Others* 2011 (1) SA 46 (CC) (S. Afr.).

12. UN General Assembly, "Universal Declaration of Human Rights," UNGA Res. 217 A (III) (1948): preamble.

13. See the World Health Organization (WHO) Commission on Social Determinants of Health, "Closing the Gap in a Generation: Health Equity Through Action on the Social Determinants of Health" (2008); and Ichiro Kawachi and Bruce Kennedy, *The Health of Nations: Why Inequality Is Harmful to Your Health* (New York: New Press, 2002).

14. See, for example, Richard Wilkinson and Kate Pickett, *The Spirit Level: Why More Equal Societies Almost Always Do Better* (London: Penguin, 2009).

15. WHO Commission on Social Determinants of Health, "Closing the Gap in a Generation: Health Equity Through Action on the Social Determinants of Health," World Health Organization (2008).

16. WHO, *Human Rights, Health and Poverty Reduction Strategies*, WHO/ETH/HDP/05.1. Draft (Geneva: World Health Organization Press, 2005), www.who.int/hhr/news/HRHPRS.pdf.

17. UN Committee on Economic, Social and Cultural Rights (CESCR), "General Comment No. 14, the Right to the Highest Attainable Standard of Health," UN Doc. No. E/C.12/2000/4 (2000): para. 16.

18. Amartya Sen and James E. Foster, *On Economic Inequality* (New York: Oxford University Press, 1997).

19. UN General Assembly, "International Covenant on Economic, Social and Cultural Rights (ICESCR)," UNGA Res. 2200, UN Doc. No. A/6316 (1966): suppl. 16, art. 2.

20. South Africa Constitution, 1996: Article 9 Equality.

21. CESCR, "General Comment No. 20, Non-Discrimination in Economic, Social and Cultural Rights," UN Doc. No. E/C.12/GC/20 (2009): para. 7.

22. *LM and Others v. Government of the Republic of Namibia* (I 1603/2008, I 3518/2008, I 3007/2008) [2012] NAHC 211 (July 30, 2012) (Namib.).

23. Catharine MacKinnon, *Sex Equality* (New York: Foundation Press, 2001).

24. Lena Lavinas, "21st Century Welfare," *New Left Review* 84 (2013): 39.

25. UN Committee on the Elimination of Racial Discrimination (CERD), "General Recommendation No. 32. The Meaning and Scope of Special Measures in the International Convention on the Elimination of All Forms of Racial Discrimination," UN Doc. No. CERD/C/GC/32 (2009); and UN General Assembly, "International Convention on the Elimination of All Forms of Racial Discrimination," UNGA Res. 2106 (1965): para. 2.

26. Karthy Govender, "The Developing Equality Jurisprudence in South Africa," *Michigan Law Review First Impressions* 107 (2009): 121.

27. CESCR, "General Comment No. 14, the Right to the Highest Attainable Standard of Health," UN Doc. No. E/C.12/2000/4 (2000): para. 12.

28. *United States v. Windsor*, 570 U.S. 12 (2013).

29. *National Legal Services Authority v. Union of India and Others*, Writ Petition (Civil) No. 604 of 2013 (India).

30. Immanuel Kant, *Critique of Practical Reason*, trans. Mary J. Gregor (Cambridge: Cambridge University Press, 1997).

31. Alicia Ely Yamin and Ole Frithjof Norheim, "Taking Equality Seriously: Applying Human Rights Frameworks to Priority Setting in Health," *Human Rights Quarterly* 36, no. 2 (2014): 315; and Trygve Ottersen et al., "Making Fair Choices on the Path to Universal Health Coverage: Final Report of the WHO Consultative Group on Equity and Universal Health Coverage," World Health Organization (2014).

32. Octavio Ferraz, "Brazil: Health Inequalities, Rights, and Courts: The Social Impact of the Judicialization of Health," in *Litigating Health Rights: Can Courts Bring More Justice to Health?*, ed. Alicia Ely Yamin and Siri Gloppen (Cambridge, Mass.: Harvard Human Rights Program Series, Harvard University Press, 2011): 76–102.

33. Judgment T-654, Corte Constitucional [C.C.] [Constitutional Court], July 8, 2004, Sentencia T-654/04, Aclaración de voto a la Sentencia T-654/04 [Concurring Opinion], Rodrigo Uprimny Yepes (Colom.).

34. Jonathan Kenneth Burns, "Mental Health and Inequity: A Human Rights Approach to Inequality, Discrimination, and Mental Disability," *Health and Human Rights* 11, no. 2 (2009): 20.

35. CESCR, "General Comment No. 20, Non-Discrimination in Economic, Social and Cultural Rights," UN Doc. No. E/C.12/GC/20 (2009): para. 8.

36. Judgment C-258, Corte Constitucional [C.C.] [Constitutional Court], May 7, 2013, Sentencia C-258/13 (Colom.): paras. 3.4.1–3.4.3.

37. UN Committee on the Elimination of Discrimination Against Women (CEDAW Committee), "Views of the Committee on the Elimination of Discrimination Against Women Under Article 7, Paragraph 3, of the Optional Protocol to the Convention on the Elimination of All Forms of Discrimination Against Women Concerning Communication No. 17/2008," UN Doc. CEDAW/C/49/D/17/2008 (2011). Alyne da Silva case.

38. CEDAW Committee, "CEDAW General Recommendation No. 25: Article 4, Paragraph 1 of the Convention (Temporary Special Measures)."

39. CESCR, "General Comment No. 20, Non-Discrimination in Economic, Social and Cultural Rights," UN Doc. No. E/C.12/GC/20 (2009): para. 8.

40. UN General Assembly, "Convention on the Rights of Persons with Disabilities," UN Doc. A/RE/61/106 (2007): art. 2.

41. *Eldridge v. British Columbia (Attorney General)*, [1997] 3 S.C.R. 624 (Can.).

42. See Aeyal M. Gross, "The Right to Health in an Era of Privatization and Globalization: National and International Perspectives," in *Implementing Social Rights*, ed. Daphne Barak-Erez and Aeyal M. Gross (Oxford: Hart Publishing, 2007): 289–339, at 310.

43. CESCR, "General Comment No. 14, the Right to the Highest Attainable Standard of Health," UN Doc. No. E/C.12/2000/4 (2000): para. 43.

44. World Health Organization, "Life Expectancy: Life Expectancy Data by Country," Global Health Observatory Data Repository, http://apps.who.int/gho/data/node.main.688?lang=en.

45. As cited in Norman Daniels, *Just Health: Meeting Health Needs Fairly* (New York: Cambridge University Press, 2008): 89.

46. Kenneth Roth, "Defending Economic, Social and Cultural Rights: Practical Issues Faced By an International Human Rights Organization," *Human Rights Quarterly* 26, no. 1 (2004).

47. Radhika Balakrishnan and Diane Elson, "Auditing Economic Policy in the Light of Obligations on Economic and Social Rights," *Essex Human Rights Review* 5, no. 1 (2008), www.pdx.edu/sites/www.pdx.edu.econ/files/Balakrishnan2.pdf.

48. WHO Commission on Social Determinants of Health, "Closing the Gap in a Generation."

49. Naoki Kondo et al., "Income Inequality, Mortality, and Self Rated Health: Meta-Analysis of Multilevel Studies," *British Medical Journal* 339, no. 102 (2009): 1.

50. Wilkinson and Pickett, *The Spirit Level*,18.

51. Ibid.

52. Kondo et al., "Income Inequality."

53. Ibid.

54. European Commission, "Demography and Inequality: How Europe's Changing Population Will Impact on Income Inequality," Employment, Social Affairs and Inclusion: Demography and Inequality (2013), http://europa.eu/epic/studies-reports/docs/eaf_policy_brief_-_demography_and_inequality_post_copy_edit_15.10.13.pdf.

55. Fernando G. De Maio, "Income Inequality Measures," *Journal of Epidemiology and Community Health* 61, no. 10 (2007): 849–52.

56. World Factbook, "Distribution of Family Income—Gini Index," Central Intelligence Agency, www.cia.gov/library/publications/the-world-factbook/fields/2172.html.

57. A. B. Atkinson, "On the Measurement of Inequality," *Journal of Economic Theory* 2 (1970): 251, cited in Larry Temkin, *Inequality* (New York: Oxford University Press, 1993): 183.

58. World Bank, "GDP per Capita (Current US$)," *World Bank Open Data* (2012), http://data.worldbank.org/indicator/ny.gdp.pcap.cd.

59. John Rawls, *A Theory of Justice* (Cambridge, Mass.: Harvard University Press, 1971); John Rawls, *Political Liberalism* (New York: Columbia University Press, 1993).

60. Rawls, *Political Liberalism*, 5–6.

61. Rawls, *Justice*.

62. Crédit Suisse, "Global Wealth Report 2013," Zurich: Crédit Suisse, https://publications.credit-suisse.com/tasks/render/file/?fileID=BCDB1364-A105-0560-1332EC9100FF5C83.

63. For a recent report on malnutrition rates in India by ActionAid, see *On the Brink: Who's Best Prepared for a Climate and Hunger Crisis?* (New Delhi: ActionAid India, 2011) www.actionaidindia.org.

64. Nancy Fraser, "Rethinking the Public Sphere: A Contribution to the Critique of Actually Existing Democracy," *Social Text* 25/26 (1990): 65.

65. Ronald Dworkin, *Justice for Hedgehogs* (Cambridge, Mass.: Harvard University Press, 2011): 375.

66. Ibid.

67. Ibid., 422.

68. Judgment C-258, Corte Constitucional [C.C.] [Constitutional Court], May 7, 2013, Sentencia C-258/13 (Colom.): paras. 3.4.2–3.4.3.

69. See, for example, Kenneth Arrow, "Extended Sympathy and the Possibility of Social Choice," *Equality and Justice in a Democratic Society* 7, no. 2 (1978): 223–37.

70. Amartya Sen, *The Idea of Justice* (Cambridge, Mass.: Harvard University Press / Belknap Press, 2009): 233.

71. Ibid., 258.

72. Ibid., 259.

73. See National Institute for Health and Care Excellence, "Measuring Effectiveness and Cost-Effectiveness: The QALY," www.nice.org.uk/proxy/?sourceUrl=http%3a%2f%2fwww.nice.org.uk%2fnewsroom%2ffeatures%2fmeasuringeffectivenessandcosteffectivenesstheqaly.jsp.

74. Jennifer Prah Ruger, "Health and Social Justice," *Lancet* 364, no. 9439 (2004): 1075–80.

75. Bouchra Assarag et al., "Postpartum Maternal Morbidity in Morocco: Self-Reported Against Diagnosed Morbidity," *Conference Paper: Global Maternal Health Conference* (2013), www.researchgate.net/publication/235673232_Postpartum_maternal_morbidity_in_Morocco_self-reported_against_diagnosed_morbidity.

76. Ruger, "Health."

77. Amartya Sen, *Resources, Values and Development* (Oxford: Blackwell, 1984): 309.

78. Will Kymlicka, *Contemporary Political Philosophy: An Introduction*, Second Edition (New York: Oxford University Press, 2002): 16.

79. Ruger, "Health"; see also Daniels, *Just Health*.

80. Daniels, *Just Health*, chapter 4.

81. Keith Syrett, *Law Legitimacy and the Rationing of Health Care: A Contextual and Comparative Perspective* (Cambridge: Cambridge University Press, 2007).

82. Nelson Mandela, *Long Walk to Freedom: The Autobiography of Nelson Mandela* (Boston: Little, Brown, 1994).

83. UN General Assembly, "General Framework Agreement for Peace in Bosnia and Herzegovina," UN Doc. A/50/79C, S/1995/999 (1995) http://peacemaker.un.org/sites/peacemaker.un.org/files/BA_951121_DaytonAgreement.pdf.

84. David Rohde, *Endgame: The Betrayal and Fall of Srebrenica, Europe's Worst Massacre Since World War II* (New York: Penguin, 1997).

85. Mitja Velikonja, *Religious Separation and Political Intolerance in Bosnia-Herzegovina* (College Station: Texas A&M University Press, 2003).

86. David Campbell, *National Deconstruction: Violence, Identity, and Justice in Bosnia* (Minneapolis: University of Minnesota Press, 1998).

87. Klaas van Dijken, "South Sudan Ravaged by Ethnic Violence," *Al Jazeera*, February 3, 2014, www.aljazeera.com/indepth/features/2014/02/south-sudan-ravaged-ethnic-violence-2014236519937368.html.

88. Jok Madut Jok and Sharon Elaine Hutchinson, "Sudan's Prolonged Second Civil War and the Militarization of Nuer and Dinka Ethnic Identities," *African Studies Review* 42, no. 2 (1999): 125–45.

Notes to Pages 205–210   281

89. The workshop "Rights-Based Approaches to Maternal Health" held in Entebbe, Uganda, February 26–March 1, 2014, was co-sponsored by the François-Xavier Bagnoud Center for Health and Human Rights at Harvard and the Center for Health, Human Rights and Development (CEHURD) in Uganda.

Chapter 8. Our Place in the World

Epigraph: Eduardo Galeano, *Upside Down: A Primer for the Looking-Glass World*, trans. Mark Fried (New York: St. Martin's Press, 2001).

1. Marcus Sanders, *Dante's Inferno* (San Francisco: Chronicle Books, 2004).

2. Aili Mari Tripp, *Donor Assistance and Political Reform in Tanzania, Working Paper No. 2012/37* (Helsinki: United Nations University World Institute for Development Economics Research (UNU–WIDER, 2012).

3. Bonny Ibhawoh and J. I. Dibua, "Deconstructing Ujamaa: The Legacy of Julius Nyerere in the Quest for Social and Economic Development in Africa," *African Journal of Political Science* 8, no. 1 (2003): 60–64.

4. Nathan Nunn, "The Long-Term Effects of Africa's Slave Trade," *Quarterly Journal of Economics* 123, no. 1 (2008): 139–40; and W. G. Clarence-Smith, ed., *The Economics of the Indian Ocean Slave Trade in the Nineteenth Century* (London: Frank Cass, 1989): 2.

5. Barak D. Hoffman, "Political Economy of Tanzania," Center for Democracy and Civil Society, Georgetown University (2013); Mark Curtis, "The One Billion Dollar Question: How Can Tanzania Stop Losing So Much Tax Revenue," Tanzania Episcopal Conference (TEC), National Muslim Council of Tanzania (BAKWATA), and Christian Council of Tanzania (CCT) (2012); and Göran Hydén and Max Mmuya, "Power and Policy Slippage in Tanzania: Discussing National Ownership of Development," Swedish International Development Cooperation Agency (Sida) Studies No. 21 (2008).

6. Barack Obama, "Remarks by the President at the Millennium Development Goals Summit in New York, New York" (September 22, 2010), www.whitehouse.gov/the-press-office/2010/09/22/remarks-president-millennium-development-goals-summit-new-york-new-york.

7. Commission on Information and Accountability for Women's and Children's Health, "Transcript of the Video Statement by H. E. Jakaya Mrisho Kikwete, President, United Republic of Tanzania," *World Health Organization* (2014), www.who.int/topics/millennium_development_goals/accountability_commission/kikwete/kikwete_transcript.pdf?ua=1.

8. Nicholas J. Kassebaum et al., "Global, Regional, and National Levels and Causes of Maternal Mortality During 1990–2013: A Systematic Analysis for the Global Burden of Disease Study 2013," *Lancet*, Early Online Publication 384 no.9947 (2014): 980-1004.

9. United Republic of Tanzania, Ministry of Health and Social Welfare, "Health Sector Public Expenditure Review, 2010/11," Directorate of Policy and Planning, Ministry of Health and Social Welfare and Health Systems 20/20 project, Abt Associates Inc. (2012).

10. Benoit Faucon, Nicholas Bariyo, and Jeanne Whalen, "Thieves Hijacking Malaria Drugs in Africa," *Wall Street Journal*, November 11, 2013, http://online.wsj.com/news/articles/SB10001424052702304672404579181632935636414.

11. Sakiko Fukuda-Parr, Alicia Ely Yamin, and Joshua Greenstein, "The Power of Numbers: A Critical Review of MDG Targets for Human Development and Human Rights," *Journal of Human Development and Capabilities* (2014): 105–17, doi: 10.1080/19452829.2013.864622; Sakiko

Fukuda-Parr and Joshua Greenstein, "Monitoring MDGs: A Human Rights Critique and Alternative," in *Millennium Development Goals and Human Rights: Past, Present and Future,* ed. Malcolm Langford, Andy Sumner, and Alicia Ely Yamin (London: Cambridge University Press, 2013): 439–60; Sakiko Fukuda-Parr and Joshua Greenstein, "How Should MDG Implementation Be Measured: Faster Progress or Meeting Targets?" Working Paper No. 63, International Policy Center for Inclusive Growth, United Nations Development Programme (UNDP) (2010); Sakiko Fukuda-Parr, "Recapturing the Narrative of International Development," Research Paper No. 2012-5, United Nations Research Institute for Social Development (UNRISD), (2012): 1–13; and David Hulme and Sakiko Fukuda-Parr, "International Norm Dynamics and 'the End of Poverty': Understanding the Millennium Development Goals (MDGs)," Working Paper No. 96, Brooks World Policy Institute, the University of Manchester (2009): 1–38.

12. United Nations, "We Can End Poverty: Millennium Development Goals and Beyond 2015," 2013, www.un.org/millenniumgoals/maternal.shtml.

13. UN General Assembly, "Integrated and Coordinated Implementation of and Follow-Up to the Outcomes of the Major UN Conferences and Summits in the Economic, Social and Related Fields; Follow-Up to the Outcome of the Millennium Summit," UN Doc. No. A/60/L.1 (2005); and Stan Bernstein (consultant to the Millennium Project's secretariat), interview by Alicia Ely Yamin, October 8–9, 2013.

14. Alicia Ely Yamin and Vanessa M. Boulanger, "Why Global Goals Matter: The Experience of Sexual and Reproductive Health and Rights in the MDGs," *Journal of Human Development and Capabilities* (2014), doi: 10.1080/19452829.2014.896322.

15. Sakiko Fukuda-Parr and Amy Orr, "The MDG Hunger Target and the Competing Frameworks of Food Security," *Journal of Human Development and Capabilities* 15, nos. 2–3 (2014): 147–60.

16. UN General Assembly, "Vienna Declaration and Programme of Action," UN Doc. A/CONF.157/23 (1993); UN Population Fund, "Report of the International Conference on Population and Development, Cairo, September 5–13, 1994," UN Doc. No. A/CONF.171/13 (1994); United Nations, "Beijing Declaration and Platform of Action," adopted at the Fourth World Conference on Women, October 27, 1995, UN Doc. A/CONF.177/20 (1995); UN General Assembly, "World Food Summit Final Report Part 1," UN Doc. WFS 96/REP Part 1 (1996); and World Education Forum, "The Dakar Framework for Action—Education for All: Meeting our Collective Commitments," UNESCO (2000).

17. World Health Organization (WHO), "Country Cooperation Strategy at a Glance: Tanzania" (2013); and Sikika, "The MoHSW's Budget Proposal 2013/14" (2013).

18. United Republic of Tanzania, Ministry of Health and Social Welfare, "Health Sector Strategic Plan III: Partnerships for Delivering the MDGs" (2008), http://hdptz.esealtd.com/fileadmin/documents/Key_Sector_Documents/Tanzania_Key_Health_Documents/Draft_Health_Sector Strategic_Plan_III__2009-2015.pdf.

19. Yamin and Boulanger, "Global Goals"; Gita Sen and Avanti Mukherjee, "No Empowerment Without Rights, No Rights Without Politics: Gender-Equality, MDGs and the Post-2015 Development Agenda," *Journal of Human Development and Capabilities* (2014), doi: 10.1080/19452829.2014.884057; Elaine Unterhalter, "Measuring Education for the Millennium Development Goals: Reflections on Targets, Indicators, and a Post-2015 Framework," *Journal of Human Development and Capabilities* (2014), doi: 10.1080/19452829.2014.880673; Elisa Díaz-Martínez and Elizabeth D. Gibbons, "The Questionable Power of the Millennium Development Goal to Reduce Child Mortality," *Journal of Human Development and Capabilities* (2014), doi: 10.1080/19452829.2013.864621; and Malcolm Langford and Inga Winkler, "Muddying the Water?

Assessing Target-Based Approaches in Development Cooperation for Water and Sanitation," *Journal of Human Development and Capabilities* (2014), doi: 10.1080/19452829.2014.896321.

20. Yamin and Boulanger, "Global Goals."

21. Alicia Ely Yamin and Kathryn L. Falb, "Counting What We Know; Knowing What to Count: Sexual and Reproductive Rights, Maternal Health, and the Millennium Development Goals," *Nordic Journal on Human Rights* 30 (2012): 353.

22. United Republic of Tanzania, Ministry of Health and Social Welfare, "Health Sector Public Expenditure Review, 2010/11."

23. Kevin E. Davis, Benedict Kingsbury, and Sally Engle Merry, "Indicators as a Technology of Global Governance," *Law and Society Review* 46 (2012): 76–77, citing James G. March and Herbert A. Simon, *Organizations* (New York: Wiley, 1958).

24. President's Emergency Program for AIDS Relief (PEPFAR), "Partnership to Fight HIV/AIDS in Tanzania," www.pepfar.gov/countries/tanzania/.

25. Nirmala Ravishankar et al., "Financing of Global Health: Tracking Development Assistance for Health from 1990 to 2007," *Lancet* 373 no. 9681 (2009): 2113–24.

26. United Republic of Tanzania, Ministry of Health and Social Welfare, "Health Sector Public Expenditure Review, 2010/11."

27. World Bank and Health Results Innovation Trust Fund, "Using Results-Based Financing to Achieve Maternal and Child Health: Progress Report" (2013), www.rbfhealth.org/system/files/HRITF%20progress%20report%202013%20Overview.pdf.

28. Benoit Faucon, Nicholas Bariyo, and Jeanne Whalen, "Thieves Hijacking Malaria Drugs in Africa," *Wall Street Journal*, November 11, 2013.

29. Siri Lange, "The Depoliticisation of Development and the Democratisation of Politics in Tanzania: Parallel Structures as Obstacles to Delivering Services to the Poor," *Journal of Development Studies* 44 (2008): 1137.

30. UN General Assembly, "International Covenant on Economic, Social and Cultural Rights (ICESCR)," UN GA Res. 2200, UN Doc. No. A/6316 (1966): art. 2(1); and UN Committee on Economic, Social and Cultural Rights (CESCR), "General Comment No. 3: The Nature of States Parties' Obligations (Art. 2, Para. 1, of the Covenant)," UN Doc. E/1991/23 (1990).

31. Benjamin Mason Meier and Ashley M. Fox, "International Obligations Through Collective Rights: Moving from Foreign Health Assistance to Global Health Governance," *Health and Human Rights* 12 (2010): 61.

32. Nirmala Ravishankar et al., "Financing of Global Health: Tracking Development Assistance for Health from 1990 to 2007," *Lancet* 373 no. 9681 (2009): 2113–24.

33. David McCoy, Sudeep Chand, and Devi Sridhar, "Global Health Funding: How Much, Where It Comes From and Where It Goes," *Health Policy and Planning* 24 (2009): 407–17; Bill and Melinda Gates Foundation, "2012 Annual Report" (2012), www.gatesfoundation.org/~/media/GFO/Documents/Annual%20Reports/2012_Gates_Foundation_Annual_Report.pdf.

34. McCoy et al., "Global Health Funding."

35. Organisation for Economic Co-Operation and Development, "Aid (ODA) by Sector and Donor [DAC5]," http://stats.oecd.org/Index.aspx?datasetcode=TABLE5.

36. Linsey McGoey, "The Philanthropic State: Market–State Hybrids in the Philanthrocapitalist Turn," *Third World Quarterly* 35, no. 1 (2014): 109–25, at 22.

37. Meier and Fox, "International Obligations," 61.

38. CESCR, "General Comment No. 14, the Right to the Highest Attainable Standard of Health," UN Doc. No. E/C.12/2000/4 (2000): para. 45.

39. UN General Assembly, "National Institutions for the Promotion and Protection of Human Rights," UN Doc. A/RES/48/134 (1993).

40. Third High Level Forum on Aid Effectiveness, "Accra Agenda for Action," (2005): para. 13(c).

41. United States Leadership Against HIV/AIDS, Tuberculosis, and Malaria Act of 2003 ("Leadership Act"), 22 U.S.C. §7601 et seq.

42. *Agency for Int'l Dev. v. Alliance for Open Soc'y Int'l, Inc.*, 570 U.S. (2013).

43. The DPG's mission is to "bring development experience and capital resources to power and energy infrastructure projects in various stages of the development cycle." Development Partners Group LLC, "Development Partners" (2009), http://developmentpartners.com/.

44. Ministry of Foreign Affairs of Denmark, DANIDA, "Danida Transparency," http://um.dk/en/danida-en/about-danida/danida-transparency/.

45. UN Commission on Human Rights, "The Right of Everyone to the Enjoyment of the Highest Attainable Standard of Physical and Mental Health: Report of the Special Rapporteur, Paul Hunt, Submitted in Accordance with Commission Resolution 2002/31," UN Doc. E/CN.4/2003/58 (2003): para. 28.

46. Matt McAllester, "America Is Stealing the World's Doctors," *New York Times*, March 7, 2012, www.nytimes.com/2012/03/11/magazine/america-is-stealing-foreign-doctors.html?pagewanted=all&_r=0.

47. Fariji Msonsa, "Where TZ Doctors Go for Greener Pastures," *The Citizen,* November 18, 2013, www.thecitizen.co.tz/News/Where-TZ-doctors-go-for-greener-pastures/-/1840392/2077472/-/item/1/-/ntb2ff/-/index.html.

48. Sikika and the Medical Association of Tanzania, "Where Are the Doctors? Tracking Study of Medical Doctors" (2013), http://sikika.or.tz/wp-content/uploads/2013/11/Practice-Status-of-Medical-Graduates-FINAL.pdf.

49. One study by Sikika and the Medical Association of Tanzania found that only 43 percent of tracked medical doctors in Tanzania are working full time in clinical settings while 14 percent are working in NGOs, 16 percent are pursuing further studies, and 12 percent work in health training or research institutions, depriving the health system of desperately needed clinical services in yet another way. See Sikaka and the Medical Association of Tanzania, "Where Are the Doctors?"

50. World Health Organization, Executive Board, "International Recruitment of Health Personnel: Draft Global Code of Practice," EB126/8 (2009), http://apps.who.int/gb/ebwha/pdf_files/EB126/B126_8-en.pdf; and the Commonwealth, "Commonwealth Code of Practice for the International Recruitment of Health Personnel" (2003).

51. Commonwealth, "Commonwealth Code of Practice for the International Recruitment of Health Personnel": art. 21.

52. Amani Siyam et al., "Monitoring the Implementation of the WHO Global Code of Practice on the International Recruitment of Health Personnel," *Bulletin of the World Health Organization* 91 (2013): 816–23.

53. CESCR, "Concluding Observations on the Fifth Periodic Report of Norway," UN Doc. E/C.12/NOR/CO/5 (2013): para. 6.

54. President, Mr. J. A. Kufuor, "Water Sector: On the Occasion of the Commissioning of the Weija Water Treatment Plant–Rehabilitation & Expansion Project" (speech, Weija, Ghana, October 18, 2001): 1.

55. Dyna Arhin-Tenkorang et al., "Report of the International Fact-Finding Mission on Water Sector Reform in Ghana," *International Fact-Finding Mission on Water Sector Reform in Ghana*

(August 2002), https://milieudefensie.nl/publicaties/rapporten/report-of-the-international-fact
-finding-mission-on-water-sector-reform-in-ghana; Christian AID and Public Citizen, "Water
Privatization in Ghana," www.citizen.org/documents/XtianAidWater.pdf.

56. CESCR, "Report on the Fifth Session, General Comment No. 3," (1991): supra note 34 at
para. 9–11; CESCR, "Report on the Fourth Session, General Comment No. 2," (1990): para. 9.

57. Committee on the Rights of the Child, "General Comment No. 16 (2013) on State Obligations
Regarding the Impact of the Business Sector on Children's Rights," UN Doc. CRC/C/GC/16 (2013).

58. Werner Biermann and Jumanne Wagao, "The Quest for Adjustment: Tanzania and the
IMF, 1980–1986," *African Studies Review* 29, no. 4 (1986): 89–103; and Roger Nord et al., "Tanzania: The Story of an African Transition," International Monetary Fund (2009).

59. Barack Obama, "Remarks by President Obama at Business Leaders Forum," (speech, Dar
es Salaam, Tanzania, July 1, 2013), www.whitehouse.gov/the-press-office/2013/07/01/remarks
-president-obama-business-leaders-forum; Barack Obama and Jakaya Kikwete of Tanzania,
"Remarks by President Obama and President Kikwete of Tanzania at Joint Press Conference,"
(speech, Dar es Salaam, Tanzania, July 1, 2013), www.whitehouse.gov/the-press-office/2013/07/01
/remarks-president-obama-and-president-kikwete-tanzania-joint-press-confe.

60. Suez Environnement (France, also known as United Water in the United States), Veolia
Environnement (France), RWE (Germany, also owns Thames Water and American Water).

61. See Oxfam America, the Coca-Cola Company, and SABMiller, "Exploring the Links Between International Business and Poverty Reduction: The Coca-Cola/SABMiller Value Chain
Impacts in Zambia and El Salvador" (2011), www.oxfamamerica.org/static/media/files/coca-cola
-sab-miller-poverty-footprint-dec-2011.pdf.

62. Tanzania National Bureau of Statistics and ICF Macro, "2010 Tanzania Demographic and
Health Survey: Key Findings" (2011), http://dhsprogram.com/pubs/pdf/SR183/SR183.pdf.

63. UN General Assembly, "Right of Everyone to the Enjoyment of the Highest Attainable
Standard of Physical and Mental Health," UN Doc. A/69/299 (2014): para. 4.

64. *All India Lawyers Union (Delhi Unit) vs. Govt of NCT Delhi & Others in WP(C)*, No.
5410/1997, High Court of Delhi at New Delhi (September 22, 2009); and case of *Matthews v. the
United Kingdom*, Eur. Ct. H.R., App. No. 24833/94 (1999).

65. Treaty Alliance, "Global Movement for a Binding Treaty," *CETIM, Dismantle Corporate
Power Campaign, ESCR-Net,FIAN, FIDH, Franciscans International, Friends of the Earth International, Transnational Institute (and others)*, www.treatymovement.com/.

66. Committee on the Rights of the Child, "General Comment No. 16 (2013) on State Obligations Regarding the Impact of the Business Sector on Children's Rights."

67. UN General Assembly, "Right of Everyone to the Enjoyment of the Highest Attainable
Standard of Physical and Mental Health," UN Doc. A/69/299 (2014).

68. See Branko Milanovic, "World Income Inequality in the Second Half of the Twentieth
Century," World Bank Paper (2001): 78, as cited in Alvaro de Vita, "Inequality and Poverty in
Global Perspective," in *Freedom from Poverty as a Human Right*, ed. Thomas Pogge (New York:
Oxford University Press, 2007): 103–32, at 104.

69. Branko Milanovic, "Global Inequality: From Class to Location, from Proletarians to
Migrants," *Global Policy* 3, no. 2 (2012): 125–34; Branko Milanovic, "Global Income Inequality:
What It Is and Why It Matters," World Bank Policy Research Working Paper No. 3865 (2006),
http://ssrn.com/abstract=922991.

70. Thomas Piketty, *Capital in the Twenty-First Century,* trans. Arthur Goldhammer (Cambridge, Mass.: Harvard University Press, 2014).

71. Marc Curtis et al., "The One Billion Dollar Question," vii.

72. Ibid.

73. Ministry of Foreign Affairs of Denmark, DANIDA, "Country Policy Paper—Tanzania" (2013).

74. Hoffman, "Political Economy."

75. World Bank, "Mobile Cellular Subscriptions (per 100 People)," *World Databank: World Development Indicators Database,* http://data.worldbank.org/topic/infrastructure.

76. World Bank, "Internet Users (per 100 People)," World Databank: World Development Indicators Database, http://data.worldbank.org/topic/infrastructure.

77. Branco Milanovic, *The Haves and Have-Nots: A Brief and Idiosyncratic History of Global Inequity* (New York: Basic Books, 2011): 174–75.

78. Eric A. Friedman et al., "Realizing the Right to Health Through a Framework Convention on Global Health? A Health and Human Rights Special Issue," *Health and Human Rights* 15, no. 1 (2013): 1–4.

79. The Lancet–University of Oslo Commission on Global Governance for Health, "The Political Origins of Health Inequity: Prospects for Change," *Lancet* 383 (2014): 660.

80. UN Commission on Human Rights, "Commission on Human Rights Resolution 2000/82," UN Doc. E/CN/4/RES/2000/82 (2000).

81. Committee on the Rights of the Child, "General Comment No. 16 (2013) on State Obligations Regarding the Impact of the Business Sector on Children's Rights"; and UN Human Rights Committee, "Concluding Observations on the Sixth Periodic Report of Germany, Adopted by the Committee at its 106th Session (October 15–November 2, 2012)," UN Doc. CCPR/C/DEU/CO/6 (2012).

82. Association of American Medical Colleges, "AAMC Physician Workforce Policy Recommendations" (2012), www.aamc.org/download/304026/data/2012aamcworkforcepolicyrecomm endations.pdf; and Association of American Medical Colleges, "Physician Shortages to Worsen Without Increases in Residency Training," www.aamc.org/download/153160/data/physician _shortages_to_worsen_without_increases_in_residency_tr.pdf.

83. Human Rights Council, Working Group on the Right to Development, "Report of the High-Level Task Force on the Implementation of the Right to Development on its Sixth Session, Addendum: Right to Development Criteria and Operational Sub-Criteria," UN Doc. A/HRC/15/WG.2/TF/2/Add.2 (2010): annex, page 9.

84. Olivier De Schutter, "Statement to the World Summit on Food Security: The Role of the Right to Food in Achieving Sustainable Global Food Security: Message of Dr. Olivier De Schutter, Special Rapporteur on the Right to Food," World Summit on Food Security (November 18, 2009).

85. Human Rights Council, Working Group on the Right to Development. See also Maria Green and Susan Randolph, "Bringing Theory into Practice: Operational Criteria for Assessing Implementation of the International Right to Development," UN Doc. A/HRC/15/WG.2/TF/CRP.5 (2010).

86. Tanganyika gained independence and then later formed a union with Zanzibar to become Tanzania.

87. Ibhawoh and Dibua, "Deconstructing Ujamaa," 60–64.

88. UN General Assembly, "The Future We Want," UN Doc. A/RES/66/288 (2012); UN General Assembly "Draft Decision Submitted by the President of the General Assembly: Open Working Group of the General Assembly on Sustainable Development Goals," UN Doc. A/67/L.48/Rev.1 (2013).

89. Hans Joachim Schellnhuber et al., *Turn Down the Heat: Climate Extremes, Regional Impacts, and the Case for Resilience* (Washington D.C.: World Bank, 2013).

90. Amartya Sen, "The Ends and Means of Sustainability," *Journal of Human Development Capabilities* 14 (2013): 1–20.

91. Brian Heap and Jennifer Kent, *Towards Sustainable Consumption: A European Perspective* (London: The Royal Society, 2000); and UN General Assembly, "The Future We Want," UN Doc. A/RES/66/288 (2012).

92. Sen, "Ends and Means," 8.

93. Ibid., 7.

94. Ibid., 10.

95. Ibid., 11.

96. Nuestro Texas Comunidad, Salud, y Familia. http://www.nuestrotexas.org.

Conclusion

Epigraphs: Miguel de Cervantes Saavedra, *Don Quixote de la Mancha*, ed. E. C. Riley, trans. Charles Jarvis (Oxford: Oxford University Press, 2008); Susan Sontag, *Regarding the Pain of Others* (New York: Picador, 2003): 73.

1. Jorge Luis Borges, *Ficciones* (New York: Grove Press, 1962): 68.

2. Risa Whitson, "Beyond the Crisis: Economic Globalization and Informal Work in Urban Argentina," *Journal of Latin American Geography* 6, no. 2 (2007): 121–36; Becky L. Jacobs, "Pesification and Economic Crisis in Argentina: The Moral Hazard Posed by a Politicized Supreme Court," *University of Miami Inter-American Law Review* 34, no. 3 (2003): 391; and William W. Burke-White, "The Argentine Financial Crisis: State Liability Under BITs and the Legitimacy of the ICSID System," *Asian Journal of WTO & International Health Law and Policy* 3, no. 1 (2008): 199–234.

3. Jan Joost Teunissen and Age Akkerman, eds., *The Crisis That Was Not Prevented: Lessons for Argentina, the IMF, and Globalisation* (The Hague: FONDAD, 2003), www.fondad.org/product_books/pdf_download/9/Fondad-Argentina-BookComplete.pdf; and Max Seitz, "The Day Argentina Hit Rock Bottom," *BBC News*, December 19, 2005, http://news.bbc.co.uk/2/hi/business/4534786.stm.

4. Roberto Mangabeira Unger, *False Necessity: Anti-Necessitarian Social Theory in the Service of Radical Democracy* (Cambridge: Cambridge University Press, 1988): xxi.

5. Amartya Sen, *The Idea of Justice* (Cambridge, Mass.: Belknap Press/Harvard University Press, 2009).

6. Lynn P. Freedman, "Achieving the MDGs: Health Systems as Core Social Institutions," *Development* 48, no. 1 (2005): 19–24.

7. Wouter Vandehole and Paul Gready, "Failures and Successes of Human Rights–Based Approaches to Development: Towards a Change Perspective," *Nordic Journal of Human Rights* 32, no. 4 (2014): 291–311.

8. Alicia Ely Yamin, "Toward Transformative Accountability: A Proposal for Rights-Based Approaches to Fulfilling Maternal Health Obligations," *Sur: An International Journal* 7, no. 12 (2010): 95–122; UN Human Rights Council, "Technical Guidance on the Application of a Human-Rights Based Approach to the Implementation of Policies and Programmes to Reduce Preventable Maternal Morbidity and Mortality." UN Doc. A/HRC/21/22 (2012).

9. Lynn Hunt, *Inventing Human Rights: A History* (New York: W.W. Norton, 2007).

10. Sen, *Idea of Justice*, 239.

11. Vandenhole and Gready, Failures and Successes."

12. Committee on the Elimination of Discrimination Against Women (CEDAW Committee), "Views of the Committee on the Elimination of Discrimination Against Women Under Article 7, Paragraph 3, of the Optional Protocol to the Convention on the Elimination of All Forms of Discrimination Against Women Concerning Communication No. 17/2008," UN Doc. CEDAW/ C/49/D/17/2008 (2011); the Center for Reproductive Rights, "Brazilian Government Gives Monetary Reparations as Part of Historic United Nations Maternal Death Case," Press Release, March 25, 2014, accessed November 14, 2014, http://reproductiverights.org/en/press-room /brazilian-government-gives-monetary-reparations-as-part-of-historic-united-nations -matern.

13. "3A Global School on Socioeconomic Rights: Course on Health Rights Litigation," Program on the Health Rights of Women and Children, FXB Center for Health and Human Rights, accessed June 4, 2014, http://fxb.harvard.edu/health-rights-of-women-and-children/; and "Courses," Global School on Socioeconomic Rights, accessed June 4, 2014, http://globalschool.co/index.php.

14. "3B Health Rights Litigation Workshops and Strategic Advisory Role," Program on the Health Rights of Women and Children, FXB Center for Health and Human Rights, accessed June 4, 2014, http://fxb.harvard.edu/health-rights-of-women-and-children/.

15. Sikika, "Health Governance and Financing, Brief No. 1 of 2012" (2012); Sikika, "Sikika Conducts SAM in Five Districts" (2014); Fariki Msonsa, "New Report Reveals Mess in Execution of Public Health Projects," *The Citizen*, February 12, 2014.

16. Flavia Bustreo et al., *Women's and Children's Health: Evidence of Impact of Human Rights* (Geneva: World Health Organization, 2013).

17. The Danish Government, *Denmark in Africa—A Continent on its Way: The Government's Priorities for Denmark's Cooperation with Sub-Saharan Africa* (Copenhagen: Royal Danish Ministry of Foreign Affairs, 2007); the Danish Government, *Right to a Better Life: Strategy for Denmark's Development Cooperation* (Copenhagen: Royal Danish Ministry of Foreign Affairs, 2012).

18. Samuel Moyn, *The Last Utopia: Human Rights in History* (Cambridge, Mass.: Harvard University Press, 2010), 4.

19. Jennifer S. Holmes, "Political Violence and Regime Change in Argentina: 1965–1976," *Terrorism and Political Violence* 13, no. 1 (2001).

20. Abimael Guzman Reynoso, *For the New Flag* (Peru: Central Committee, Communist Party of Peru, 1981).

21. Nils Jacobsen, *Mirages of Transition: The Peruvian Altiplano, 1780–1930* (Berkeley: University of California Press, 1993).

22. Marisa Mealy and Carol Shaw Austad, *"Sendero Luminoso* (Shining Path) and the Conflict in Peru," in *Handbook of Ethical Conflict: International Perspectives*, ed. Dan Landis and Rosita D. Albert (New York: Springer, 2012): 553–83.

23. Crane Brinton, *The Anatomy of Revolution*, revised ed. (New York: Vintage Books, 1957), 251. First edition, 1938.

24. Mark Perry, "A Fire in the Minds of Arabs: The Arab Spring in Revolutionary History," *Insight Turkey* 16, no. 1 (2014): 27–34.

25. Brinton, *Anatomy*.

26. Upendra Baxi, "Taking Suffering Seriously: Social Action Litigation in the Supreme Court of India," *Third World Legal Studies* 4, no. 6 (1985): 132.

27. UN General Assembly, "Universal Declaration of Human Rights," UNGA Res. 217 A (III), (1948), preamble.

28. Unger, *False Necessity*, 363.

29. Roberto Mangabeira Unger, *What Should the Left Propose* (New York: Verso, 2005): 32.

30. Michael Neocosmos, "Civil Society, Citizenship and the Politics of the Impossible: Rethinking Militancy in Africa Today," *Interface: A Journal for and About Social Movements* 1, no. 2 (2009): 263–34, at 278.

31. Unger, *What Should the Left Propose*, 32.

32. Unger, *False Necessity*, xxi.

33. Ibid., lxxii.

34. Ronald Dworkin, *Justice for Hedgehogs* (Cambridge, Mass.: Harvard University Press, 2011); Ronald Dworkin, *Life's Dominion: An Argument About Abortion, Euthanasia, and Individual Freedom* (New York: Knopf, 1993).

35. *Petition Number 16*, CEHURD (2011); "Current Projects: 3. Constitutional Petition 16/2010," CEHURD, accessed June 5, 2014, www.cehurd.org/projects/current-projects/; and *CEHURD et al. v. Attorney General* [Constitution Court], Petition No. 16 of 2011 (Ugan.), www.iser-uganda.org/images/stories/Downloads/Ruling_on_Maternal_Health.pdf.

36. See Unger, *False Necessity*, 1.

Glossary

1. UN Committee on Economic, Social and Cultural Rights (CESCR), "General Comment No. 14, the Right to the Highest Attainable Standard of Health," UN Doc. E/C.12/2000/4 (2000): para. 12.

2. "Human Rights Committee: Monitoring Civil and Political Rights," United Nations Human Rights, Office of the High Commissioner for Human Rights (OHCHR), accessed June 2, 2014, www.ohchr.org/EN/HRBodies/CCPR/Pages/CCPRIndex.aspx.

3. "Committee on Economic, Social and Cultural Rights: Monitoring the Economic, Social and Cultural Rights," United Nations Human Rights, OHCHR, accessed June 4, 2014, www.ohchr.org/EN/HRBodies/CESCR/Pages/CESCRIntro.aspx.

4. "Committee on the Elimination of Discrimination Against Women," United Nations Human Rights, OHCHR, accessed June 4, 2014, www.ohchr.org/EN/HRBodies/CEDAW/Pages/CEDAWIndex.aspx.

5. UN General Assembly, "Convention against Torture and Other Cruel, Inhuman or Degrading Treatment or Punishment," UN Doc. A/RES/39/46 (1981).

6. UN General Assembly, "Convention on the Elimination of All Forms of Discrimination Against Women," UN Doc. A/RES/4/180 (1979).

7. UN General Assembly, "Convention on the Rights of the Child," November 20, 1989, UN Doc. A/RES/44/25 (1989).

8. UN General Assembly, "Convention on the Rights of Persons with Disabilities," UN Doc. A/RE/ 61/106 (2007).

9. "Cost Effectiveness Analysis," Centers for Disease Control and Prevention (CDC), accessed June 2, 2014, www.cdc.gov/owcd/eet/costeffect2/fixed/1.html.

10. "Health Economics and Modeling Unit (HEMU)," Division of Preparedness and Emerging Infections (DPEI) at the CDC, accessed June 4, 2014, www.cdc.gov/ncezid/dpei/hemu/.

11. "Metrics: Disability-Adjusted Life Year (DALY)," World Health Organization (WHO), accessed June 2, 2014, www.who.int/healthinfo/global_burden_disease/metrics_daly/en/.

12. Human Rights Centre Clinic, *Disaggregated Data and Human Rights: Law, Policy and Practice* (Colchester, UK: University of Essex, 2013), 7, www.humanrightsatlas.org/wp-content/uploads/2013/12/Disaggregated-Data-and-Human-Rights-Law-Policy-and-Practice.pdf.

13. Nancy Krieger, "Proximal, Distal, and the Politics of Causation: What's Level Got to Do with It?" *American Journal of Public Health* 98, no. 2 (2008): 221–30.

14. "Frequently Asked Questions on Economic, Social, and Cultural Rights," OHCHR, accessed June 2, 2014, www.ohchr.org/Documents/Issues/ESCR/FAQ%20on%20ESCR-en.pdf.

15. WHO, UN Population Fund (UNFPA), UNICEF, and Averting Maternal Death and Disability (AMDD), *Monitoring Emergency Obstetric Care: A Handbook* (Geneva: WHO, 2009), http://whqlibdoc.who.int/publications/2009/9789241547734_eng.pdf?ua=1.

16. "Human Rights Bodies—General Comments," United Nations Human Rights, OHCHR, accessed June 4, 2014, www2.ohchr.org/english/bodies/treaty/comments.htm.

17. "Measuring Inequality," World Bank, 2014, accessed June 5, 2014, http://web.worldbank.org/.

18. "GINI Index," The World Bank, 2014, accessed June 2, 2014, http://data.worldbank.org/indicator/SI.POV.GINI.

19. "Human Rights Committee: Monitoring Civil and Political Rights," United Nations Human Rights, OHCHR, accessed June 4, 2014, www.ohchr.org/EN/HRBodies/CCPR/Pages/CCPRIndex.aspx.

20. "United Nations Human Rights Council: Welcome to the Human Rights Council," United Nations Human Rights, OHCHR, accessed June 4, 2014, www.ohchr.org/EN/HRBodies/HRC/Pages/AboutCouncil.aspx.

21. UN General Assembly, "International Covenant on Economic, Social and Cultural Rights (ICESCR)," UNGA Res. 2200, UN Doc. No. A/6316 (1966).

22. Octavio L. Motta Ferraz, "Brazil: Health Inequalities, Rights, and Courts: The Social Impact of the Judicialization of Health," in *Litigating Health Rights: Can Courts Bring More Justice to Health?* ed. Alicia Ely Yamin and Siri Gloppen (Cambridge, Mass.: Harvard Human Rights Program Series, Harvard University Press, 2011), 76.

23. Andrew Barry, Thomas Osborne, and Nikolas S. Rose, eds., *Foucault and Political Reason: Liberalism, Neo-Liberalism, and Rationalities of Government* (Chicago: University of Chicago Press, 1996), 22.

24. Jeffrey H. Reiman, *Critical Moral Liberalism: Theory and Practice* (Lanham, Md.: Rowman & Littlefield, 1997), ix; Barry et al., *Foucault,* 22.

25. Ruth W. Grant, *John Locke's Liberalism,* (Chicago: University of Chicago Press, 2010), 196.

26. "Maternal Mortality Ratio (per 100,000 Live Births)," WHO, accessed June 2, 2014, www.who.int/healthinfo/statistics/indmaternalmortality/en/.

27. World Health Organization, *International Classification of Diseases and Related Health Problems—10th Rvision* (Geneva: WHO, 1992).

28. UN General Assembly, "United Nations Millennium Declaration," UN Doc. A/55/L.2 (2000); and "The Millennium Declaration and the MDGs," United Nations Development Group, accessed June 4, 2014, www.undg.org/content/achieving_the_mdgs/millennium_declaration_and_the_mdgs.

29. "Millennium Development Goals and Beyond 2015," United Nations, accessed June 4, 2014, www.un.org/millenniumgoals.

30. Barry et al, *Foucault,* 22–23.

31. "Official Development Assistance—Definition and Coverage," Organisation for Economic Co-operation and Development (OECD), accessed June 2, 2014, www.oecd.org/dac/stats/official developmentassistancedefinitionandcoverage.htm.

32. "Roles and Types of NHRIs," International Coordinating Committee of National Institutions for the Promotion and Protection of Human Rights (ICC), accessed June 4, 2014, http://nhri.ohchr.org/EN/AboutUs/Pages/RolesTypesNHRIs.aspx.

33. Carlos Sánchez Mejorada, "The Writ of Amparo: Mexican Procedure to Protect Human Rights," *Annals of the American Academy of Political and Social Science* 243 (1946): 107–11.

34. "Protracted Labor," *The Merck Manual for Healthcare Professionals*, accessed June 2, 2014, www.merckmanuals.com/professional/gynecology_and_obstetrics/abnormalities_and_complications_of_labor_and_delivery/protracted_labor.html.

35. Nancy Krieger, "Proximal, Distal, and the Politics of Causation: What's Level Got to Do with It?" *American Journal of Public Health* 98, no. 2 (2008): 221–30.

36. Alan J. Krupnik, *Valuing Health Outcomes: Policy Choices and Technical Issues* (Washington, D.C.: Resources for the Future, 2004).

37. "Maternal, Newborn, Child and Adolescent Health: Skilled Birth Attendants," World Health Organization, accessed June 2, 2014, www.who.int/maternal_child_adolescent/topics/maternal/skilled_birth/en/.

38. "Social Determinants of Health," World Health Organization, accessed June 2, 2014, www.who.int/social_determinants/en/.

39. "Colombia: Political Constitution of Colombia," World Intellectual Property Organization, accessed June 4, 2014, www.wipo.int/wipolex/en/text.jsp?file_id=198962.

40. "Special Rapporteur on the Promotion and Protection of the Right of Freedom of Opinion and Expression," OHCHR, accessed June 2, 2014, www.ohchr.org/EN/ISSUES/FREEDOMOPINION/Pages/OpinionIndex.aspx.

41. "Definitions," UN Treaty Collection, accessed June 4, 2014, https://treaties.un.org/pages/Overview.aspx?path=overview/definition/page1_en.xml#signatories.

42. "Sustainable Development Goals," UN Sustainable Development Knowledge Platform, accessed June 2, 2014, http://sustainabledevelopment.un.org/?menu=1300.

43. "Human Rights Bodies," United Nations Human Rights, OHCHR, accessed June 4, 2014, www.ohchr.org/EN/HRBODIES/Pages/HumanRightsBodies.aspx.

44. UN General Assembly, "Universal Declaration of Human Rights," UNGA Res. 217 A (III), (1948), preamble, www.un.org/Overview/rights.html.

45. Richard A. Posner, "Utilitarianism, Economics, and Legal Theory," *Journal of Legal Studies* 8 (1979): 103–40.

46. Hagan Schultz-Forberg, "Welfare State," *Encyclopedia of Global Studies*, ed. Helmut K. Anheier, Mark Jurgensmeyer, and Victor Faessel (Thousand Oaks, Calif.: Sage, 2012), 1783–88.

Glossary

AAAQ—A framework set out by the Committee on Economic, Social and Cultural Rights to ensure that aspects of health facilities, goods, and services are to be made available, accessible, acceptable, and of adequate quality for the entire population on the basis of nondiscrimination.[1] The same framework has been applied to other rights under the International Covenant on Economic, Social and Cultural Rights.

civil and political (CP) rights—Human rights concerning individual autonomy and participation in government, defined in international law by the International Covenant on Civil and Political Rights (ICCPR) and other treaties; for example, the right to life, equality before the law, and freedom of expression.[2]

Committee on Economic, Social and Cultural Rights (CESCR)—The treaty-based body of independent experts established in 1985 to monitor the implementation of the International Covenant on Economic, Social and Cultural Rights by its states' parties.[3]

Committee on the Elimination of Discrimination Against Women (CEDAW Committee)—The treaty-based body of independent experts established in 1982 that monitors the implementation of the Convention on the Elimination of All Forms of Discrimination Against Women.[4]

Convention Against Torture—A multilateral treaty promulgated by the United Nations in 1984, which entered into force in 1987, to ensure that no person shall be subjected to torture or to cruel, inhuman or degrading treatment or punishment.[5]

Convention on the Elimination of All Forms of Discrimination Against Women (CEDAW)—A multilateral treaty promulgated by the United Nations in 1979, which entered into force in 1981, to ensure the equality of economic, social, cultural, civil, and political rights of women.[6]

Convention on the Rights of the Child—A multilateral treaty promulgated by the United Nations in 1989, which entered into force in 1990, to promote the economic, social, cultural, civil, and political rights of children.[7]

Convention on the Rights of Persons with Disabilities (CRPD)—A multilateral treaty promulgated by the United Nations in 2006, which entered into force in 2008, to promote, protect, and ensure the full and equal enjoyment of all human rights and fundamental freedoms by persons with disabilities.[8]

cost-effectiveness analysis (CEA)—A form of economic analysis that compares the relative costs and effects (or outcomes) of two or more plans of action.[9]

cost-utility analysis— A form of cost-effectiveness analysis in which the outcomes are valued in terms of utility or quality, using nonmonetary units such as the quality-adjusted life year (QALY) or the disability-adjusted life year (DALY).[10]

disability-adjusted life year (DALY)—A measure of overall disease burden, expressed in number of years of life lost because of ill-health, disability, or early death.[11]

disaggregated data—Data that has been broken down, or is possible to break down, into smaller, specific subgroups with the same identifiable criteria (for example, sex, nationality, or ethnicity).[12]

distal cause—Upstream societal influences that shape downstream (proximate) exposures, thereby affecting population health.[13]

economic, social, and cultural (ESC) rights—A group of human rights concerning the workplace, social security, family life, cultural life, and access to an adequate standard of living, among other things, defined in international law by the International Covenant on Economic, Social and Cultural Rights and other treaties; for example, the right to health, housing, and education.[14]

emergency obstetric care (EmOC)—Emergency care given to pregnant or laboring mothers in case of major complications. This care includes six signal functions for basic services and two additional signal functions for comprehensive services.[15]

general comment or general recommendation—The format by which each human rights treaty body publishes its interpretation of the content of human rights provisions. The Committee on the Elimination of Racial Discrimination (CERD) and the CEDAW Committee refer to their general comments as general recommendations.[16]

Gini coefficient—A measure of income inequality of a nation's residents, defined as a ratio with values between 0 and 1, with values approaching 1 representing greater inequality within a nation.[17]

Gini index—The Gini coefficient multiplied by 100, with 0 representing perfect equality and 100 representing perfect inequality.[18]

Human Rights Committee—The treaty-based body of independent experts that monitors the implementation of the International Covenant on Civil and Political Rights by its states' parties.[19]

Human Rights Council (HRC)—The charter-based "inter-governmental body within the United Nations system responsible for strengthening the promotion and protection of human rights around the globe and for addressing situations of human rights violations and make [sic] recommendations on them." This body replaced the former United Nations Commission on Human Rights in 2006.[20]

International Conference on Population and Development (ICPD)—A conference coordinated by the United Nations in Cairo, Egypt in September 1994 during which 20,000 delegates from governments, UN agencies, NGOs, and the media discussed issues including immigration, infant mortality, birth control, family planning, education of women, and protection for women from unsafe abortion services. The Program of Action that resulted from the conference is the steering document for the United Nations Population Fund (UNFPA).

International Covenant on Economic, Social and Cultural Rights (ICESCR)—A multilateral treaty promulgated by the United Nations in 1966, which entered into force in 1976, committing states' parties to the pursuit of the economic, social, and cultural rights of its citizens.[21]

judicialization (of health rights)—To bring debates about health rights under the remit of the courts.[22]

laissez-faire state—Theory of state in which regulation of private commercial activities should be minimized on the grounds that individuals will preserve their autonomy and benefit more by limiting political interference with the market.[23]

liberalism—A moral philosophy that believes in the right of individuals to live as they choose as long as this right is respected in others and in economic terms; the belief in limiting government or public interference with private choices and individual autonomy.[24]

liberal state—Theory of a societally driven democratic state emerging in the nineteenth century in which the state held responsibility for protecting the rights of its citizens but otherwise respected standards set by the natural law regarding human freedom, reason and, will.[25]

maternal mortality—Death of a woman while pregnant or within forty-two days of termination of pregnancy, irrespective of the duration and site of the pregnancy, from any cause related to or aggravated by the pregnancy or its management but not from accidental or incidental causes.[26] Late maternal mortality includes death of the women up to a year after termination of the pregnancy.[27]

Millennium Declaration—A declaration adopted in 2000 by the UN General Assembly following the UN Millennium Summit to address development challenges faced globally and to outline responses to these challenges.[28]

Millennium Development Goals (MDGs)—Eight international goals established to measure the achievement of the Millennium Declaration with a target date of achievement of 2015. The goals are as follows: (1) Eradicate extreme poverty and hunger; (2) achieve universal primary education; (3) promote gender equality and empower women; (4) reduce child mortality; (5) improve maternal health; (6) combat HIV/AIDS, malaria, and other diseases; (7) ensure environmental sustainability; and (8) develop a global partnership for development.[29]

neoliberalism—A modern form of liberalism, extending from the traditional liberal philosophy that supports laissez-faire economics and enhancing the role of the private sector.[30]

official development assistance (ODA)—Development assistance provided by official agencies, including state and local governments, administered for the economic development and social welfare of the countries that receive it.[31]

Ombuds Office—A form of national human rights institution (NHRI) in which a public agency is mandated to investigate the complaints of citizens against government agencies; address discrimination; and promote the protection of civil, political, economic, social, and cultural rights.[32]

protection writs (*amparos* or *tutelas*)—A remedy or an action for the protection of individual constitutional rights.[33]

protracted labor—Abnormally slow cervical dilation or fetal descent during active labor.[34]

proximate cause—Downstream physical, behavioral, psychosocial, and biological exposures that operate directly on or within the body.[35]

quality-adjusted life years (QALYs)—A measure of disease burden used in assessing the value of a medical intervention that takes into consideration both the quality and the quantity of life lived.[36]

skilled birth attendant (SBA)—An accredited health professional, such as a midwife, doctor, or nurse, who has been educated and trained to proficiency in the skills needed to manage normal (uncomplicated) pregnancies, childbirth, and the immediate postnatal period, as well as the identification, management, and referral of complications in pregnant women and newborns.[37]

social determinants of health—"The conditions in which people are born, grow, live, work and age . . . shaped by the distribution of money, power and resources at global, national and local levels" that influence health outcomes or access to health care.[38]

"social state of law" (*estado social de derecho*)—Defined by the Constitution of Colombia as "a unitary, decentralized, democratic, participatory, and pluralistic Republic, with autonomous territorial entities, founded on respect for human dignity, work and the solidarity of the persons composing it, and the prevalence of the general interest."[39]

special rapporteur—Independent expert who is given a specific mandate from the UN Human Rights Council to investigate, monitor, and propose solutions to certain human rights issues (for example, special rapporteur on the Right to Health).[40]

state party—States that have expressed their consent to be bound by a treaty, where a treaty is in force for such states.[41]

Sustainable Development Goals (SDGs)—International development goals that will succeed the Millennium Development Goals after 2015. The term emerged from an agreement made at the United Nations Conference on Sustainable Development held in Rio de Janeiro in 2012 (Rio+20).[42]

Treaty-Monitoring Committee—A committee of independent experts established in accordance with the provisions of a treaty it is meant to monitor.[43]

Universal Declaration of Human Rights—Promulgated by the UN General Assembly in 1948, following World War II and the creation of the United Nations, this document set forth a standard of fundamental human rights to be universally protected.[44]

utilitarianism—An ethical theory that holds that the moral worth of an action (or a practice, an institution, a law, and so on) should be judged by its ability to promote happiness in society or, in economic terms, to maximize utility.[45]

welfare state—An evolution of the traditional liberal state by which government practice aims to provide social justice and equal opportunity to its citizens by way of conscious government intervention into the market through taxes, regulations, redistributions, and interest negotiations.[46]

Index

judicial remedies and litigation (*continued*)
Costa Rican Supreme Court, 91; as
"dialogical remedies," 124, 142, 167;
European Court of Human Rights, 153;
Ferraz on "first-come first-served"
approaches, 189; and formal equality,
189–90; HIV/AIDS issues, 61, 91, 141, 148, 149,
215–16; Indian Supreme Court, 66, 94, 140,
144, 189; Inter-American Court of Human
Rights, 31; judicial review and the standard
of reasonableness, 141–42; the judicialization
of health rights, 123, 141, 189; LGBT rights,
31, 94, 188–89; material and symbolic effects
of judicial decisions, 142–43, *143f*; misuses
of, 141; people with disabilities, 192; South
African Constitutional Court, 32, 66, 91, 118,
121, 148–49, 184; state constitutions and
state-level courts, 61, 140–41; U.S. Supreme
Court, 66, 94, 188, 215–16, 259n49
justice: Rawls's prioritarian theory of
distributive justice, 196–97, 199; and wealth
equality, 195–97; women's health as
reflections of patterns of, 6–7, 232–33

Kant, Immanuel, 28–29, 31, 57, 234
Kenya: Constitution (2010), 242; decentrali-
zation of government responsibilities
for health, 164; extreme poverty in, 54;
women's involuntary sterilization based on
HIV status, 54, 163, 166
Kessy, Egbert, 217
Khan, Irene, 131
Kikwete, Jakaya, 208–9
Kilimanjaro Christian Medical University
College (Tanzania), 217
King, Martin Luther, Jr., 99
KL v. Peru, 39
Kleinman, Arthur, 81
Kony, Joseph, 248
Kothari, Uma, 170
Krieger, Nancy, 86

laissez-faire state, 64–65
Lancet, 4, 182, 214
Lancet–University of Oslo Commission on
Global Governance for Health, 88, 223
Lange, Siri, 213
Latin America: conditional cash transfers
(CCTs), 69–70, 187; legacy of revolutionary
movements in, 244–46; magical realist
literature, 99, 263n2

Latin American Committee for the Defense of
the Rights of Women (CLADEM Perú), 177
lawalawa (Swahili word), 83
LGBT (lesbian, gay, bisexual, and transgender) persons and rights, 93–95; anti-LGBT
legislation in Uganda, 94–95; Argentina,
94; *Atala* decision on parental custody in
Chile, 31; criminalized homosexual
activity, 89–90; and formal equality,
188–89; HIV/AIDS rates, 95; Indian
Supreme Court's NALSA decision on
rights of intersex people, 94, 189; legal
recognition of transgender people, 94;
same-sex marriage in the U.S., 94, 188. *See
also* MSM
liberalism and liberal rights paradigm: and
assaults on human dignity in the private
sphere, 42–44; and decentralization of
government responsibilities for health,
163–65; distinguishing between CP rights
and ESC rights, 63, 235; individual
responsibility and health, 84–85;
neoliberal economic policies, 19, 62–65,
139, 235; progressive critiques, 165–66,
170–71; the public sphere in the traditional
liberal state, 42–44; Rawls's prioritarian
theory of distributive justice, 196–97, 199;
rights based on individual autonomy in the
public sphere, 32, 42–43; understanding of
power and political participation in health,
161–66, 170–71. *See also* neoliberalism
Liberia, Ebola crisis in, 20, 155, 156
Link, Bruce, 78
litigation. *See* judicial remedies and litigation
London, Leslie, 136
Lord's Resistance Army (LRA) (Uganda), 248
Lukes, Steven, 45, 173

MacKinnon, Catharine, 187
MacNaughton, Gillian, 187
Maine, Deborah, 108
Malawi: children's HIV/AIDS deaths, 70;
extreme poverty in, 70–72; witchcraft/
curse explanations for maternal
deaths, 83
Mamérita Mestanza v. Peru, 177
Mandela, Nelson, 25, 49, 202
"manifest injustice," 5, 233, 240
Mann, Jonathan, xii, 58, 85; three dimensions
of links between health and human rights,
13, 36–38, 163

Acknowledgments

This book could not have been written without the inspiration, support, and guidance of a great number of people, to whom I am enormously grateful and deeply indebted.

Writing a book can be a solitary exercise, but ideas do not live alone and the creative process never takes place in a vacuum. I have benefitted enormously from the insights and encouragement of extraordinary friends and colleagues with a wide array of different disciplinary as well as personal perspectives. These include Siri Gloppen, Ole Frithjof Norheim, Manuel José Cepeda, Sakiko Fukuda-Parr, Malcolm Langford, Camila Gianella, Chris Desmond, Carmel Williams, Masuma Mamdani, Ibadat Dhillon, Heather Adams, Aline Newton, Michelle DeLong, and Mary Plummer, as well as many others, who may not even know how much their intellectual guidance and support meant at critical points in framing and writing this book.

Rebecca Cantor, Melanie Baskind, Alexandra Goodwin, Angela Duger, Emily Maistrellis, Melanie Norton, and Allyson Baughman not only diligently read through countless iterations of chapters and subchapters and tracked down references with unfailing good humor and dedication, but also provided me with essential feedback at different points throughout the process.

Susan Holman's devoted reading of the manuscript was critical to pushing me gently along the way.

Peter Agree, Editor-in-Chief at the University of Pennsylvania Press, provided encouragement from the beginning, and infinite patience throughout the process of making this book a reality. I am also ever grateful to Bert Lockwood, series editor of Pennsylvania Studies in Human Rights at Penn

Press, for literally decades of professional encouragement and his wonderful enthusiasm for the idea of this book.

The peer reviewers' enthusiasm, coupled with constructive and deeply informed critiques from different disciplinary perspectives, encouraged me to make significant improvements to the manuscript.

Jennifer Leaning, the director of the FXB Center for Health and Human Rights at Harvard University, generously supported me through three years of directing a program for Harvard from East Africa, which was critical in enabling me to write this book.

But writing the book is only part of the story, and of the stories collected here. I have shared this journey over the years with many extraordinary individuals, with whom I have cried tears of joy as well as frustration, rage and sadness, but in the end who have inspired me through their commitment and example to know that another world is possible. In Mexico I worked closely with, among others, Pilar Noriega and Teresa Jardí, who are two of the most courageous people I have ever known. In Peru, I continued to be inspired by the integrity and courage of women who took the human rights admonition to "speak truth to power" seriously, including the late Giulia Tamayo—who eventually was forced to leave the country because of her work exposing the forced sterilizations of thousands of indigenous women. The examples taken from Peru were based on many different collaborations with Mario Rios, Ariel Frisancho, Luz Estrada, Tiffany Moore, and Marion Brown, among others.

My research in Colombia, over a number of years, would have been impossible without Oscar Parra Vera from whom I have learned far more than I have taught him.

In carrying out research and investigations for various projects over years in Sub-Saharan Africa, I am grateful to Jane Shuma, Mitike Molla, Junior Bazile, Lucia Knight, and Tania Bernath, among many others. And it was, and continues to be, an enormous privilege to work with Allan Maleche, Catherine Mumma, Moses Mulumba, David Kabanda, and Nakibuuka Noor, among others, who are committed to making health rights real in East Africa, and who inspire me by their example as to what is possible.

I am indebted to the late Patwant Singh and his sister, Rasil Basu, for inviting me to the Kabliji Rural Health Centre in Haryana, India, which changed my life.

I am thankful to Eric Rosenthal for including me in many fact-finding delegations of Disability Rights International, including the one in Argentina referred to in this book, and from whom I have learned much about advocacy for the rights and dignity of persons with disabilities.

Paul Farmer, generous friend and profound inspiration, laid the seeds for this book when he asked me to become an editor of the newly revamped *Health and Human Rights* journal and to help readers understand what it would mean to apply a human rights framework to health.

I am grateful to the entire *Health and Human Rights Journal* team, including Jim Yong Kim, Evan Lyon, Vivek Maru, Alexander Irwin, Ann Barger Hannum, Susan Holman, Catlin Rockman, Arlan Fuller, and Patricia Spellman. Without that early experience of working on the synthesis articles for the journal, this book might not have come to fruition.

I have also had the privilege of working closely with both the first and second Special Rapporteurs on the Right to Health, Paul Hunt and Anand Grover, respectively, and I am greatly indebted to those collaborations for raising my awareness of diverse issues in relation to normative frameworks as well as impacts of applying rights frameworks to health.

I was also tremendously fortunate that in consulting on the "UN Technical Guidance on the Application of Rights-Based Frameworks to Health in the Context of Reducing Preventable Maternal Morbidity and Mortality," my contact at the Office of the UN High Commissioner for Human Rights was Lucinda O'Hanlon, whose unflagging commitment to promoting understanding of sexual and reproductive health in terms of rights fueled my own determination to complete this book.

I would never have been in a position to develop the linkages between maternal health and human rights without the mentorship of both Deborah Maine and Lynn Freedman, with whom I had the enormous privilege of working at Columbia University, and from whom I have continued to learn over the years.

I am, as ever, grateful to my partner, Jeremy, who heard the stories recounted here as they were happening, saw how they affected me, and unfailingly encouraged me to share them with others.

I will be forever indebted to my sons, Nico and Sam, who sacrificed my time and presence, not just while I was writing this book but over many years of their childhoods, when I was documenting the effects of the absence of a mother on other people's children. That they both are now also deeply committed to seeing the world transformed is the greatest affirmation possible for a mother, and gives me hope for a future that does not merely repeat the past.

And, finally, I am profoundly humbled by and thankful to all of the people whose stories I share in these pages, who have shown me the myriad textures of suffering, as well as the true meaning of human rights and dignity, and to whom this book is dedicated.